Reimbursement Management

Improving the Success and Profitability
of Your Practice

Coker Group

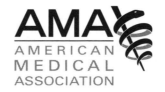

Executive Vice President, Chief Executive Officer: Michael D. Maves, MD, MBA
Chief Operating Officer: Bernard L. Hengesbaugh
Senior Vice President, Publishing and Business Services: Robert A. Musacchio, PhD
Vice President, Business Operations: Vanessa Hayden
Publisher, AMA Publications and Clinical Solutions: Mary Lou White
Senior Acquisitions Editor: Elise Schumacher
Continuity Editor: Carol Brockman
Manager, Book and Product Development and Production: Nancy Baker
Senior Developmental Editor: Michael Ryder
Production Specialist: Meghan Anderson
Director of Sales, Business Products: Mark Daniels
Manager, Marketing and Strategic Planning: Erin Kalitowski
Marketing Manager: Lori Hollacher
Content Reviewers:
  Carol Scheele, Jennifer L. Shevchek, Steve Ellwing, Karen Kmetik

Copyright © 2011 by the American Medical Association. All rights reserved.

Printed in the United States of America.

US public laws and federal rules and regulations included in this publication are in the public domain. However, the arrangement, compilation, organization, and history of, and references to, such laws and regulations, along with all CPT data and other materials are subject to the above copyright notice.

Internet address: www.ama-assn.org

> The American Medical Association ("AMA") and its authors and editors have consulted sources believed to be knowledgeable in their fields. However, neither the AMA nor its authors or editors warrant that the information is in every respect accurate and/or complete. The AMA, its authors, and editors assume no responsibility for use of the information contained in this publication. Neither the AMA, its authors, or editors shall be responsible for, and expressly disclaims liability for, damages of any kind arising out of the use of, reference to, or reliance on the content of this publication. This publication is for informational purposes only. The AMA does not provide medical, legal, financial, or other professional advice, and readers are encouraged to consult a professional advisor for such advice.

The contents of this publication represent the views of the author[s] and should not be construed to be the views or policy of the AMA, or of the institution with which the author[s] may be affiliated, unless this is clearly specified.

Additional copies of this book may be ordered by calling 800 621-8335 or from the secure AMA Web site at www.amabookstore.com. Refer to product number OP091910.

BP77:10-P-089:10/10

Library of Congress Cataloging-in-Publication Data

Reimbursement management : improving the success and profitability of your practice/Coker Group.

p. ; cm.

Includes bibliographical references.

Summary: "This book provides current resources for supporting the medical practice through reimbursement management. Resources include a comprehensive Glossary, Online Resources, Medicare Intermediaries by State, Prompt Pay Statutes and Regulations, Refund Recoupment Statutes, and multiple sample letters for dealing with reimbursement challenges and issues"—Provided by publisher.

ISBN 978-1-60359-293-2

1. Medicine—Practice—Economic aspects—United States. 2. Medicine—Practice—United States—Management. I. Coker Group. II. American Medical Association.

[DNLM: 1. Practice Management, Medical—economics—United States. 2. Practice Management, Medical—organization & administration—United States. 3. Reimbursement Mechanisms—United States. W 80]

R728.R46 2011

610.68—dc22

2010035299

CONTENTS

Preface xi

Acknowledgements xiii

Introduction xv

About the Contributors xvii

About Coker Group xxi

1 Health Insurance Basics 1

Introduction 3

Types of Health Insurance Plans 3
 Indemnity, or Fee-for-Service, Plans 3
 Managed Care Plans 3
 Financial Instruments for Health Care Reimbursement 5

Types of Health Insurance Providers 5
 Employer-Provided Health Insurance Plans 6
 Individually Purchased Health Insurance Plans 6
 Federal Employees Health Benefits Program 6
 Medicare and Medicaid 6
 Children's Health Insurance Program 8
 Indian Health Services 9
 TRICARE 9
 Veterans Administration 9
 Workers' Compensation Insurance 9
 Automobile Insurance 10
 Liability and Casualty Insurance 10

Reimbursement Terminology Overview 10
 ICD-9-CM and CPT® 10
 Resource-Based Relative Value Scale 10
 Medicare Reimbursement Standards and Arrangements 11
 Deductible 12
 Copayment 12
 Co-insurance 12

      Out-of-Pocket Maximum   13
      Covered Services, Exclusions, and Limitations   13
      Primary and Secondary Insurance, and Coordination of Benefits   13
      Pre-certification   13
      Insurance Verification   13
      Primary Physician Referral   14
      In-Network and Out-of-Network Payment Schedules   14
      Capitation and Capitated Contracts   14

   Claim Submission Terminology Overview   14
      Intermediaries and Carriers   14
      Third-Party Administrators   15
      Computerized Billing Systems and Electronic Claims   15
      Electronic Clearinghouse   15
      Electronic Payment Posting and Manual Payment Posting   15
      Lockbox Payments   16

   Credentialing   16

   Conclusion   16

2 Getting Paid What You Deserve: Strategies for Payer Contracting and Optimal Reimbursement   19

   Introduction   19

   Basics of Negotiating Strategy   20

   The Negotiation Process   22
      Evaluating the Plan   22
      Identify the Deal-Breakers   25

   Recognizing the Do's and Don'ts of Contracting   26

   Operations and Administration of the Process   28

   Conclusion   29

3 Pay for Performance and Quality Initiatives   31

   Introduction   32

   Quality   33
      Aligning Forces for Quality   33
      National Committee for Quality Assurance   34
      Agency for Healthcare Research and Quality   34

Health Plans 35
Conclusions 36

Pay for Performance 36
Professional Organizations 36
Government Programs 40
Conclusions 44

Physician Quality Reporting Initiative 45
Background Information 45
Eligible Providers 46
Incentive Payment 47
2010 PQRI Program: Reporting 47
2010 PQRI: Measures 48
Claims-Based Reporting 49
Maximizing Success Within the PQRI Program 50
Available PQRI Resources 52
Group Practice Reporting Option 52
Conclusions 53

Conclusion 54

4 Basics of Coding 57

Introduction 57

CPT Procedure Coding 61
Using the CPT Codebook 63
CPT Modifiers 64
Evaluation and Management Coding 65

ICD-9-CM Diagnosis Coding 71

ICD-10-CM 72

Conclusion 73

5 Revenue Cycle Management: Front-End Processes 75

Introduction 76

Scheduling Patient Appointments 76
Capturing Demographic Information 76
Verifying the Demographic Information 77
Conducting Authorizations and Pre-Certifications 78
Confirming the Appointment 78

    Communicating Office Policies 79
    Managing Missed Appointments 79

Registering the Patient 79
    Complying with Identity and Privacy Regulations 80
    Obtaining Consent for Treatment 82
    Collecting From the Patient at Registration 83

Checking Out the Patient 83
    Surveying Patient Satisfaction 83
    Creating First Impressions 84
    Using Electronic Records in Patient Visits 84

Completing the End-of-the-Day Processes 84
    Balancing Receipts and Verifying Charges 85
    Contacting No-Show Patients 85

Conclusion 85

6 Back-Office Processes 87

Introduction 88

Charge Capture and Entry 88
    In-Office Charges 88
    In-Office Ancillary Charges 88
    Hospital charges 89

Claims Submission 89
    Claims Scrubbing 89
    Electronic Clearinghouse 90
    Prompt-Pay Laws and Clean-Claim Laws 90

Remittances and Explanation of Benefits 91
    Lockbox Services 91
    Cash Posting and Contract Monitoring 91
    Balancing 92
    Zero Payments 92
    Denied Claims 92
    Secondary Insurance 92
    Cycle Billing 93

Forms of Payment 93

Insurance Claims Follow-Up 93
    Contacting Payers 94
    Patient Follow-Up 94
    Bankruptcy 95

Selecting a Collection Agency   95
   Bad Debt   95
   Right to Cure   96
   Monitoring the Collection Agency   96
   Legal Action   96

Conclusion   97

7 Appeals and Reviews   99

Introduction   99

Managing Appeals and Reviews   100

Know What Payer Contracts Allow   100
   External Resources   101
   Administrative Manuals   101
   Negotiated Reimbursement Rates   102
   Changes to Employer-Sponsored Health Plans   105

Internal Payer Processes and Timelines for Claim Processing   105
   Clean Claims Criteria   106
   Coding Expert's Role in the Appeals Process   108
   Billing Systems   109

The Appeals Processing   110
   Key Components of an Appeals Program   111
   Appealing Claims   113

Conclusion   115

8 Benchmarking and Monitoring Reimbursement   117

Introduction   118

Financial Measures of Tracking Reimbursement and Efficiency   118
   Benchmarks   119
   Budgeting   123

Monitoring and Trending   128
   Importance of Constant Review   129
   Monitoring Key Statistics   129
   Dashboard Reports   130

Conclusion   134

9 Billing and Reimbursement for Ancillary Services   135

Introduction   135

What Are Ancillary Services?   136

When to Provide Services and Who Provides Services   137

Be Aware (or Beware) of Stark   139

Negotiate Separately Within the Managed Care Contracts for Services Normally Provided by Physician   141

Monitor Usage, Cost to Deliver, and Revenue Generated   142
    Additional Resources on Billing and Reimbursement for Ancillary Services   143

Conclusion   143

10 Compliance Programs   145

Introduction   146

Sanction Authorities   147
    False Claims Act   147
    The Anti-Kickback Statute   148
    The Physician Self-Referral Act   150
    Health Insurance Portability and Accountability Act   152
    Red Flags Rule   153
    Commercial Insurer Fraud and Abuse Programs   154

Who Else is Watching   155
    Medicare Claims Review Programs   156

Developing an Effective Plan   160
    Designating a Compliance Officer   160
    Implementing Written Policies and Standards of Conduct   161
    Conducting Effective Training and Education   164
    Developing Effective Lines of Communication   167

Enforcing Standards Through Well-Published Disciplinary Guidelines   168
    Responding Promptly to Detected Offenses and Developing   170
    Conducting Internal Monitoring and Auditing   174

Conclusion   181

11 Information Technology and Reimbursement: The Role of Information Systems in the Revenue Cycle   185

Introduction   186

Revenue-Enhancing Features   186
   Electronic Health Records Charge Capture   186
   Portability Devices for Providers   187
   Patient Portal Access and Kiosks   187
   Real-Time Insurance Verification   188
   Reporting Tools   188
   Telephone and Email Reminder Systems   188
   Automated Advanced Beneficiary Notice Checking   189
   Simplification of Documentation   189

Best of Breed Versus One Throat to Choke   189

Managing a Conversion Successfully   190
   Assembling an Implementation Team   191
   Establishing Buy-In   193
   The Implementation Plan   194
   EHR Implementation Strategy   196
   Transforming Workflow   199

Conclusion   206

Appendix A   Online Resources   207

Appendix B   Section I—Medicare Part A Intermediary and Part B Carrier by State   213

Appendix C   Prompt Pay Statutes and Regulations by State   225

Appendix D   Refund Recoupment Statutes by State   239

Appendix E   15 Steps to Protect Your Practice from Abusive Payment Tactics   265

Appendix F   Disclosure of Security Breach by State   267

Appendix G   Sample Appeals Letters   273

Glossary   285

Index   299

PREFACE

THE AMERICAN MEDICAL ASSOCIATION has continually supported the physician in the management of reimbursement for the services performed in providing patient care. Over the years, the path to reimbursement has become increasingly complex. Government and private payers have grown more demanding in their expectations. Compliance with multiple rules and regulations have ratcheted up notch by notch to the point that the exposure to liability, penalties, and non-payment are continual hazards experienced in the medical practice.

In its role as consultants to physicians on the business-side of medical practice, Coker Group strives to educate physicians and their staff on best practices for managing reimbursement. The purpose of this book is to address the background of the insurance systems and to lay out the details required to maneuver through the mine fields that reimbursement presents. The objective is for the correct coding and billing of every service and for expeditious collections for professional services rendered.

We hope that *Reimbursement Management* becomes and continues to be a relevant and helpful resource to physicians and their staff.

ACKNOWLEDGEMENTS

THIS BOOK IS A result of the contributions, support, and assistance of many people. First, the AMA staff pursued a resource for continuing education on managing reimbursement. Marsha Mildred, Suzanne Fraker, Elise Schumacher, and Carol Brockman took this project from the point of recognizing and fulfilling a need, through development, and finally through production. Michael Rider was instrumental in shepherding the manuscript through all the stages of editing and publishing.

Coker Group, equally committed to achieving the goals and expectations in skillful management of reimbursement, derived expertise from several areas of practice administration and financial management. Contributors include Jeannie Cagle, Jeffery Daigrepont, Aimee Greeter, Deborah Hill, Barbara Landes, Rick Langosch, Priscilla Moore, Crystal Reeves, John Reiboldt, and Kay Stanley.

Finally, we extend great appreciation to all the many physicians and their staff that the AMA and Coker Group serve. We want you and your practices to thrive and to flourish as you continue to deliver the highest quality of health care in an environment that is financially stable and secure.

INTRODUCTION

"**THAT OUGHT TO BE** taught in medical school," is a comment often heard when physicians lament over the complexity of medical practice management. Operating a successful business is the one aspect of medicine that medical students, interns, and residents scarcely consider during the intense education that primarily encompasses the best clinical information available. After all, if you are intelligent enough to become a physician, you are smart enough to run a medical practice, right? Well, it takes a different set of knowledge and an immense amount of time to do both. As a result, most busy physicians rely on their practice staff to oversee reimbursement aspects for the services that the physician renders, yet both play significant roles in managing the revenue cycle.

This book begins by introducing health insurance basics, laying the foundation for the remaining chapters. In the current environment, physicians are compelled to contract with payers; thus, the next topic addresses getting the most out of negotiations and contracting with the insurance companies. Pay for performance and quality initiatives are vital aspects of reimbursement, requiring an explanation of current programs and information on how they fit now and in the future of the medical practice.

The physician's goal is to take care of the patient's health needs. However, a medical practice requires financial resources to run effectively, and financial reimbursement is the source of revenue. Who can afford to practice medicine without suitable compensation? Chapter 4 presents essential information on coding, which is the backbone of the reimbursement system.

The revenue cycle is a confluence of front-end and back-office processes. The details of each step in sequence are addressed in Chapters 5 and 6. The mechanisms of the revenue cycle continue by addressing the importance of appeals and reviews—a necessary aspect of reimbursement covered in Chapter 7. Chapter 8 provides guidance through benchmarking and monitoring reimbursement with the goal to achieve best practices and better performance.

Most physicians provide ancillary services as a means for improving patient convenience and for enhancing reimbursement. Chapter 9 provides a current perspective on ancillary services and addresses measures necessary to ensure that the practice obtains suitable reimbursement.

Compliance is a confusing area, generating many questions about what needs to be done to become or remain compliant. Compliance violations can cost organizations huge sums of money and massive penalties. Chapter 10 provides a much-needed overview and establishes practical guidelines for developing an effective compliance plan for protecting the practice.

Information technology plays a vital role in the revenue cycle, which is the topic addressed in Chapter 11. This how-to chapter is rich with sound advice on the challenging questions regarding selection, conversion, and implementation of information systems.

Lastly, this book provides current resources for supporting the medical practice through reimbursement management. Resources include a comprehensive Glossary, Online Resources, Medicare Intermediaries by State, Prompt Pay Statutes and Regulations, Refund Recoupment Statutes, 15 Steps to Protect Your Practice from Abusive Payment Tactics, Disclosure of Security Breach, and multiple sample letters for dealing with reimbursement challenges and issues.

Reimbursement management is a complex topic requiring ongoing education as the payment systems continually evolve. Along with providing high quality patient care, the goal of every physician should be to take responsibility for having the right staff in place and for providing the necessary training and resources for keeping on top of the reimbursement process. This book will help to achieve that end.

ABOUT THE CONTRIBUTORS

Jeannie Cagle The role of Jeannie Cagle in practice management consulting includes working with physicians in completing coding analyses, medical chart audits, practice assessments, and in human resource management. Her engagements by hospitals and practices encompass coordination of compliance audits for medical necessity reviews and corporate integrity agreements, including serving as an Internal Review Officer (IRO). Analyzing EMR software from a coding perspective and conducting return-on-investment analyses for implementation of EMR software in medical practices are also projects that Ms Cagle manages. Ms Cagle is a strong educator and instructor in a variety of areas. An experienced public speaker who incorporates a practical and keen approach to tedious subjects, her current emphasis is on physician education and training in coding and compliance issues. A graduate of Harding University with a Bachelor of Science in Nursing, and a Registered Nurse, Ms Cagle is certified by the American Academy of Professional Coders.

Aimee Greeter Aimee Greeter is a senior associate in the financial services service line within Coker. She works on a variety of consulting projects, including financial consulting, hospital accounts, practice management initiatives, as well as research and writing for various client projects. In her most recent engagement, Ms Greeter coordinated post-merger integration efforts for a faith-based hospital system, with a particular focus on human resources and supply chain management. Prior to joining Coker, Ms Greeter worked at the Centers for Disease Control and Prevention (CDC) in Atlanta, Georgia, where she conducted extensive research on health care related projects. Ms Greeter holds a Master of Public Health (MPH) in Health Policy and Management from the Rollins School of Public Health at Emory University. She is an honors graduate of Michigan State University, where she attained a Bachelor of Science (BS) in Human Biology.

Deborah Hill Deborah B Hill serves as a manager in the practice management area, responsible for managing the delivery of services to physicians, both through client hospitals and to individual practices. Her broad experience encompasses the following areas: billing management, network contract negotiations, referral resource network, coding and consulting services, coding compliance management, negotiation of vendor contracts, EMR implementation, and provider enrollment and credentialing. Ms Hill holds an MBA in Healthcare Administration and a BBA in Management. Additionally, she is a Certified Professional Coder by the American Academy of Professional Coders, and a Certified Medical Practice Executive by the American College of Medical Practice Executives.

Christine Ingram Christine Ingram, vice president, has amassed expertise in all areas of practice management, using her skills and experience to assist Coker's clients with operational and financial issues. Since joining Coker Group in 2006, Ms Ingram's assignments encompass serving as Interim Executive Director of a hospital-owned employed physician network, located in the Midwest. In the Northeast, she serves as project director to achieve a performance turnaround for a hospital's employed physician network. Projects in the West and Southwest include numerous operational assessments and assistance with mergers. Her work crosses all specialties including multispecialty, cardiology, pain management, and urology. Ms Ingram holds a Masters in Healthcare Management from Troy State University, and a BS in Health Care Management from Clayton College and State University. She is a member of MGMA, ACHE, and Georgia Association of Healthcare Executives.

Rick Langosch Rick Langosch, a senior vice president, works with hospital clients to realize sustainable improvements at the organizational, departmental, and services level. Coker Group's Hospital Strategies consulting practice provides timely and responsive solutions to its hospital clients in Service Line Analysis, Staffing/Productivity Benchmarking and Analysis, Interim Management, and RAC Audit Readiness. A seasoned healthcare executive, with over 25 years of experience managing operations and finance in hospitals and physician practices, Mr Langosch has held a wide range of financial, operational, and information technology responsibilities, including multi-hospital ownership and hospital senior management positions. He uses that experience to assist Coker clients in developing a specific implementation strategy that will produce improved performance and drive profitability for their organizations. Langosch is a graduate of Eastern Illinois University in Charleston, Illinois, and he is a Fellow with the Healthcare Financial Management Association. He is active with the Georgia Chapter of HFMA.

John P Reiboldt John Reiboldt is a managing director with Coker Capital Advisors. Prior to co-founding Coker Capital Advisors, Mr Reiboldt spent more than 10 years with Coker Group, founded the firm's financial services group, which provided mergers and acquisitions and strategic financial advisory services to the health care industry. While leading the financial services group, Mr Reiboldt executed numerous transactions and advisory assignments across a wide variety of health care subsectors, both domestically and internationally. In addition to his role with Coker Capital Advisors. Mr Reiboldt earned his Bachelor of Business

Administration in Economics at the University of Mississippi and his Master of Business Administration with a concentration in Finance from The Robinson College of Business at Georgia State University.

Crystal Reeves With over 28 years experience in health care and medical practice management, both in primary care and multi-specialty practices, Ms Reeves is a recognized leader in medical practice management in areas pertaining to implementing and refining billing and collection services, improving operations, and physician and staff education.
Ms Reeves is a sought-after speaker and consultant presenting seminars nationwide on coding and reimbursement, documentation guidelines, front desk operations, and customer service. She is a regular speaker at MGMA and other associations at the national and state levels.
Ms Reeves is certified by the American Academy of Professional Coders and has achieved the status of Certified Medical Practice Executive through the Medical Group Management Association's American College of Medical Practice Executives. In addition, she has attained recognition from the American Academy of Professional Coders for coding proficiency in the specialty of oncology.

Yong Zhang Yong Zhang is a senior associate with Coker Capital Advisors. Prior to joining Coker Capital Advisors, Ms Zhang spent four years with Coker Group, a leading management and strategic consulting firm focused on the health care and life sciences industries. During her tenure with Coker Group, Ms Zhang worked for the firm's financial services group where she assisted in mergers and acquisitions, valuations and fairness opinions, and numerous advisory assignments across a wide spectrum of health care subsectors. Ms Zhang earned her Bachelor of Accounting at Fudan University in Shanghai, China and her Master of Accountancy from the University of Georgia. Prior to her position at Coker Group, Ms Zhang was an accountant at General Motors of China. Ms Zhang is in the process of completing her Chartered Financial Analyst (CFA) designation, Accredited Senior Appraiser (ASA) designation, and is in the final stages of obtaining her Certified Public Accountant (CPA) designation. Ms Zhang is fluent in Chinese.

ABOUT COKER GROUP

COKER GROUP, A LEADER in health care consulting, help providers achieve improved financial and operational results through sound business principles. The consulting team members are proficient, trustworthy professionals with expertise and strengths in various areas. Coker Group represents three service lines: Coker Consulting, Coker Capital Advisors, and Coker Technology. Through these service areas, Coker consultants enable providers to concentrate on patient care.

Coker Group's nationwide client base includes major health systems, hospitals, physician and specialty groups, and solo practitioners in a full spectrum of engagements. Coker Group's has gained reputation since 1987 for thorough, efficient, and cost-conscious work to benefit its clients financially and operationally. The firm prides themselves on their client profile of recognized and respected health care professionals through the industry. The firm's exceptional consulting team has health care, technical, financial, and business knowledge and offers comprehensive programs, services, and training to yield long-term solutions and turnarounds. Coker staff members are devoted to helping health care providers face today's challenges for tomorrow's successes.

Service areas include:

- Capital advisory and strategic financial advisory and analysis
- Strategic planning/business planning
- Practice operational assessments
- Physician network development
- Disengagements of practices and network unwinds
- Hospital-physician alignment
- Practice management, billing and collections reviews, chart audits
- Compensation
- Post-merger integration implementation
- Hospital services, medical staff development
- Executive search
- Interim and long-term network management

- Practice appraisals
- Practice start-ups
- Buy/sell and equity analysis
- Group formation and dissolution
- Practice acquisition, mergers, and due diligence
- Compensation reviews, FMV opinion services, and call coverage compensation
- HIPAA assessments and compliance
- MSA development
- Revenue cycle management and procedural coding analysis
- Compliance plans
- Policy and procedure manuals
- Medication and expert witnessing
- Strategic information technology planning and review, including EMR
- HIT software/hardware vendor vetting and procurement
- Contract negotiations
- Project management
- Managed IT services
- Educational programs, workshops, and training

For more information, please contact:

Coker Group
1000 Mansell Exchange West
Suite 310
Alpharetta, GA 30022
800-345-5829
www.cokergroup.com

CHAPTER 1
Health Insurance Basics

OUTLINE

I. Introduction
II. Types of Health Insurance Plans
    A. Indemnity, or Fee-for-Service, Plans
    B. Managed Care Plans
        1. Health Maintenance Organizations (HMOs)
        2. Preferred Provider Organizations (PPOs)
        3. Point of Service (POS) Plans
    C. Financial Instruments for Health Care Reimbursement
        1. Health Reimbursement Accounts (HRAs)
        2. Health Savings Accounts (HSAs) and High-Deductible Plans
III. Types of Health Insurance Providers
    A. Employer-Provided Health Insurance Plans (Self-Insured and Purchased)
    B. Individually Purchased Health Insurance Plans
    C. Federal Employees Health Benefits Program
    D. Medicare and Medicaid
        1. Medicare Parts A and B
            a. Part A
            b. Part B
        2. Medicare Part D
        3. Medicare Advantage Plans
        4. Medicare Supplemental Plans
        5. Dual Eligibility—Medicare and Medicaid Recipients
        6. Railroad Retirement Health Insurance
        7. Employer or Union Coverage and Medicare
        8. Medicare Open Enrollment Advantage and Medicare Drug Programs
        9. Medicaid

- E. Children's Health Insurance Program (CHIP)
- F. Indian Health Services
- G. TRICARE
- H. Veterans Administration
- I. Workers' Compensation Insurance
- J. Automobile Insurance
- K. Liability and Casualty Insurance
- IV. Reimbursement Terminology Overview
    - A. ICD-9-CM and CPT®
    - B. Resource-Based Relative Value Scale (RBRVS)
    - C. Medicare Reimbursement Standards and Arrangements
        1. Medicare Allowed Amount or Medicare Payment Schedule
        2. Participation and Nonparticipation with Medicare
        3. Medicare Limiting Charge
        4. Usual and Customary Payment Schedules
        5. Standard Charge Fee Schedule
        6. Contractual Adjustments
        7. Payment Schedules
    - D. Deductible
    - E. Copayment
    - F. Co-Insurance
    - G. Out-of Pocket-Maximum
    - H. Covered Services, Exclusions, and Limitations
    - I. Primary and Secondary Insurance, and Coordination of Benefits
    - J. Pre-Certification
    - K. Insurance Verification
    - L. Primary Physician Referral
    - M. In-Network and Out-of-Network Payment Schedules
    - N. Capitation and Capitated Contracts
- V. Claim Submission Terminology Overview
    - A. Intermediaries and Carriers
    - B. Third-Party Administrators (TPAs)
    - C. Computerized Billing Systems and Electronic Claims
    - D. Electronic Clearinghouse
    - E. Electronic Payment Posting and Manual Payment Posting
    - F. Lockbox Payments
- VI. Credentialing
- VII. Conclusion

Introduction

Many insurance companies sell different types of individual and group plans, and many employers offer these different plans to their employees. These plans have varying degrees of coverage, referral restrictions, and payment schedules. As a result, health insurance plans are always changing and patients frequently have a hard time understanding what their health plans cover.

Most physicians in the United States treat patients who have some type of medical insurance, and most patients expect their physician's office staff to file health insurance claims, on their behalf, for at least a portion of the payment charged for a medical service. In most cases, insurance payments account for the majority of payment received by a medical practice.

Consequently, a medical practice that devotes time and personnel to verifying and understanding each patient's particular insurance coverage can increase collections and cash flow. As the first step to gaining that understanding, this chapter broadly defines the most common types of insurance plans, discusses the different kinds of insurance providers, and reviews basic terminology and billing procedures that must be in place for effective billing and collections in a medical practice.

Types of Health Insurance Plans

There are hundreds of different health insurance plans in the United States. Although each plan is different, most health insurance plans fall into two major categories: indemnity plans and managed care plans.

Indemnity, or Fee-for-Service, Plans

Indemnity, or fee-for-service (FFS), plans usually pay for medical services provided by any licensed medical provider at either a fixed rate (sometimes called a usual and customary payment schedule) or a percentage of the fee charged. These plans offer insured patients the widest range of choice when choosing a physician or deciding when they wish to see a specialist. However, these plans can be very expensive to purchase.

Managed Care Plans

Managed care plans are built on contractual agreements between an insurance company and physicians, hospitals, and ancillary service providers in order to offer services to an insured population of patients, using a contracted payment schedule or payment plan. Managed care plans help an insurance company control costs and usually can be purchased at a lower premium.

There are three major categories of managed care plans:

- health maintenance organizations (HMOs),
- preferred provider organizations (PPOs), and
- point-of-service (POS) plans.

Each plan establishes contracts with physicians, hospitals, ancillary service providers, and prescription drug providers to create a network of medical services. Patients are encouraged to use this network for all of their medical care.

There are always exceptions, but in most cases, an HMO places severe restrictions on a patient's ability to go out of network for care and will not pay for any nonemergency service provided outside of the HMO network. A POS offers more flexibility to the patient in choosing providers, and a PPO offers the most choice. Often, PPO and POS plans have a two-tiered payment schedule that pays more to in-network providers than to out-of-network providers.

Health Maintenance Organizations (HMOs)

An HMO is a comprehensive health care system, or an organized group of physicians and providers, who contract with an insurance company to provide services to a specific group of insured individuals or families. In some cases, the physicians are employees of the HMO and, in some situations, they contract with the HMO to provide services.

Often, an HMO will pay contract physicians a fixed or "capitated" amount per month, per member, regardless of the number of patients requiring medical care. Most HMO plans assign a primary care physician (PCP) for each patient. Patients are usually seen first by the PCP, who coordinates care and referrals to specialists within the HMO, if needed. Sometimes this arrangement is referred to as using a "gatekeeper."

Preferred Provider Organizations (PPOs)

A PPO is made up of physicians and physician groups who agree to accept a predetermined payment schedule when treating an insured patient covered by that particular insurance plan. Usually, the insured patient can see any physician approved by the plan without a referral from a PCP.

Point-of-Service (POS) Plans

A POS plan is similar to a PPO except that the patient has an identified PCP who coordinates the patient's care and makes any necessary referrals to specialists within the POS plan network. Aside from certain exceptions, the patient cannot see a specialist without a referral from his or her PCP.

Financial Instruments for Health Care Reimbursement

Although they are not considered health insurance plans, two financial instruments are used by many employers and individuals to help pay for medical costs. They are described in the following paragraphs.

Health Reimbursement Accounts (HRAs)

The first is a health reimbursement account (HRA), sometimes called a flexible spending account (FSA). These accounts allow an employee to set aside part of his or her earnings to pay for health insurance deductibles, copayments, co-insurance, and other approved medical expenses on a pretax basis. These accounts have a potential downside, in that the employee must spend all of the set-aside funds every year or lose those funds entirely. This is referred to as "use it or lose it."

Health Savings Accounts (HSAs) and High-Deductible Plans

The second is a health savings account (HSA), which can be used only if the insured person has an approved high-deductible health insurance plan. The deductible amounts must be at least $2,300 for families and $1,150 for individuals. Either an individual or an employer can establish an HSA, and contributions are allowed to accumulate from year to year, as long as they are used for designated medical expenses.

Types of Health Insurance Providers

Health care insurance coverage is attainable through various means and encompasses a variety of providers. This section gives a brief description of the sources and plans generally available to consumers.

Employer-Provided Health Insurance Plans (Self-Insured and Purchased)

Most Americans are covered by group coverage plans that are provided through their employer, a professional organization, or a union. These plans accept all qualified employees and their dependents without pre-existing condition clauses. Employers and employees usually share in the cost of the premiums, and many employers offer more than one type of plan (PPO, HMO, POS) from which employees may choose.

Most employers purchase this insurance from a private insurance company. Some employers are "self-insured," meaning that they pay for claims out of their own reserves. However, they usually purchase backup insurance, or re-insurance, from an insurance company for catastrophic claims and they usually hire an outside health care administrator or insurance company to process and pay claims for them.

Individually Purchased Health Insurance Plans

Insurance companies also sell individual policies for people who are not covered through a group plan. These policies vary in type (FFS, PPO, HMO), costs, and benefits provided.

Federal Employees Health Benefits Program

The Federal Employees Health Benefits (FEHB) Program administers health insurance programs for federal employees, dependents, retirees, and their survivors, and offers several different health insurance plans including FFS, HMO, PPO, and high-deductible plans.

Medicare and Medicaid

Medicare and Medicaid were signed into law in 1965 under Title XVIII and Title XIX of the Social Security Act. These two programs are often confused with each other but they are distinct and separate programs with major differences. Both programs are administered through the U.S. Department of Health and Human Services in the Centers for Medicare and Medicaid Services (CMS).

Medicare Parts A and B

The original Medicare (Parts A and B) provides health insurance to most Americans over age 65, to some under age 65 with certain disabilities, and to people of all ages with end-stage renal disease. Broadly, Medicare Parts A and B pay for the following types of medical services.

Part A. Medicare Part A pays for eligible hospital stays, skilled nursing facility care, home health care, and hospice care. Part A is provided at no cost to most Americans over age 65 because of Medicare taxes that were previously paid by the retiree or their spouse.

Part B. Medicare Part B pays for eligible physician services for office visits and surgeries, diagnostic tests, clinical laboratory services, home health care, and outpatient hospital services. Medicare Part B enrollees pay a monthly premium for coverage.

Medicare Part D

Medicare Part D, the Medicare prescription drug benefit, became effective January 1, 2006, as an addition to the Medicare program. Medicare recipients pay a monthly premium for individual prescription drug insurance policies from approved private insurance companies. The plans vary widely in cost, coverage, and design, but all plans must meet or exceed guidelines established by the Medicare program.

Medicare Advantage Plans

Medicare Advantage plans, sometimes called Medicare Part C, are managed care health plans that are administered by private insurance companies and are similar to HMO, PPO, and POS plans. There are also Medicare Advantage plans that are private FFS plans. Advantage plans provide the benefits of both Part A and Part B services, and some plans include a prescription drug benefit as well. Some Advantage plans charge recipients an additional monthly premium.

Medicare Supplemental Plans

Medicare supplemental plans, or Medigap plans, are supplemental insurance policies purchased to pay for the gaps in Part A and Part B Medicare, such as deductibles and co-insurance. Except in Massachusetts, Minnesota, and Wisconsin, there are up to 12 standardized Medigap policies labeled Medigap Plan A through Plan L. Medigap policies only work with original Medicare. Not all insurance companies offer all 12 plans, but all 12 plans are the same, no matter which insurance company offers the plan.

Dual Eligibility—Medicare and Medicaid Recipients

Some Medicare patients, especially those in financial need, qualify for different levels of state Medicaid programs, which can act as a supplement to their Medicare, because they cannot afford to pay the premium for Medicare Part B or for a Medigap policy. These patients are referred to as "dual eligibles."

Railroad Retirement Health Insurance

Railroad retirement health insurance, or Railroad Medicare, provides the same coverage as original Medicare Part A and Part B but is administered through the Railroad Retirement Board.

Employer or Union Coverage and Medicare

Some individuals are not covered by Medicare Part B, even though they are age 65, because they are still insured by an employer group health plan. This usually occurs when the insured or his or her spouse is still working. Many employer and union contracts also provide supplemental and/or prescription benefits for retired persons who have original Medicare.

Medicare Open Enrollment Advantage and Medicare Drug Programs

Medicare recipients are allowed to make certain changes every year during an open enrollment period (November 15 through December 31 of each year). With certain restrictions, this enables recipients to change prescription drug plans and switch between original Medicare coverage and Medicare Advantage plans or change from one Advantage plan to another.

Medicaid

Medicaid is also administered through CMS, but it is a joint federal and state program that serves low-income families with dependent children and certain qualified aged, blind, and disabled persons. Medicaid eligibility requirements and benefits vary from state to state.

Children's Health Insurance Program (CHIP)

The Children's Health Insurance Program (CHIP) is jointly financed by the federal and state governments and is administered by the states. Within broad federal guidelines, each state determines the design of its program, eligibility groups, benefit packages, payment levels for coverage, and administrative and operating procedures.

Indian Health Services

The Indian Health Service (IHS) is an agency within the U.S. Department of Health and Human Services that is responsible for providing medical and public health services to American Indians and Alaska natives. The IHS also coordinates with many state health care programs, such as Medicaid, CHIP, and early-detection and screening programs. The IHS owns and manages numerous hospitals and medical clinics and employs more than 15,000 physicians, nurses, pharmacists, dentists, and other heath care professionals. In some areas, the IHS contracts with private physicians and hospitals through its Contract Health Service (CHS) Program, to provide medical services unavailable within the IHS system.

TRICARE

TRICARE, formerly known as CHAMPUS (Civilian Health and Medical Program for Uniformed Services), is a component of the military health system. It offers several health care plans to active-duty military service members, National Guard and Reserve members, retirees, their families, survivors, and certain former spouses. TRICARE contracts with certain civilian medical facilities and providers to augment its medical delivery system.

Veterans Administration

The Veterans Administration (VA) provides medical care to veterans of the armed services. It is composed of a network of more than 150 hospitals and hundreds more community-based outpatient clinics. Like the TRICARE network, the VA also employs its own physicians, nurses, and health care professionals. In some cases, the VA contracts with civilian medical facilities and providers.

Workers' Compensation Insurance

All 50 states have laws that require employers to purchase workers' compensation insurance to protect employees who are injured on the job. It is designed to pay medical bills and pay the employee for lost wages due to an injury. In most cases, workers' compensation insurance is purchased from private insurance companies, but the policies are regulated through the state department of labor. Rules vary from state to state about how and when an injury must be reported, who makes the choice of physician, referrals to specialists, and how payment amounts are determined.

Automobile Insurance

Auto insurance policies usually include coverage for bodily injury for a person hurt in an auto accident. The specifics of coverage and payments vary from policy to policy and are also affected by different state regulations.

Liability and Casualty Insurance

Liability and casualty insurance refers to a broad range of policies that protect an individual or business from the risk that they may be sued and held legally liable for malpractice or negligence resulting in a loss or injury.

Reimbursement Terminology Overview

Medical practices have a language of their own that includes many confusing abbreviations, as well as other terms that warrant explanation. This section briefly introduces some common terminology that is essential to understanding and managing reimbursement functions. Later chapters cover these concepts in more detail.

ICD-9-CM and CPT®

To bill insurance companies, physicians use two primary coding systems that assign a unique number to every disease or condition a patient might have and to every procedure a physician performs. The *International Classification of Diseases, 9th Revision, Clinical Modification* (ICD-9-CM) describes diagnosis codes, and the Current Procedural Terminology (CPT®) describes procedures.

Resource-Based Relative Value Scale (RBRVS)

In 1992, Medicare began using the resource-based relative value scale (RBRVS) to determine payments for physicians' services. This system assigns a value to every CPT code and multiplies it by a dollar amount to determine what the payment will be for that CPT code. The dollar amounts vary from region to region in the United States due to health care cost differences in different parts of the country.

Medicare Reimbursement Standards and Arrangements

A working knowledge of the following terms is fundamental for the reimbursement of health care services. In addition to Medicare standards, some terms in this section also apply to reimbursement from other insurance plans.

Medicare Allowed Amount or Medicare Payment Schedule

The RBRVS information, which is updated and published every year by Medicare, determines the Medicare payment schedule, or Medicare allowed amount, for every CPT code.

Participation and Nonparticipation with Medicare

Physicians have the option to receive reimbursement for services provided to Medicare patients in one of two ways: as a participating physician or as a nonparticipating physician.

When a physician agrees to participate with Medicare, he or she agrees to accept the Medicare allowed amount as payment in full for his service to all patients with original Medicare. After the patient's deductible has been met, Medicare pays 80% of the allowed amount and the patient is responsible for paying the remaining 20% (co-insurance).

Medicare Limiting Charge

If a physician elects to be nonparticipating with Medicare, he or she must agree to accept the Medicare limiting charge, or 115% of the Medicare allowed amount, as payment in full from patients with original Medicare. For nonparticipating physicians, Medicare will only pay 95% of the 80% payment and the patient is responsible for the remaining balance.

Usual and Customary Payment Schedules

Most insurance companies use the RBRVS and Medicare allowable payment schedule when determining their various payment schedules. In some cases, policies describe their payment schedules as "usual and customary." In some managed care contracts, payment is determined at a percent times the Medicare allowable. An example might be 125% of the Medicare allowable.

Standard Charge Fee Schedule

Although insurance plans pay different amounts for services, a medical practice should have only one standard fee schedule, or standard charge. Often this fee schedule is based on a number times the Medicare allowable, such as 2 × (allowable).

Contractual Adjustments

Because of federal law in the case of Medicare and contractual agreements with insurance companies, physicians agree to make contractual adjustments to their standard charge when receiving payment.

Payment Schedules

In order to monitor the accuracy of payments received, a practice must have up-to-date payment schedules from all payers. The practice can then monitor the accuracy of the Medicare and insurance payments received.

Deductible

The deductible is the dollar amount an insured person is required to pay before the insurance company will pay anything. Often there is an individual deductible amount and a family deductible amount stated in a health insurance policy.

Copayment

A copayment is a specific dollar amount, defined in the insurance policy that the patient is required to pay at the time a service is rendered. Many health insurance plans use this feature, and it is also used in some Medicare Advantage plans, and also by Medicaid and TRICARE.

Co-Insurance

Co-insurance is the percentage a patient is required to pay a physician or medical provider for covered services.

Out-of-Pocket Maximum

Out-of-pocket maximum is the total dollar amount an insured person or family is required to pay in a year for covered health care services under a policy. This is the total of the deductible and co-insurance. An out-of-pocket maximum does not include co-payments.

Covered Services, Exclusions, and Limitations

Insurance policies usually specify a list of covered services and also spell out what services will not be covered. For example, some policies do not pay for certain procedures, such as elective cosmetic surgery, maternity care, or acupuncture treatments. In addition, some policies place limits on the number of treatments or services used in a year, such as routine mammograms or physical therapy visits. Also, some policies place a dollar cap on the amount to be paid for certain types of care, such as preventive care or annual physicals.

Primary and Secondary Insurance, and Coordination of Benefits

Many patients are covered by two or more insurance policies. For example, a patient might have original Medicare and a Medigap policy. In this case, Medicare is the primary insurance and the Medigap policy is the secondary. Medicare is billed first. After Medicare pays and the Medicare adjustments are made, the Medigap policy pays. Generally, all health insurance policies have provisions that do not allow for a duplication of payment for the same service.

Pre-Certification

To control costs, most public and private insurers require that certain services be pre-approved, or pre-certified, by the insurance company before the service is performed. If pre-certification is not obtained, payment will be denied. This applies to most nonemergency hospitalizations and surgeries and many outpatient procedures and diagnostic tests.

Insurance Verification

Insurance verification refers to a medical practice's verification of a patient's insurance coverage prior to treating the patient.

Primary Physician Referral

In many managed care insurance plans, such as HMO and POS plans, before a patient can be seen by a specialist, the PCP must make a formal referral to the second physician according to the procedures spelled out in the plan or contractual agreement.

In-Network and Out-of-Network Payment Schedules

Many managed care contracts provide insured patients with a choice of seeing physicians both inside and outside of the managed care network. However, the plan usually pays less for services provided by an out-of-network physician. This means that the amount the patient pays is greater. For example, the insurance payment to an in-network physician might be 80% of the approved payment and only 70% to an out-of-network physician.

Capitation and Capitated Contracts

Capitation is a system used to pay health care providers who contract with an HMO; it is usually a fixed dollar amount per enrolled member, per month. The physician agrees to see any patient who is covered under the contract and does not charge the patient, except for the plan's approved copayment amount. These contracts are usually for a certain population of patients that live in a specific geographic area.

Claim Submission Terminology Overview

The following paragraphs provide a basic introduction to terminology used in claims submission.

Intermediaries and Carriers

Medicare, Railroad Medicare, and many other government-funded insurance programs do not pay for medical services directly. They contract with an intermediary, or carrier, to process and pay claims for them. A complete listing of the insurance companies used by Medicare can be found on the Medicare Website at www.cms.hhs.gov/contractinggeneralinformation.

Third-Party Administrators (TPAs)

A third-party administrator (TPA) is a company that processes insurance claims on behalf of another entity. For example, a large business may be self-insured for its employees' health insurance payments but will contract with a third party (sometimes an insurance company) to administer its health insurance plans and other employee benefits.

Computerized Billing Systems and Electronic Claims

Using a computerized billing system and filing claims electronically can speed up reimbursement and help a practice monitor the accuracy of payments. A practice can also use computer software programs that verify a patient's insurance before the patient is seen, automatically check for errors in procedure codes and diagnosis codes, provide reports to assist in follow-up and collections, and create billing notices for patients.

In the United States, a majority of health insurance claims are now billed electronically. Medicare requires that all physicians submit Medicare claims electronically, except for certain defined small providers.

Depending on size, type, and preferences, a medical practice can choose between purchasing and operating its own in-house billing system or utilizing a medical practice billing company to bill insurance claims for them.

Electronic Clearinghouse

Most claims are sent to the different insurance carriers through an intermediary called an electronic clearinghouse. A clearinghouse can expedite claims by checking them for completeness and accuracy before they are sent on to the insurance company.

Electronic Payment Posting and Manual Payment Posting

When a payment is received for a medical service, it must be posted to the correct patient's account in the billing system. Many practices use electronic payment posting, which is usually offered through a clearinghouse or directly from an insurance carrier. Other practices choose to have billing employees manually enter payment data into the billing system.

Even when a practice uses all available electronic posting services available, there is still a need for manually posting copayments and personal payments into the billing system. It is also necessary to review the accuracy of all electronic payment postings due to possible errors.

Lockbox Payments

Many medical practices have payments mailed to a lockbox at their banking institution rather than to the practice address. This ensures that money is deposited immediately into the practice's bank account and payments are then posted from copies of checks rather than live checks.

Credentialing

Credentialing refers to the process of review and verification of a physician or medical practice by an insurance company or a managed care organization. For all in-network providers, the managed care organization will verify such items as current professional licenses, Drug Enforcement Administration and controlled drug substance certificates, the physician's education, postgraduate training, hospital staff privileges, and professional liability insurance. Several vendors provide software programs to assist physicians in streamlining the credentialing process.

Conclusion

Medical insurance is a complicated topic. It is a highly regulated field with many different plans, payers, definitions, and rules. And the rules and regulations change often and will continue to do so as the health care delivery system in our country changes. To understand insurance, you must stay up-to-date with these changes. The wise use of continuing education resources can help a practice stay abreast of new regulations. It is also important to communicate changes in insurance requirements to clinical staff in a medical practice. Accurate billing relies on accurate clinical documentation and often on documented communication with a patient.

Even for an experienced medical office employee, it can be a challenge to maintain a complete understanding of health insurance. So, it is easy to see why many patients have a difficult time understanding their own insurance coverage. By verifying a prospective patient's insurance coverage, a medical practice can help explain to a patient what the insurance company will pay and what the patient will owe for services. While this may appear to make good business sense, it is also a service to the patient and can enhance the patient care experience.

The following chapters provide an in-depth look at the terms introduced in this chapter in order to bring proficiency to managing the reimbursement process.

CHAPTER 2
Getting Paid What You Deserve

Strategies for Payer Contracting and Optimal Reimbursement

OUTLINE

I. Introduction
II. Basics of Negotiating Strategy
III. The Negotiation Process
    A. Evaluating the Plan
        1. Step One: Gather Information
        2. Step Two: Review the Contract Revisions
        3. Step Three: Investigate Utilization Review and Quality Assurance
        4. Step Four: Analyze the Plan Reimbursement
        5. Step Five: Make Recommendation to the Decision Maker
    B. Identify the Deal-Breakers
IV. The Do's and Don'ts of Contracting
V. Operations and Administration of the Process
VI. Conclusion

Introduction

Few health care entities contract with managed care organizations (MCOs) in order to gain access to a high volume of patients. Managed care contracts are reimbursement vehicles designed by insurers to manage the costs of care through negotiated rates. Physicians and hospitals are compelled to participate in managed care plans in exchange for the patients each payer represents. Medical practices, however, frequently forfeit available reimbursement due to lack of information about the specifics of managed care contracts and the requirements of each plan. Realistically, without adequate reimbursement for services, many practices are unsustainable over the long term. This chapter addresses strategies for getting paid at reasonable rates for the services the practice renders—money the practice deserves to make.

Basics of Negotiating Strategy

A reimbursement strategy for arriving at an acceptable middle ground with MCOs begins by laying initial ground work. The three guiding principles that form the foundation for negotiation are: (1) devote resources adequate to accomplish the task; (2) define the competition and know the market share; and (3) consistently remember that volume matters to payers, in that loss of membership can destabilize a plan more rapidly than financial loss.

Managed care contract negotiations, which typically occur annually, require preparation, organization, and consideration of all opportunities available to increase negotiating leverage. A good place to start is to gather all historical data available that support the strengths of the organization and all data that may support any historical performance problems with the MCO. Effective negotiation requires adequate time to prepare. As an illustration, if the contract renewal date of the MCO is December 31, preparation should begin well in advance. Begin by gathering information in early summer and setting meetings to discuss the terms of the contract. All arrangements and details must be discussed and in place by the fall in order for the contract to be effective by January 1. Each MCO will prepare to negotiate with employers during the fall so that by November/December, the MCO can wrap up negotiations for January 1 implementation. The important element of preparation is to allow adequate time to avoid being shut out by the MCOs' deadlines of having to negotiate with employers at the end of the year.

The negotiating team should involve the right people at the right time. The individual responsible for overall contract negotiations will assume the negotiating team lead; room should be left for an individual at a higher rank who may need to be brought in at the right time, particularly if negotiations stall. The practice's negotiating team leadership should possess the following "know" factors:

- Know the deal breakers.
- Know which issues are negotiable and which ones have an established conclusion.
- Know the organization's volumes and capacity.

- Know costs and the breakeven point.
- Know MCO comparisons.
  - Chart the volume of each plan.
  - Chart the bottom line of each plan.
  - Establish a goal to eliminate the below-cost plan(s).
- Know where patients are going (out-migration).
- Know why participants are going (quality of service, other participating providers).

The more you know about the MCO, the better equipped you will be during negotiations. Preparation involves determining historical member volumes by product type and the related reimbursement levels by product type. It also involves knowing about the plan's operational performance history. Ask these questions: Does the plan have the ability to provide timely and accurate data? Have the plan representatives been responsive? Is there a level of burden regarding authorization and referral requirements? It is important to know the MCO's chain of command and, most important, to establish a relationship with the plan representative, even though the representative's role is rarely more than a messenger. Knowledge of the MCO chain of command will make it easier to contact the decision maker and achieve a positive outcome. Because it would not be to their advantage, this individual may be the person the payer would not want you to contact. Conversely, it would not be to the practice negotiator's advantage to engage in dialogue with the MCO's decision maker prematurely, as it may be the only opportunity to influence this key person.

The long-term relationship should never be ignored in order to gain leverage in the short term; further, sometimes having no relationship is better than having a bad relationship. It is important to work hard to know the numbers and know the basis of the plan's numbers and specifically how the MCO calculated what it is bringing to the table. On behalf of the practice, the negotiators should not be afraid to ask for benefits that are essential for the organization's survival. Subsequently, the practice's negotiators should make an effort not to be the first to concede on major issues, as this is part of the give-and-take negotiating strategy. By planning for a negotiating strategy, the practice's negotiator can determine what the practice wants out of the discussions and establish risk limitations.

MCOs commonly indicate that they are unable to move on certain fees because they are "national." The immediate response to this MCO strategy should be to identify what they cannot move on and then aggressively negotiate on other parts. For example, if the MCO says that they cannot move on Evaluation and Management (E/M) codes because they are set at the national level, the immediate response should be to look at all individual procedures that are not in the E/M section of the contract and negotiate better rates for those procedures.

Another common MCO strategy is to express a take-it-or-leave-it position. When this discussion ensues (and usually emotions rise), it is best to be reluctant to accept this way of thinking. Some reasonable responses include, "My understanding is that we were both working toward a partnership" or "I perceive you are not negotiating in good faith." The goal is to not be reluctant to state the issues and call the bluff and, at the same time, acknowledge when the practice cannot just walk away from the deal. One successful strategy is to ask for something, thus giving the appearance of negotiating. For example, if you first gave consideration to your fee structure and knew that it was solid and reasonable, you could ask for a percent of charges to gain the benefit, even though you are well aware that the MCO is negotiating toward a fixed rate schedule. Here the objective is to ask for something and yet appear to be willing to go with the MCO view of a fixed rate, even though you have not conceded anything. In the event that the negotiations drag on and the proposed changes seemingly are not being heard, consider other strategies, such as asking for a shorter contract, possibly six months, or walking away (reaching no agreement and not signing).

Every effort should be made to back away from confrontation in negotiations and move to another element of the contract, such as volumes, outcomes, or history, thus, pulling the discussion away from only rates.

The negotiating team should be led by the organization's most seasoned managed care leader; the business office manager should be involved throughout the negotiations to ensure that the contract can be effectively implemented. Legal counsel and a business advisor, such as a consultant or financial advisor, should also be on the negotiating team.

The Negotiation Process

Nothing can take the place of being organized responsive and having an agreed-upon strategy prior to negotiations. This section focuses on the evaluation process.

Evaluating the Plan

To prepare the negotiating team, each plan should be evaluated separately. The following steps should be considered when evaluating each plan.

Step One: Gather information

- Make a list of all the plans the practice is considering.
- Call the health plans or the third-party organization (TPO) that administers other plans not contracted with by the practice, eg, Blue Cross, Aetna, Prudential. Tell them that the practice

is considering participation and ask for credentialing applications and a contract.

- Ask for a list of all physicians in the market area who are participating in the plan (or access it via the plan Website).
- Inquire about market share and program growth.
- Inquire regarding a list of employers in the market area that offer the plan.
- Obtain the plan's standard payment rates (see Figure 2-1).

Step Two: Review the Contract Revisions

Look specifically at certain provisions and make sure you have an understanding of and agreements with these provisions. Essential elements include:

- applicability to MCO products;
- claim submission and payment, definitions, amendment, termination;

MEMORANDUM

TO: Managed Care Provider
FROM: ENT Associates
RE: Your Proposed Contract

We have reviewed the terms of your proposed contract and are interested in joining your plan. Prior to signing, we would like to know your proposed payment for the following codes:

CPT Code	Our Fee ($)
99203	70
99204	100
99205	130
99212	30
99213	48.50
99214	72.50
99242	85

CPT Code	Our Fee ($)
99243	110
99244	140
30420	2750
31250	150
31252	500
42415	2300

FIGURE 2-1 Memorandum to the Managed Care Provider.

- retrospective denial and refunds;
- access to books and records;
- audits and reconciliation;
- appeals and dispute resolution; and
- code edits*.

Step Three: Investigate Utilization Review and Quality Assurance

The evaluation should investigate utilization review (UR) and quality assurance. Ask these questions:

- Is there a peer review or performance rating system?
- What services/procedures need to be preauthorized?
- Are there clinical guidelines that impact the practice?
- Are there standards and procedures for peer review that address quality assurance and cost containment?
- Does the plan have its own UR department or does it subcontract for UR and peer review?

Step Four: Analyze the Plan Reimbursement

In considering what is being offered by the plan, look at the methodology used, gain understanding of the weighted average of the plan, and perform a break-even analysis to determine the dollar impact the practice is negotiating against. Table 2-1 illustrates how to determine a plan's weight average. It is critical to use the procedure frequency report when evaluating how one plan measures up to others. You must be aware of which Current Procedural Terminology (CPT®) codes have the highest utilization and be able to document fees in order to compare each plans ultimate reimbursement. In addition to calculating conversion factors and comparing fees against Medicare and the plan's fees, the usefulness during negotiations becomes apparent when you determine this weighted average reimbursement.

Follow these steps when completing the calculations:

1. Multiply both the physician charges and payer reimbursements by the frequency at which these procedures are performed.
2. Calculate the total gross charges and total gross payments for all CPT codes.
3. Divide the total gross payments into total gross charges to determine the weighted percentage of reimbursement for each plan.

---

*The Medicare Code Editor (MCE) detects and reports errors in the coding claims data. An example is available at http://www.cms.hhs.gov/AcuteInpatientPPS/downloads/MCEonIPPSUserGuide.pdf. Accessed March 23, 2010.

TABLE 2-1 Chart for Determining Weight Average of the Plan

CPT Code (A)	Your Fee (B)	Medicare wRVU (F)	RBRVS Individual Conversion Factors (G)	RBRVS Conversion Factor @ $____ (H)
99201		0.45		
99202		0.88		
99203		1.34		
99204		2.30		
99205		3.00		
99211		0.17		
99212		0.45		
99213		0.92		
99214		1.42		
99215		2.00		
99241		0.64		
99242		1.34		

The goal of many practices is to have a minimum of 70% reimbursement on their fees (this would equal a 30% discount rate).

Step Five: Make Recommendation to the Decision Maker

The final step in evaluating the plan is to summarize recommendations for the decision maker. Put the summarized conclusion in a written format and clearly show all financial indicators that were used, an assessment of the MCO, an operational impact as well as a legal assessment, and, finally, what is recommended upon entering into negotiations.

Identify the Deal-Breakers

When planning for the negotiating process, be aware of several areas that are considered to be deal-breakers. MCOs will attempt to influence certain items that could tip the scales unfairly in their favor. Those at the practice level must know costs; subsequently, any agreed-upon fees and reimbursement must at least equal all of the practice's costs, including direct and indirect overhead costs. Another potential deal-breaker, particularly in a solo or small practice, would be if the considered fees do not result in an acceptable bottom line to the physician(s). Caution should be taken by any practice that assumes the obligations of the MCO (nonfinancial considerations such as undue reporting mechanisms or laborious and burdensome quality measures in order to meet certain proposed fees). Similarly, do not negotiate contract terms that are purely alterable at the MCO's will, such as any unilateral amendments that consider only the MCO. Another example of this is when an MCO attempts to influence contract terms whereby the practice does not have the opportunity to appeal adverse decisions, such as utilization review and quality assurance inquiries.

What are considered tie-breakers in the negotiating process? At this point assume that the practice's negotiators have prepared adequately for the negotiating process and have significantly influenced a decision that the practice can live with. The rates may be acceptable, but be cautious of anything that limits the ability to bill beyond 90 days after the service date, as well as an MCO's ability to assign without providing a notice or gaining approval from the practice. Both of these items would be seen as "non-rate items" even though they affect cash flow. Another tie-breaker would be if the MCO demands that they have the ability to deny payment retroactively; this does not solidify considerations of accounts receivable and cash. On the other hand, certain nonfinancial items that could be viewed as to the practice's benefit might be negotiated, such as exclusivity in the market or specific agreement that the payment period is less than 30 days. In contrast, an MCO could state in writing that the payment period may be allowed to go beyond 45 days.

The Do's and Don'ts of Contracting

To negotiate favorable contracts with each plan, the following essential elements must be kept in mind. Someone on the negotiating team, ideally the leader, must have a working knowledge and understanding of both incremental and replacement pricing strategies. Incremental pricing is aligned to cost (a bottom-line consideration), and replacement pricing is pricing as it relates to revenue (volume consideration). To influence the strategy to the practice's benefit, one may only be concerned with the actual dollar impact to the bottom-line incremental. Conversely, the practice negotiators may want to negotiate so as to significantly increase volumes due to clear capacity opportunities within the entity. When a capitation contract is on the table, the negotiating team must initially establish a basis for performing a cost accounting exercise for each procedure the practice performs. One benefit of a capitation contract being offered is that certain market information may become available that might not be apparent with other contract strategies.

The following checklist will help in influencing favorable contracts that are beneficial to the practice:

- Define utilization management and credentialing.
- Know the size and any limits on access of the provider network.
- Assure data are in agreement (practice versus MCO).
- Verify plan data independently.
- Define services (seizing every opportunity to be reimbursed).
- Consider scenarios for location of services to be rendered.
- Establish arbitration procedures.
- Assess impact of copayment levels on capitation rates.
- Include methodology for dealing with noncompliant members.
- Use market rates in absence of good historical data.
- Include, provisions for contracts that do not get renegotiated before the end of the contract term.
- Review stop-loss attachment.
- Include-mechanism for reconciling stop-loss payments to actual experience.
- Nail down provisions for additions and deletions to the plan.
- Place all services offered on the table and gain price agreement.

The following due-diligence steps should be considered ideally before, but no later than during, the negotiating process:

- Discover the ownership/form of organization.
- Understand the organization's history.
- Know what type of relationship the practice is entering into.
- Get a list of corporate and local officers and management.
- Have copies of the agreement, fee schedule, referenced attachments and exhibits, including policies and procedures manuals.
- Maximize the use of your information technology department.
- Collect geographic, membership, and covered lives demographics.
- Identify the current provider network.
- Know the major employer groups.
- Conduct a reference check on the MCO.
- Discuss the MCO's marketing plan.
- Look into opportunities for "designated provider" status.
- Question the claim billing system.

- Know the provider's representatives for claims management issues and general contract issues.
- Know the required primary care physicians approvals.
- Understand the procedures for out-of-plan approval.
- Ask for a copy of the grievance or dispute procedure.
- Learn what documentation is available.
- Assess how the MCO's required procedures vary from your current procedures.
- Evaluate the marketing materials that are given to members.
- Get written confirmation of all explanations and agreements.
- Review the hold harmless/indemnification clause.
- Go through a legal review.

Operations and Administration of the Process

Assuming that the contract negotiating process was well-planned and allowed for discussion of key matters and that a reasonable and favorable process took place, much work still remains pertaining to the specific plan. All levels of management and staff must now consider how to effectively administer the contract terms. All staff should realize that when adequate reimbursement does not seem apparent, it is acceptable to encourage the patient to go back to his or her employer or those responsible for the contract. Likewise, the patient should be shown the appropriate portion of his or her bill and expect prompt payment. Many practices are reluctant to share difficult news with patients, even though it is the employer, not the practice, that sets the parameters for payment and, specifically, their deductible and copayment. In many cases, the practice does not set the rules for selection of a patient's employer's plan, and practice staff cannot get involved in the emotions that patients experience as a result of certain outcomes. In considering operations and administration of the reimbursement process, management should be willing to consider a reduction of certain services or procedures that clearly lose money (eg, MCO rates do not even meet the direct cost).

Although this chapter has provided documentation relative to the dollars and cents of running a practice, the underlying principle is that service to patients and the community must come first. All plans should be administered in a way that encourages patients to use the practice's services regardless of the difficulty in administering certain contracts. The goal is to administer all contracts so as to achieve volumes that are close to what can be handled effectively from a capacity standpoint. Likewise, some contracts may be subject to nonrenewal because volumes are unacceptable and select MCOs have not been consistent in offering acceptable rates. Another example of administering to near capacity would be to reduce volumes on certain days. If Wednesday is consistently a slow day, it is acceptable and actually advisable to reduce service hours on that day such that the remaining weekdays can be administered near capacity. The administrative process should include renewal reminders for all MCO contracts to allow adequate time to prepare for renegotiations and consider a plan's effect on the practice.

Conclusion

While performing the difficult task of negotiating meaningful contracts with MCOs, the negotiation team should embrace the attitude that the practice's business is important to the MCO. The MCO would not be in business if it did not have satisfactory arrangements with every entity with which it contracts. In other words, the practice should acknowledge its leverage and should not give up. Negotiators must be well prepared, confident in the numbers they have generated, and willing to manage the practice to near capacity. The negotiating process and strategy is as important as any other job within the practice. Accordingly, time must be set aside to prepare and get organized and to achieve effective communications with others. In this case, the MCO representative should become a valued partner in medical practice administration.

Following are some helpful resources for developing negotiation skills and strategies:

Fisher R, Ury W. *Getting to Yes: Negotiation Agreement Without Giving In*, 2nd ed. New York: Penguin Group; 1991.

Laubach CL. *Mastering the Negotiation Process: A Practical Guide for the Healthcare Executive*. Ann Arbor: Health Administration Press; 2002.

Lax DA, Sebenius JK. *3-d Negotiation: Powerful Tools to Change the Game in Your Most Important Deals*. Boston: Harvard Business Press; 2006.

Mnookin R. *Bargaining with the Devil: When to Negotiate, When to Fight*. New York: Simon & Schuster; 2010.

Shell GR. *Bargaining for Advantage: Negotiation Strategies for Reasonable People*, 2nd ed. New York: Penguin Group; 2006.

CHAPTER 3
Pay for Performance and Quality Initiatives

OUTLINE

I. Introduction
II. Quality
    A. Aligning Forces for Quality
    B. National Committee for Quality Assurance
    C. Agency for Healthcare Research and Quality
    D. Health Plans
    E. Conclusions
III. Pay for Performance
    A. Professional Organizations
        1. Institute of Medicine
        2. Medical Group Management Association
        3. American Academy of Family Physicians
        4. American Medical Association
    B. Government Programs
        1. Centers for Medicare and Medicaid Services
        2. Physician Group Practice Demonstration
        3. Premier Hospital Quality Incentive
        4. Medicare Care Management Performance
        5. Medicare Health Care Quality Program
        6. Chronic Care Improvement Program
        7. End Stage Renal Disease Quality Initiative
        8. Disease Management for Severely Chronically Ill
        9. Care Management for High Cost Beneficiaries
    C. Conclusions

IV. Physician Quality Reporting Initiative
   A. Background Information
   B. Eligible Providers
   C. Incentive Payment
   D. 2010 PQRI Program: Reporting
   E. 2010 PQRI: Measures
   F. Claims-Based Reporting
   G. Maximizing Success Within the PQRI Program
   H. Available PQRI Resources
   I. Group Practice Reporting Option
   J. Conclusions
V. Conclusion

> P4P programs are designed to offer financial incentives to physicians for providing evidenced-based care, achieving favorable patient outcomes and/or improving patient satisfaction.
>
> —*Ready or not, pay for performance is here,* MGMA Connexion, October 2005[1]

Introduction

Pay for performance (P4P) and quality programs are relative newcomers to the health care industry. In some industries, such as manufacturing, products are routinely tested for adherence to quality protocols. The same has historically not been true within service-based industries, including health care. In the past, clinicians offered their services, and patients trusted that the care they received was of the highest possible quality. Today, various government agencies, along with public and private organizations, are working to measure the quality of services provided to patients, compare them to best practices, publicize scores specific to individual physicians and hospitals, and even provide monetary and other rewards for providers whose care meets specific guidelines.

This chapter discusses the opportunities to participate in programs designed to improve quality that have developed within the realm of quality, including opportunities for hospitals, practices, and providers to participate in established P4P programs.

Also discussed in this chapter are the nuances of the Centers for Medicare and Medicaid Services' (CMS') Physician Quality Reporting Initiative (PQRI). This is a relatively new program, inaugurated in 2007, that provides an incentive payment to Medicare providers for reporting on clinically relevant quality measures.

Quality

Although quality is an increasingly important component within health care today, it has not always been such an integral part of the industry. However, several organizations have truly championed the quality effort and driven it to the forefront of health care. Their efforts include the Aligning Forces for Quality Project, the National Committee for Quality Assurance, and the Agency for Healthcare Research and Quality. In addition, health plans and commercial payers have begun to embrace and implement quality-focused initiatives and have raised awareness on the part of both physicians and patients. The impact of each of these efforts is the subject of this section.

Aligning Forces for Quality

The Aligning Forces for Quality (AF4Q) initiative, which is funded by the Robert Wood Johnson Foundation (RWJF), began in 2006 and aims to:

- help physicians and nurses improve the quality of care for patients,
- engage people more fully in their own health care experiences,
- make data on physicians' performance available to the public, and
- reduce inequality in care for patients of different races and ethnicities.[2]

The first phase of the AF4Q initiative focused on implementing health care systems in areas where such services were not currently available. AFQ4 considered this phase such a success that the initial scope was expanded in June 2008 to focus on the role of nursing, inpatient care, and the gaps in health care that exist from both a racial and ethnic perspective.[3] There are now three focus areas within the initiative, including quality improvement, consumer engagement, and performance measurement/public reporting.

Currently there are 17 communities or states throughout the United States participating in the initiative, including Albuquerque, N.M.; Boston, Mass.; Central Indiana; Cincinnati, Ohio; Cleveland, Ohio; Detroit, Mich.; Humboldt County, Calif.; Kansas City, Mo.; Maine; Memphis, Tenn.; Minnesota; Puget Sound, Wash.; South Central Pennsylvania; West Michigan; Western New York; Willamette Valley, Ore.; and Wisconsin. These regions account for 12.5% of the total U.S. population and represent not only a cross section of the nation's population but also a comprehensive subset of health care stakeholders, including providers (physicians and nurses), hospitals, patients, health plans, purchasers, and consumer groups. One tenet of the AF4Q program is that a community-based approach is necessary to effect the change that is necessary to develop and maximize the U.S. health care system.

The RWJF has committed up to $300 million in efforts to ensure that the highest possible quality of health care is being provided in America and that there is equality among all Americans in regards to the health care that is accessed and received.

National Committee for Quality Assurance

Another entity that strives to drive the quality initiative within the health care industry is the National Committee for Quality Assurance (NCQA). NCQA's mission and vision are clear: its mission is to improve the quality of health care and its vision is to transform health care quality through measurement, transparency, and accountability.[4] One way that NCQA addresses its mission is through accreditation, certification, and recognition programs. As part of these programs, NCQA collects data relative to health care delivery, outcomes, and overall quality of care. This information is then made available to a wide public audience, including patients, physicians, and health plans, who can use this data to make informed decisions related to health care. NCQA began its accreditation process in 1991; they currently have six accreditation programs, including disease management, health plan accreditation, wellness and health promotion, managed behavioral health care organization, new health plan, and quality plus. In addition, they have several certification programs, including multicultural health care, physician organizations, health information products, credentials verification organizations, physician and hospital quality, organization certification, and disease management. NCQA also has a number of recognition programs, including patient-centered medical home, back pain recognition, diabetes recognition, heart/stroke recognition, and physician practice connections. NCQA designation requires significant effort and denotes a marked effort to meet its standards.

One of the most widespread impacts of NCQA is in its continuous evaluation of the Healthcare Effectiveness Data and Information Set (HEDIS) measures. HEDIS is used by more than 90% of America's health plans to measure performance on a variety of health issues.[5] Although initially designed for health plan evaluation, NCQA now works in conjunction with the Physician Consortium for Performance Improvement founded by the American Medical Association to identify measures for physician use. Each year, NCQA's Committee on Performance Measurement (CPM) analyzes the current and potential measures and renders a decision on what measures should be included within HEDIS for the following year. In 2010, HEDIS includes 71 measures across several key areas, including asthma, heart attack, high blood pressure, diabetes, breast cancer, and depression.

Agency for Healthcare Research and Quality

There has been an increase in governmental participation in quality initiatives, including efforts by the Agency for Healthcare Research and Quality (AHRQ), an organization within the U.S. Department of Health and Human Services (HHS). One of AHRQ's quality-minded initiatives is the Consumer Assessment of Healthcare Providers and Systems (CAHPS). This program helps to develop and promote standardized consumer surveys that can be used to assess various aspects of health care. The two overarching goals of the program are to:

- develop standardized patient questionnaires that can be used to compare results across sponsors and over time; and
- generate tools and resources that sponsors can use to produce understandable and usable comparative information for both consumers and health care providers.[6]

Interestingly, even the name CAHPS represents the movement that has taken place within the health care industry. Originally defined as the Consumer Assessment of Health Plans Study when the program began in October 1995, as research and interest in quality initiatives grew from considering only health plans to a vast expanse of health care providers, AHRQ recognized this shift and grew with it. The program is currently in its third stage, known as CAHPS3. In the first stage, CAHPS1, the program focused on developing tools that consumers could use to evaluate their experiences with health plans. In CAHPS2, the second stage of the program, the focus expanded to developing survey tools that were also relevant to medical groups and individual providers. Now, in CAHPS3, the objectives center on the tools necessary to support the use of surveys that have already been created. Data collected from the three stages of the program are catalogued in the National CAHPS Benchmarking Database, which is accessible to the public at www.cahps.ahrq.gov/CAHPSIDB/Default.aspx.

Health Plans

Health plans were some of the first institutions to be assessed in terms of the quality of care they offered to patients, largely as a result of programs such as NCQA and CAHPS. However, health plans have become more accepting of quality initiatives and more proactive in their program planning surrounding quality. Some major health plans, such as Aetna, CIGNA, and Blue Cross Blue Shield, have elected to participate in the larger, established quality programs. For example, CIGNA participates in the NCQA accreditation program. It has been awarded "excellent status" according to the Managed Care Organization standards and "distinguished status" according to the Quality Plus standards. Other health plans have developed their own comprehensive quality plans, which aim to positively influence the delivery of health care services. For example, in 2006, Blue Cross Blue Shield implemented their Blue Distinction program, which recognizes facilities that meet objective, evidence-based thresholds for clinical quality. The goals of the program are to encourage providers to improve the overall quality and delivery of health care to achieve better overall outcomes for patients and to support consumers as they identify medical facilities that best meet their needs.[7] The program awards the Centers for Specialty Care designation to facilities within six key areas that meet rigorous criteria related to quality. The targeted areas include bariatric surgery, cardiac care, complex and rare cancers, knee and hip replacement, spine surgery, and transplants. There are currently 1,600 centers throughout the United States that have earned this recognition.

Conclusions

The focus on quality initiatives is continually evolving within the health care industry and it has significantly increased based on the work completed by programs and organizations such as the AF4Q, NCQA, and AQHR. Continuing to engage individual physicians as well as larger health plans as they relates to quality will be important in building new and more successful health improvement programs.

Pay for Performance

The increased focus on quality within the health care industry has led to the development of many related initiatives, including pay for performance (P4P). Different stakeholders within the health care industry have influenced the P4P landscape, including professional organizations and governmental programs. The various roles these entities play are defined in this section.

Professional Organizations

Several professional organizations have been influential in the development of the P4P process, including the Institute of Medicine (IOM), the Medical Group Management Association (MGMA), the American Academy of Family Physicians (AAFP), and the American Medical Association (AMA). (Note: The AMA neither supports nor approves of P4P, but does have a strict policy of "do's and don'ts" when it is being utilized.)

Institute of Medicine

In 2001, the Institute of Medicine (IOM) released its landmark report, "Crossing the Quality Chasm: A New Health Care System for the 21st Century," which called for significant change to the U.S. health care system.[8] One well-known quote from that report, "Between the health care we have and the care we could have lies not just a gap, but a chasm," is cited often when P4P is discussed. Within this report, the IOM developed 10 principles that they believe should form the basis for health care redesign:

1. Care is based on continuous healing relationships.
2. Care is customized according to patient needs and values.
3. The patient is the source of control.
4. Knowledge is shared and information flows freely.
5. Decision making is evidence-based.
6. Safety is a system property.
7. Transparency is necessary.
8. Needs are anticipated.
9. Waste is continuously decreased.
10. Cooperation among clinicians is a priority.

These 10 principles along with the entire IOM report and subsequent updates have generated a great deal of conversation regarding P4P. IOM continues to issue reports related to quality performance and improvement, with almost 600 reports published to date.

Medical Group Management Association

The Medical Group Management Association (MGMA) has taken steps to develop standards relating to P4P. In February 2005, the MGMA board of directors approved and released a position paper titled, "Principles for Pay-for-Performance Programs and Recommendations for Medical Group Practices," which established nine principles for evaluating participation in P4P, including the following:

1. The primary goal of P4P programs must be improving health quality and safety.
2. Medical group practice participation in P4P programs must be voluntary.
3. Practicing physicians and physician professional organizations must be involved in the design of P4P programs.
4. Physician performance measures used in P4P programs must be evidence-based, broadly accepted, clinically relevant, continually updated, and developed by practicing physicians.
5. Physician performance data must be fully adjusted for sample size and case-mix composition, including factors of age/sex distribution, severity of illness, number of co-morbid conditions, and other features of physician practice and patient population that may influence results.

6. P4P programs must reward physician participation, including physician use of electronic health records and decision-support tools.
7. A Medicare P4P program must not be budget-neutral within the Medicare physician payment system or subject to artificial Medicare payment volume controls, such as the sustainable growth rate (SGR).
8. P4P programs must reimburse physicians for any administrative burden for collecting and reporting data to payers.
9. Physicians must have the ability to review and correct performance data.

The MGMA's position paper, similar to the IOM report, established clear principles to guide the development of P4P initiatives. It was also a reminder to the health care community that P4P remained an issue, and even four years after the release of the IOM report, much work was yet to be done to ensure that patients were receiving the highest quality care as part of a system that valued safety *and* cost control.[9]

American Academy of Family Physicians

The American Academy of Family Physicians (AAFP) has taken a progressive yet structured approach to P4P. As taken from its "Policy Statement on Pay for Performance," the AAFP supports P4P under the following stipulations:

1. P4P programs should provide incentives to physician practices for:
    a. the adoption and utilization of health information technologies;
    b. the implementation of systems to improve the quality of patient care and patient safety;
    c. adhering to evidence-based clinical guidelines;
    d. improving performance and meeting performance targets;
    e. improving patient access to appropriate and timely care; and
    f. measuring and attempting to improve patient acceptance and satisfaction with their care.
2. P4P programs should be consolidated across employers and health plans to make the payment meaningful and the program more manageable for physician practices.
3. P4P incentive programs should utilize new money funded by using a portion of the projected total system savings. There should be no reduction in existing fees for service paid to physicians as a result of implementing a P4P program.
4. The financial rewards to physician practices must be more than sufficient to both recoup the additional administrative costs to participate in the program (data collection and measurement) and provide significant incentive.

5. The program cannot create incentives that place physicians at odds with their patients, eg, incentives to fragment care or deselect certain patients. If a physician is inappropriately deselecting non-adherent patients solely for financial reasons and this can be demonstrated through appropriate documentation, the physician may forfeit his or her pay-for-performance incentives. Case-mix evaluation and appropriate adjustments, including known clinical and socioeconomic factors, should be employed to allow fair comparisons of different practices.
6. Programs should minimize administrative, financial, and technological barriers to participation.
7. The P4P entity should notify the patients affected, provide related self-care information, and reinforce patient responsibilities in achieving the desired health outcomes.
8. When evidence is lacking regarding the value of a particular diagnostic or therapeutic intervention, acknowledge that physicians' judgment, patient's preference, and the costs associated with various options may be the best measures of the appropriateness of a given intervention for P4P purposes.
9. Patient cases should be removed from the performance measure(s) being assessed ("denominator exclusion") when a physician can demonstrate that attempts have been made to provide patients support to follow recommended care and they have subsequently not followed such recommendations, the recommendations are inappropriate for this patient due to other clinical or socioeconomic considerations, or the patient is unable to comply.
10. Programs should be designed to include practices of all sizes.[10]

The AAFP works collaboratively with a number of other professional organizations and governmental agencies on quality and P4P initiatives, including the AMA's Physician Consortium for Performance Improvement.

American Medical Association

In 2000, the American Medical Association (AMA) convened the Physician Consortium for Performance Improvement (PCPI) to develop clinical performance measures that are patient-focused and that can be implemented to improve patient outcomes. The PCPI actively engages all stakeholders, including payers, patient advocates, and other organizations that are committed to high-quality care. The PCPI has grown more than 130% since its inception and is currently comprised of more than 170 member organizations, including national medical specialty and state medical societies, other health care professional organizations, the Council of Medical Specialty Societies, the American Board of Medical Specialties and its member boards, experts in methodology and data collection, the Agency for Healthcare Research and Quality, and CMS.

The PCPI has experienced many successes during its 10-year tenure. By the end of 2009, there were 270 PCPI measures within 43 measure sets. The organization has set a goal to develop at least six new measure sets in 2010, including adult sinusitis, back pain management, dementia, diagnostic imaging, maternity care, and percutaneous coronary intervention.[11]

As the leading developer of physician-level measures, it is recommended that the PCPI be recognized as such in CMS' plan to ensure that clinically relevant quality measures are accurately specified and adequately tested for inclusion in the meaningful-use program. The PCPI incorporates all critical factors in the measure-development process and is also committed to maintaining its portfolio of measures. It operates through a transparent, consensus-based process for developing physician-level measures and has worked aggressively to develop more than 270 physician performance measures and specifications covering 43 clinical topics and conditions. These measures are available for implementation, and many have been adopted by CMS for use in CMS quality improvement demonstration projects and the PQRI. In addition, the PCPI ensures that measures (1) are evidence-based and developed with cross-specialty representation and consensus; (2) include enhanced relevance to clinical practice; and (3) that the measure developer is committed to maintaining its measures. Any incentive program must use measures that meet these criteria.

Like other organizations previously discussed, AMA has been integral in creating and publicizing their standards for P4P programs. The association has published these views in "Principles for Pay-for-Performance Programs" and "Guidelines for Pay-for-Performance Programs" (both are available at www.ama-assn.org/ama/pub/advocacy/current-topics-advocacy/private-sector-advocacy/practice-data-ranking/pay-for-performance.shtml). The AMA's principles for P4P programs are as follows:

1. Ensure quality of care.
2. Foster the patient/physician relationship.
3. Offer voluntary physician participation.
4. Use accurate data and fair reporting.
5. Provide fair and equitable program incentives.

Government Programs

Centers for Medicare and Medicaid Services

As P4P became a larger focus within the nation's health care delivery system, Centers for Medicare and Medicaid Services (CMS) took action and implemented various quality programs to encourage improved quality care in health care settings where Medicare beneficiaries receive services. These settings include physician offices, ambulatory care facilities, hospitals, nursing homes, home health agencies, and dialysis facilities. Many of these programs were implemented after HHS and CMS announced the creation of a large-scale quality initiative in November 2001. According to CMS, the "initiative is intended to (a) empower consumers with quality of care information to make more informed decisions about their health care, and (b) encourage providers and clinicians to improve the quality of health care."[12] The initiative was launched in November 2002 for nursing homes and was expanded to home health agencies and hospitals in 2003. In 2004, it was expanded again to include end stage renal disease (ESRD) efforts. Several of the programs created through the initiative are discussed below.

Physician Group Practice Demonstration

CMS is working with physician practices to evaluate quality-based incentive payments. The Physician Group Practice (PGP) Demonstration is one example. This was the first P4P initiative for physicians under the Medicare program and includes 10 large (200+ physicians) group practices throughout the United States. The program rewards physicians for improving the quality and efficiency of health care delivered to Medicare beneficiaries. By the third year of the initiative, all 10 physician groups had achieved benchmark performance on 28 or more of the 32 measures, and two practices achieved benchmark performance on all 32 performance measures, including areas related to diabetes, congestive heart failure, coronary disease, cancer screening, and hypertension. As a result of their participation within the program, five groups will have received a total of $25.3 million, their portion of the $32.3 million in Medicare savings that were generated in year 3 alone.[13]

Premier Hospital Quality Incentive

One CMS quality program related to hospital care is the Premier Hospital Quality Incentive (PHQI). In 2003, CMS partnered with Premier, Inc., to implement and manage the PHQI, which "recognizes and provides financial rewards to hospitals that demonstrate high quality performance in a number of areas of acute care."[14] Under this program, hospitals are paid bonuses for achieving high performance in the treatment of the following five clinical conditions:

1. Acute myocardial infarction
2. Heart failure
3. Pneumonia
4. Coronary artery bypass graft
5. Hip and knee replacements

One outcome of the project is a publically available Web tool, Hospital Compare (available at www.hospitalcompare.hhs.gov), that includes information on the quality of care being provided in hospitals throughout the United States. Debuted in April 2005, Hospital Compare aims to be an informational resource for health care consumers. Currently, the hospital quality measures reported within Hospital Compare fall into one of six categories:

1. Acute myocardial infarction
2. Heart failure
3. Pneumonia
4. Surgical care improvement project
5. Hospital consumer assessment of health care providers and systems
6. Children's asthma care[15]

During the project's first four years (2003–2007), CMS paid more than $36.5 million to the top-performing hospitals, including payments of $12 million to 225 hospitals in year 4 (which ended in October 2007).[16] The program's successes have resulted in expansion from its initial three-year demonstration period, to allow CMS to test new incentive models and additional ways to improve patient care.[17]

Medicare Care Management Performance

The Medicare Care Management Performance (MCMP) demonstration project recognizes and provides financial rewards to physicians who demonstrate high-quality performance in numerous areas of acute care. The project tests methods to promote the use of health information technology to help improve quality of care for chronically ill Medicare beneficiaries. These include areas of diabetes, heart failure, coronary artery disease, and preventative care. Enacted through Section 649 of the Medicare Prescription Drug, Improvement, and Modernization Act of 2003 (MMA), the program was implemented on July 1, 2007, in both rural and urban sites in Arkansas, California, Massachusetts, and Utah. Unlike the PGP demonstration, the focus of this program is on small to medium-sized physician practices. The first incentive payments under the MCMP were made in spring 2008 and totaled $1.5 million. In total, 88% of participating practices received the maximum potential payment for which they were eligible. In the second year, the practices were incentivized on the performance of the quality measures, not simply on whether or not they were reported, and this will likely continue until the program ends on June 30, 2010.

Medicare Health Care Quality Program

Other physician-based programs include the Medicare Health Care Quality Program, a five-year program to enhance quality while improving patient safety, encourage shared decision-making, and cultivate the use of culturally and ethnically appropriate care. This program, enacted through Section 646 of the MMA, includes physician practices, integrated health systems, and regional physician coalitions.

Another initiative, the Physician Quality Reporting Initiative, which is discussed in detail later in this chapter, has become one of the most expansive physician quality initiatives.

Chronic Care Improvement Program

Specific programs exist to address disease management. From 1999 to 2009, CMS conducted seven disease management demonstrations that included 35 programs and more than 300,000 beneficiaries. One such program, the Chronic Care Improvement Program (CCIP; later changed to the Medicare Health Support Program [MHSP]), was implemented to test a population-based model of disease management for advanced congestive heart failure and/or complex diabetes. It was implemented between August 2005 and January 2006 by various health care agencies in nine sites, including Humana, Inc. (South and Central Florida), CIGNA Health Support, LLC (Georgia), XLHealth Corporation (Tennessee), McKesson Health Solutions (Mississippi), Health Dialog Services Corporation (Pennsylvania), Aetna Life Insurance Company, LLC (Illinois), LifeMasters Supported SelfCare (Oklahoma), United (New York), and American Healthways (Washington, D.C., and Maryland). After several of the agencies requested early termination and preliminary results demonstrated a greater cost than potential savings, CMS announced in January 2008 that the program would be discontinued at the end of its three-year pilot period.

End Stage Renal Disease Quality Initiative

Although the potential of the MHSP program was not maximized, CMS also implemented several other programs that target quality for disease management, including those within the End Stage Renal Disease Quality Initiative (ESRDQI). The ESRDQI is a wide-reaching program that includes several different components, including the Dialysis Facility Compare (accessible at www.medicare.gov), the Fistula First Breakthrough Initiative, and the ESRD Disease Management Demonstration. The demonstration program, which began in summer 2005 and lasted for four years, tested a case-mix–adjusted payment system for a larger scope of ESRD services. Organizations that served ESRD patients were eligible to receive payment to test the effectiveness of various disease management models aimed at increasing quality and controlling cost.

Disease Management for Severely Chronically Ill

Another program, the Disease Management for Severely Chronically Ill, tested whether disease management and prescription drug coverage in a fee-for-service environment will improve health outcomes and reduce costs for the severely chronically ill. The conditions considered within the program included congestive heart failure, diabetes, and coronary artery disease, among others. Participants in this program, which began in February 2004, include XLHealth (Texas), CorSolutions (Louisiana), and HeartPartners (California and Arizona). Next, the Disease Management for Chronically Ill Dual Eligible Beneficiaries provided disease management services to Medicaid- and Medicare-eligible enrollees who suffer from congestive heart failure, diabetes, or coronary heart disease.

Care Management for High Cost Beneficiaries

The Care Management for High Cost Beneficiaries (CMHCB) program provides care management for the high-cost and high-risk Medicare fee-for-service (FFS) population, those beneficiaries who have multiple chronic diseases and typically incur higher Medicare costs. Six organizations from across the United States were part of the original three-year pilot; all organizations focused on congestive heart failure, diabetes, and chronic kidney disease. In January 2009, three participants in this program (Key to Better Health, Massachusetts General Care Management program, and Health Hero Network) received a three-year extension based on their success in managing costs during the initial demonstration and in meeting or exceeding the savings target that was part of the demonstration agreement. The intent is for these three organizations to continue to maximize savings and assist CMS in determining if the program can be replicated in other areas and for a larger overall audience.[18]

Conclusions

P4P has been greatly influenced by academic institutions, professional organizations, governmental agencies, and health plans. These groups have researched much of the theory behind P4P programs and have taken action by implementing various programs, while taking steps to demand better transparency and accuracy in the physician ratings used by other such programs, to encourage physicians, medical practices, and hospitals to move toward higher-quality patient care and lower costs. These stakeholders have acted on the recognition that the U.S. health care system must be improved in order to remain sustainable and that quality and cost are two of the key metrics that will "make or break" the system in the long term. To that end, physicians, health care organizations, third-party payers, and the government must continue to explore, test, and improve the transparency and problematic accuracy ratings used in P4P models to determine the most efficient way in which to structure, implement, and manage such programs. These programs may have the potential to significantly impact the health care industry in a significant fashion, but only if the physician quality and cost efficiency ratings accurately reflect physicians' practices.

Physician Quality Reporting Initiative

The Physician Quality Reporting Initiative (PQRI) is one of the government's most recognized physician health care quality programs; it has grown both in scale and size since its inception in 2007. This section provides information regarding the program's history and current status as well as useful information to assist physicians in maximizing their potential for successful reporting.

Background Information

PQRI is a voluntary reporting program designed to improve quality through the use of performance measures related to a variety of clinical conditions. Established by CMS in July 2007, the program was originally enacted through the Tax Relief and Healthcare Act of 2006 (TRHCA), which was signed by President Bush on December 20, 2006. Overall, PQRI was built on and ultimately replaced the 2006 Physician Voluntary Reporting Program (PVRP). Although established as a smaller-scale, temporary program, continuation of PQRI was allowed when President Bush signed the Medicare, Medicaid, and SCHIP Extension Act of 2007 (Extension Act) on December 29, 2007; it was further revised under the Medicare Improvements for Patients and Providers Act of 2008 (MIPPA).

CMS states that one goal of the PQRI program is to transform Medicare from a passive payer to an active health care purchaser. Central to this is the transition from paying for procedure (vis-à-vis the physician fee schedule), to payment based on the quality of services being provided. CMS wishes to increase the value of the services Medicare patients receive and as directed by congressional statute are implementing incentive programs that encourage physicians to report on quality performance measures.

The 2007 PQRI had a six-month reporting period from July 1, 2007 through December 31, 2007. As a result of significant problems associated with the program's initial analytics, significant changes were made to the program in order to improve its overall structure and program design. Figure 3-1 gives a snapshot of the current program. In 2008 and 2009, the program ran for a full year, from January 1 to December 31, and this will continue in 2010. During the first three years, participation in the program was completely voluntary. However, based on health reform legislation, there will be penalties for not successfully participating in PQRI beginning in 2015. Specifically, in 2015, practices will receive a -1.5% penalty for not successfully participating, and this will increase to a -2% penalty in 2016 and beyond.

$35,432	Average medical group incentive in 2008 for completing Medicare's PQRI
48	Percentage of medical groups able to download the feedback report to determine PQRI performance
67	Percentage of medical groups "dissatisfied" or "very dissatisfied" with feedback report's effectiveness in providing guidance
60	Percentage of medical groups "dissatisfied" or "very dissatisfied" with the report's presentation of the performance
9	Average hours to download feedback report

Source:
Medical Group Management Association.
Lewis, Morgan, "PQRI//By The Numbers," *Medical Economics*, Vol. 87 No. 6, March 19, 2010, p. 13.

FIGURE 3-1 PQRI by the Numbers

Eligible Providers

The following providers are currently eligible to participate in PQRI:

Medicare Physicians
- Doctor of Medicine
- Doctor of Osteopathy
- Doctor of Podiatric Medicine
- Doctor of Optometry
- Doctor of Oral Surgery
- Doctor of Dental Medicine
- Doctor of Chiropractic

Practitioners
- Physician Assistant
- Nurse Practitioner
- Clinical Nurse Specialist
- Certified Registered Nurse Anesthetist (and Anesthesiologist Assistant)
- Certified Nurse Midwife
- Clinical Social Worker
- Clinical Psychologist
- Registered Dietician
- Nutrition Professional
- Audiologists

Therapists
- Physical Therapist
- Occupational Therapist
- Qualified Speech-Language Therapist

Because PQRI is based on professional services that are paid under or based on the Medicare physician fee schedule (PFS), providers who perform services that are payable under methods other than PFS do not qualify for PQRI. This includes providers who perform services in federally qualified health centers, independent diagnostic testing facilities, independent laboratories, hospitals, rural health clinics, and ambulatory surgery center facilities, among other locations. In addition, durable medical equipment (DME) suppliers are not eligible for PQRI because DME is not paid for under the PFS.

Incentive Payment

In 2007, eligible providers could receive an incentive payment equal to 1.5% of estimated total "allowed charges," for all covered services payable under the Medicare Part B PFS. "Allowed charges" refers to total charges including beneficiary deductible and copayment, not only the 80% paid by Medicare or the portion covered by Medicare when they are the secondary payer.

Also in 2007, bonuses were subject to a cap, which was designed to encourage greater measure reporting. The cap was primarily used when a participant reported relatively few instances of quality measures. It was calculated at the end of the reporting period by multiplying the national average per measure payment amount (national total charges associated with quality measures/national total instances of reporting) by 300% and then multiplying by the individual provider's instances of reporting quality data, provided it did not exceed 1.5% of the individual provider's total Medicare charges for the reporting period. However, in 2008, the cap was removed, and was not included in future program years.

In 2009, the incentive bonus payment was increased to 2% of Medicare Part B allowed charges. This will continue in the 2010 program. [Note: Incentive payment information for 2009 and 2010 may be outdated by the time this book is published, because the 2011 program will incorporate many changes as a result of health reform legislation.]

Financial incentives for the current year are paid the following year as a lump-sum bonus payment. Bonuses paid to the practice are done so at the taxpayer identification number (TIN) level, either electronically or by check, depending on how the TIN typically receives payment for Medicare Part B PFS covered services. For example, if CMS determines that an eligible provider has reported on fewer than three quality measures when they could have reported on a greater number, the provider is considered ineligible and will not receive a bonus payment.

2010 PQRI Program: Reporting

In 2010, there will be two reporting periods: January 1 through December 31 and July 1 through December 31. For the first time, there will be three methods of reporting: claims based, through a qualified registry, and using a qualified electronic health record (EHR). However, the new EHR reporting mechanism, may be used for reporting individual measures only and is only valid for the full-year reporting period. (For a list of qualified registries and EHR vendors for the 2010 program, consult www.cms.hhs.gov/PQRI/20_AlternativeReportingMechanisms.asp#TopOfPage.)

To receive an incentive payment, a provider must successfully report on either individual measures or measure groups. To report on individual measures, a provider may use any of the three reporting mechanisms for the full-year reporting period and either the claims-based or registry reporting method for the half-year reporting period. In both periods, there are two criteria for satisfactory reporting of individual measures. The first includes reporting at least three PQRI measures (or, for claims-based reporting only, one to two measures if fewer than three apply). It is important to note that eligible providers who report on fewer than three measures may be held to the measure applicability validation process to ensure that providers are reporting on all applicable measures. (For further detail on the validation process, consult www.cms.hhs.gov/PQRI/25_AnalysisAndPayment.asp#TopOfPage.) The second criterion for satisfactory reporting includes reporting each measure for at least 80% of applicable Medicare Part B FFS patients seen during the reporting period.

If an eligible provider elects to report on measures groups in 2010, they can only use the claims-based or registry reporting options (EHR reporting is currently not an option). The criteria for reporting measures groups for the full-year period include reporting at least one PQRI measures group and reporting each measures group for at least 30 patients seen during the reporting report. This marks a change from previous years, wherein reporting on consecutive patients was necessary. In addition, it is important to note that if a provider reports using the Medicare Part B claims, the patients must all be Medicare Part B FFS patients. However, if a provider reports using a registry, the patients do not need to be exclusively Medicare Part B FFS patients. The second method a provider can use is reporting on a measures group for the full program year on at least 80% of their applicable Medicare Part B FFS patients. This option is available through claims or registry based reporting.

If an eligible provider elects to report on measures groups for the partial-year reporting period, they must meet the following criteria: report at least one PQRI measures groups, report each measures group for at least 80% of applicable Medicare Part B FFS patients seen during the reporting period, and report each measures group for at least eight Medicare Part B FFS patients seen during the reporting period.

2010 PQRI Program: Measures

In 2010, the program contains 175 individual measures, including 46 registry-only measures, 10 measures for EHR-based reporting, and 30 new measures from the 2009 PQRI program. The 30 new measures are related to a variety of clinical issues, including stroke and stroke rehabilitation, referral for otologic evaluation, cataracts, coronary artery disease, heart failure, oncology, HIV/AIDS, ischemic vascular disease, and functional communication. There were also six new measures groups, including coronary artery disease, heart failure, ischemic vascular disease, hepatitis C, HIV/AIDS, and community-acquired pneumonia. These new measures groups are in addition to the seven measures groups from 2009, which include diabetes mellitus, chronic kidney disease, preventative care, coronary artery bypass graft surgery, rheumatoid arthritis, perioperative care, and back pain (the four quality measures related to back pain are reportable as a measures group only and cannot be reported as individual measures). In addition, the 2010 program included the retirement of four measures. (For a complete description of measures specifications, consult www.cms.hhs.gov/PQRI/15_MeasuresCodes.asp#TopOfPage.)[19]

Measures are developed through a number of organizations, including the AMA convened Physician Consortium for Performance Improvement (PCPI). Other participating organizations include Quality Insights of Pennsylvania, AQA (formerly the Ambulatory Care Quality Alliance), and the American Podiatric Medical Association. The National Quality Forum, a private, nonprofit organization has been tasked by Congress to endorse measures for use in public and private health program, including Medicare and Medicaid.

Claims-Based Reporting

Claims-based reporting was the original method of reporting designed during the inaugural 2007 PQRI program and remains a viable method of reporting in 2010. For claims-based reporting, eligible providers use Medicare Part B claims to submit billable services for allowable charges. In general, each measure that can be reported has two major components: the numerator, which specifies the clinical action that must be completed for reporting and performance (specified by Current Procedural Terminology (CPT®) Category II or G-codes), and the denominator, which describes the eligible patient population that corresponds with the numerator (specified by ICD-9-CM and CPT Category I codes). Each measure also includes a reporting frequency and a performance timeframe. Whether the frequency is reported one time only, once per each procedure performed, or once per each acute episode is distinct for each measure. The performance timeframe is defined in each measure's description and is unique to that measure and it is distinct from reporting frequency. Common timeframes are "within 12 months" or "most recent."

Claims-based reporting is implemented via the paper-based CMS 1500 claim form or an electronic transaction claim 837-P. CPT Category II code(s) (or the G-code(s)) must be reported on the same claim as patient diagnosis and services to which the quality data code applies. Providers should append the appropriate CPT Level II or G-codes to the CMS 1500 or 837-P form used to report the service for which the measures are appropriate. In addition, modifiers may be used with Category II codes to substantiate documentation. They are also used to indicate that a service specified in the performance measure was considered but not provided due to medical, patient, or system reasons. Modifiers serve as denominator exceptions; however, not all performance measures have exceptions, so it is important to determine such for compliance with the reporting standards.

There are several technology-related issues that arise with claims-based reporting. First, it is important to ensure that a provider's computerized practice management system can accept CPT Level II or G-codes. These codes are alpha-numeric, and some systems will not accept them. Additionally, if an eligible provider chooses to use a clearinghouse or scrubbing service to submit their bills, they must be sure that the service can accept CPT Level II or G-codes, as some cannot. Another potential technology problem is that some systems will not accept a zero dollar amount in the field following a CPT code. If that is the case, it is easily solved by inserting a small dollar amount, eg, $0.01. In reality, if a provider's practice management billing system or clearinghouse will not accept CPT Level II or G-codes, it may cost more to modify the system than they could recover in the bonus payment. If a provider must collect data by abstracting medical charts, the costs may also outweigh the potential incentive payment. Every provider must assess their current situation to determine whether or not participating is a realistic venture for them.

More information is available regarding claims-based reporting, as it was most applicable to providers in initial program years. However, providers must consider each reporting mechanism currently available, along with their practice patterns and availability of technology, before ultimately selecting the reporting mechanism to use.

Maximizing Success Within the PQRI Program

Payment for participation in PQRI is based on successful reporting on the first attempt. That is, there is not an opportunity to receive feedback on submitted reports and then resubmit applicable patient records within the same program year. Therefore, it is imperative that eligible providers adequately prepare and plan for their participation in the PQRI program. To maximize the potential for successful reporting, the first step an eligible provider should take is to determine the measures that apply to them. It is important that all applicable measures be identified for the provider in question so that reporting can be completed with maximum efficiency. In several of the reporting methods, any three of the measures that relate to a provider must be reported. If they are not, it will likely be vetted during the measure applicability validation process, and the provider will be ineligible for an incentive payment. CMS advises, "at a minimum, the following factors should be considered when selecting measures for reporting:

- Clinical conditions usually treated
- Types of care typically provided (eg, preventive, chronic, acute)
- Settings where care is usually delivered (eg, office, ED, surgical suite)
- Quality improvement goals for 2010."

Currently, the measures are not broken down by specialty. However, professional organizations may be an asset in isolating applicable measures. For example, the American College of Cardiology has posted a work sheet on their Website (www.acc.org/) to help eligible providers within this specialty identify pertinent measures. If such a resource is not available, an eligible provider can determine the measures that apply to them by looking through each of the 175 measures and isolating those that are clinically relevant.

The second step to maximizing the potential for successful reporting is improving data collection techniques data collection. Data collection for this program can be timely and costly if not adequately addressed prior to program participation. For the applicable reporting mechanism, data may be collected using electronic, paper, or administrative methods. Electronic methods, if available, may prove to be the most efficient. EHRs may allow for some data to be entered by a provider during a patient visit, while other data may be entered from laboratory reports, radiology reports, or other reports from health care institutions where patients receive care. The use of standardized, industry-wide codes can make querying in an EHR possible. (If standardized codes are not yet available, eligible providers should work with their EHR vendors to allow this capability.) If EHR is not available and paper medical records must be used, the data must be abstracted from existing records. PCPI, a measure developer of many PQRI measures, provides definitions to help an abstractor find required data elements in a medical record. Providers may want to consult this resource as part of their preparation for reporting.

Reporting for PQRI can be made easier by working with EHR vendors. The vendors can modify and individualize an existing system to meet a provider's needs. Practice management needs to be involved if utilization of EHR is not an option. A third-party vendor may be required if a provider is unable to complete reporting using any other method. However, the cost of this must be carefully weighed because providers are not guaranteed an incentive payment simply for reporting. (would reconsider the strong focus on the EHR reporting mechanism.

The third step to consider is the importance of reporting correctly the first time. For example, for claims-based reporting, if quality data are not submitted on the same claim as the applicable patient diagnosis, service and procedure codes will not count toward successful reporting or for calculation of a potential bonus payment. It is not possible to resubmit claims. So if a claim is submitted incorrectly, it is impossible to go back and correct it. Coders continue to be an essential component of the process because they can train providers on the specifics of coding elements necessary for accurate reporting. Additionally, for claims-based reporting, coders can pull the "numerator" and "denominator" from patient records to assist with the reporting process.

Overall, participation in the PQRI program requires a significant amount of advance planning and diligent documentation throughout the reporting period. One way to help drive success may be to utilize financial incentives for participation vis-à-vis the potential 2% bonus provided by Medicare. However, eligible physicians must remain aware that reporting alone does not automatically warrant the bonus payment. Rather, it is tied to a successful reporting attempt, which will only come with proper planning and execution.

Available PQRI Resources

For each of the measures within the PQRI program, the AMA, in collaboration with CMS, Mathematica Policy Research Inc., and the National Committee for Quality Assurance, provides a participation tool kit including:

- measure description,
- background information,
- data collection, and
- coding specifications.

For the 2010 PQRI program, AMA has resources available that focus specifically on individual measures (www.ama-assn.org/ama/pub/physician-resources/clinical-practice-improvement/clinical-quality/participation-tools-individual-2010.shtml) as well as group measures (www.ama-assn.org/ama/pub/physician-resources/clinical-practice-improvement/clinical-quality/participation-tools-measure-groups-2010.shtml).

In addition to the AMA, a plethora of resources regarding the PQRI program can be found through professional organizations. Consult Appendix A for a listing of professional organizations and their Websites, as applicable.

Group Practice Reporting Option

For the first time, a Group Practice Reporting Option (GPRO) is now available for participants in the 2010 PQRI program.[20] Based on stipulations within the MIPPA, by January 1, 2010, CMS was required to establish a program wherein eligible providers in a group setting could report on quality measures. As such, the GPRO was established, based on the CMS Physician Group Practice and Medicare Care Management Performance demonstration programs. To participate in the GPRO, a group practice must meet the following criteria and then ultimately be selected to participate:

- Have greater than or equal to 200 individual eligible providers.
- Self-nominate by January 31, 2010.
- Have an active IACS (Individuals Authorized Access to the CMS Computer Services) account.
- Provide information regarding the practice's TIN and the National Provider Identification (NPI) numbers for all eligible providers participating.
- Agree to participate in all mandatory training sessions.
- Have billed Medicare Part A and Part B on or after January 1, 2009, and prior to October 29, 2009.

The reporting period for the 2010 GPRO is January 1, 2010 through December 31, 2010, and the GPRO excludes individual eligible providers that bill under the same TIN as the group practice from also participating in PQRI.

The reporting mechanism is such that in 2011, group practices will be asked to complete a prepopulated data collection tool provided by CMS for a specific set of Medicare beneficiaries that received services during the reporting period. To successfully report, the practice must report on all 26 measures included in this tool, which are focused on clinical issues such as diabetes, heart failure, coronary artery disease, hypertension, and preventative care. In addition, the practice must complete the tool for the first 411 consecutively ranked and assigned beneficiaries for each measure or disease module. If there are fewer than 411 eligible beneficiaries, the group is then required to report on 100% of assigned beneficiaries. If the practice successfully reports, they will be eligible for an incentive payment equal to 2% of the group practice's total estimated Medicare Part B allowed charges for services provided during the reporting period. For additional information on the PGRO, consult www.cms.hhs.gov/PQRI/22_Group_Practice_Reporting_Option.asp#TopOfPage.

The inclusion of a group reporting option marks another significant change in the scale of the PQRI program, one that may encourage greater participation.

Conclusions

The PQRI program has helped drive quality-measure reporting within the health care industry. Continual improvements to and expansion of the PQRI program are encouraging additional providers to participate, allowing additional methods for use in reporting, and providing larger incentives for providers that do successfully participate. Physician practices should carefully consider both the costs and rewards of participation and identify or develop the necessary infrastructure to measure the quality of patient care and report it accurately.

Conclusion

A book on managing reimbursement should encompass the vital topics of pay for performance and quality initiatives. However, the relatively brief history of these programs makes it difficult to understand exactly how these major initiatives will impact the bottom line of the practice. The overview provided in this chapter lays the groundwork for capitalizing on quality performance programs in the future.

References

1. Jessee WF. "Ready or not, pay for performance is here," *MGMA Connexion*. Medical Group Management Association (October 2005). Accessed 1/26/2010. at http://findarticles.com/p/articles/mi_qa4083/is_200510/ai_n15716199/.
2. Aligning Forces for Quality Website. Accessed 5/20/2010 at www.forces4quality.org/sites/default/files/AF4Q_Brochure_r3.pdf.
3. Aligning Forces for Quality Website. Accessed 5/20/2010 at www.forces4quality.org/sites/default/files/AF4Q_Backgrounder_r1.pdf.
4. National Committee for Quality Assurance Website. Accessed 5/20/2010 at www.ncqa.org/tabid/675/Default.aspx.
5. National Committee for Quality Assurance. What Is HEDIS? Accessed 5/20/2010 at www.ncqa.org/tabid/187/Default.aspx.
6. Agency for Healthcare Research and Quality. The CAHPS Program. Accessed 5/20/2010 at www.cahps.ahrq.gov/content/cahpsOverview/OVER_Program.asp?p=101&s=12.
7. BlueCross BlueShield Association. Fact Sheet: Blue Distinction. Accessed 5/20/2010 at www.bcbs.com/innovations/bluedistinction/blue-distinction-fact-sheet.pdf.
8. Committee on Quality of Health Care in America, Institute of Medicine, *Crossing the Quality Chasm: A New Health System for the 21st Century*. Washington, D.C.: National Academies Press; 2001.

9. Medical Group Management Association. "Principles for Pay-for-Performance Programs and Recommendations for Medical Group Practices." February 2005. Accessed 1/21/2010 at ftp://ftp.mgma.com/pub/WEBMISC/PressRoom/position-paper_PFP.pdf.
10. American Academy of Family Physicians. Pay-For-Performance. Accessed 5/20/2010 at www.aafp.org/online/en/home/policy/policies/p/payforperformance.html.
11. American Medical Association. 2009 PCPI Report. Accessed 5/20/2010 at www.ama-assn.org/ama1/pub/upload/mm/370/pcpi-report-2009.pdf.
12. Centers for Medicare and Medicaid Services. Hospital Quality Initiative Overview. July 2008. Accessed 1/19/2010 at http://www.cms.hhs.gov/HospitalQualityInits/Downloads/Hospitaloverview.pdf.
13. CMS Media Affairs Office. "Medicare Demonstrations Show Paying for Quality Pays Off." August 17, 2009. Accessed 1/19/2010 at http://www.cms.hhs.gov/HospitalQualityInits/Downloads/HospitalPremierPressReleases20090817.pdf.
14. Premier Hospital Quality Incentive Demonstration—Rewarding Superior Quality Care Fact Sheet. July 2009. Accessed 1/19/2010 at http://www.cms.hhs.gov/HospitalQualityInits/downloads/HospitalPremierFactSheet200907.pdf.
15. U.S. Department of Health and Human Services. Hospital Compare. Accessed 1/26/2010 at www.hospitalcompare.hhs.gov/Hospital/Search/Welcome.asp?version=default&browser=IE%7C8%7CWinXP&language=English&defaultstatus=0&MBPProviderID=&TargetPage=&ComingFromMBP=&CookiesEnabled Status=&TID=&StateAbbr=&ZIP=&State=&pagelist=Home.
16. Centers for Medicare and Medicaid Services. "Medicare Demonstrations Show Paying for Quality Health Care Pays Off." August 17, 2009. Accessed 5/20/2010 at www.cms.gov/HospitalQualityInits/downloads/HospitalPremierPressReleases20090817.pdf.
17. Premier, Inc. CMS/Premier Hospital Quality Incentive Demonstration (HQID). Accessed 5/20/2010 at www.premierinc.com/p4p/hqi/.
18. CMS Office of Public Affairs. "Medicare Extends Demonstration to Improve Care of High Cost Patients and Create Savings." January 13, 2009. Accessed 5/21/2010 at http://www.cms.gov/apps/media/press/release.asp?Counter=3399&intNumPerPage=10&checkDate=&checkKey=&srchType=1&numDays=3500&srchOpt=0&srchData=&keywordType=All&chkNewsType=1,+2,+3,+4,+5&intPage=&showAll=&pYear=&year=&desc=&cboOrder=date.
19. Centers for Medicare and Medicaid Services. "2010 Physician Quality Reporting Initiative Implementation Guide." November 13, 2009. Accessed 5/21/2010 at http://www.facs.org/ahp/pqri/2010/2010implementationguide.pdf.
20. Centers for Medicare and Medicaid Services. "Physician Quality Reporting Initiative (PQRI) National Provider Call." November 10, 2009. Accessed 1/24/2010 at http://www.cms.hhs.gov/PQRI/04_CMSSponsoredCalls.asp#TopOfPage.

CHAPTER 4

Basics of Coding

OUTLINE

I. Introduction
II. CPT® Procedure Coding
    A. Using the CPT codebook
    B. CPT Modifiers
    C. Evaluation and Management Coding
        1. Documentation Guidelines
        2. E/M Code Components
            a. History
            b. Examination
            c. Medical Decision Making
        3. Documentation Based on Time
        4. Consultations
        5. Preventive Services
III. ICD-9-CM Diagnosis Coding
IV. ICD-10-CM
V. Conclusion

Introduction

The number one goal of every physician practice is to effectively take care of their patients' health needs. This is certainly a worthy goal, but it must be remembered that the medical practice is also a business in need of financial reimbursement for the services it provides. The medical coding system is used to ensure payment to the medical practice. Simply stated, coding uses numbers to tell a story. Imagine how difficult payment would be without a standardized system of reporting.

The physician and practice staff must invest time and energy into understanding the three coding systems most commonly used by physicians in the United States: Current Procedural Terminology (CPT®),[1] the Healthcare Common Procedure Coding System (HCPCS) Level II codes,[2] and the *International Classification of Diseases, 9th Revision, Clinical Modification* (ICD-9-CM).[3] (Note: ICD-10 is scheduled to be implemented October 1, 2013.) Each system tells a different portion of the coding story in order for a practice to be properly reimbursed for the services provided.

In simplest terms,

- CPT tells the payer *what* you did.
- ICD-9-CM tells a payer *why* you did it.

HCPCS Level II codes are used to report services such as durable medical equipment, prosthetics, orthotics, medications, medical supplies, ambulance services, and other services not described in CPT. Unlike CPT and ICD-9-CM, these codes are not used on every medical claim. HCPCS Level II codes are five-digit alphanumeric codes that begin with the letters A through V. These codes are used by all Medicare carriers (Part B) and intermediaries (Part A) and by Medicaid in all states. Although they are written by the government, it has become more and more common for commercial carriers to use them as well, particularly for injectable medications.

For proper medical coding to take place, the physician and staff must understand the coding guidelines; the physician then performs the service for the patient and documents what took place (according to the guidelines); the appropriate codes are assigned based on the service provided; a bill is sent for what was documented; and the reimbursement is received for the service provided. Most physicians graduate from residency programs with very little coding knowledge, yet they are expected to accurately use these codes on their first day of practice. Not only is there a specific language of coding that must be mastered but the guidelines are constantly being updated and changed. As these changes become more complicated, the physician practice must develop systems and strategies to ensure they meet medical coding guidelines and insurance and billing procedures.

To keep up to date with the basics of coding and all related updates, the following is recommended:

- Every new provider joining a practice, whether straight from residency or from another entity, should have initial coding training based on CPT and ICD-9-CM coding basics, with an emphasis on Evaluation and Management (E/M) codes and medical necessity. The *Medicare Claims Processing Manual* says that medical necessity is the "overarching criterion for payment in addition to the individual requirements of a CPT code."[4] Never assume a physician does not need initial training; if he or she is already proficient in coding, training will serve as a great reminder and ensure the physician starts out on the right foot. If the physician is undereducated with regard to coding, training will give him or her a basis from which to start coding.

- Buy new coding books or access online coding sources each year. Although new coding books are expensive, the use of outdated codes leads to denials with no reimbursement. When the new CPT codebook is received, look at Appendix B, Summary of Additions, Deletions, and Revisions, to see which codes affect your practice. The ICD-9-CM changes are found in the front of the book in a section titled "2010 ICD-9-CM Code Changes." (Note: The title may vary depending on the book publisher.)

- Once the new and changed codes for the year have been reviewed, update encounter forms, billing software, and practice cheat sheets. New CPT codes go into effect January 1 of each year and ICD-9-CM codes go into effect October 1. Any deleted codes used after these dates may result in a denial—there is no grace period for using the correct code.

- Be sure the physician and staff are provided additional resources to stay up to date on coding changes, such as newsletters, Websites, seminars, and supporting publications.

- Beware of "coding folklore," which is information that has been handed down from one person to another and because of that is assumed to be accurate. Always use an official source, such as the Centers for Medicare and Medicaid Services (CMS) or the American Medical Association (AMA), to verify any changes or updates you receive. When interacting with a private payer, always ask for information verification in writing or access and print the payer's online resources and policies.

- Be proactive and check with your most frequently billed claims for updates and changes yearly, using their client communications, a customer service representative, and/or Websites. Though it may be initially time-consuming, it will save time in the long run in fewer denials to review.

- Continuing education is imperative for both physicians and the staff. Make it a part of the practice culture to regularly give coding updates. Ongoing chart reviews to monitor correct assignment of CPT codes as well as ICD-9-CM codes via physician education is a great way to ensure that the physicians are complying with coding guidelines.

Correct coding is a balancing act between being properly reimbursed for services rendered and staying within guidelines for compliance. Many physicians are concerned about being audited and choose lower codes, based on fear. Other physicians feel their work and documentation is sufficient, so they use higher codes that are not supported in order to receive what they believe is proper reimbursement for their work. The first view poses a financial risk because the full reimbursement will not be received. The second perspective poses the risk that the coding will be audited and the documentation will be considered not in compliance with established guidelines. A healthy balance of both is needed, along with proper understanding of the guidelines to ensure every reimbursement is received without violating any of the published coding rules. It is much like the wings of an airplane; one is not more important than the other, but if one is out of alignment, the entire airplane is harmed.

All physicians as well as their staff should follow the guidelines outlined in Figure 4-1, published by CMS and available on the CMS Website, in order to understand the basic foundation for correct documentation. Many a great physician may only feel it necessary to

---

To ensure that medical record documentation is accurate, the following principles should be followed:

- The medical record should be complete and legible.
- The documentation of each patient encounter should include:
  - Reason for the encounter and relevant history, physical examination findings, and prior diagnostic test results.
  - Assessment, clinical impression, or diagnosis.
  - Medical plan of care.
  - Date and legible identity of the observer.
- If not documented, the rationale for ordering diagnostic and other ancillary services should be easily inferred.
- Past and present diagnoses should be accessible to the treating and/or consulting physician.
- Appropriate health risk factors should be identified.
- The patient's progress, response to and changes in treatment, and revision of diagnosis should be documented.
- The Current Procedural Terminology (CPT) and *International Classification of Diseases, 9th Edition, Clinical Modification* (ICD-9-CM) codes reported on the health insurance claim form or billing statement should be supported by the documentation in the medical record.

Centers for Medicare & Medicaid Services, Evaluation & Management Services Guide, 2009; 7:4

FIGURE 4-1 Medical Record Documentation.

document a brief note; however, if the notes are too brief and poorly documented, the quality of the work will not be reflected adequately and the work will not be judged appropriately. Even careful documentation of an encounter will not protect a physician from an audit if the physician cannot prove a service was medically necessary. The old adage "If it's not documented, it wasn't done" is true in the world of medical coding, particularly in the case of an audit or malpractice claim.[5]

In this chapter, the organization, format, and coding guidelines for CPT are discussed, including modifiers and E/M codes. There is also an overview of ICD-9-CM coding guidelines, format, and medical necessity. In addition, an update on the status of ICD-10-CM is included. This is not an exhaustive analysis of the coding system but rather a basic description with directions for finding further information that will be necessary to ensure correct coding.

CPT® Procedure Coding

The AMA published its first edition of *Current Procedural Terminology (CPT)* in 1966, with CMS adopting the coding system for reporting physician's services for most government programs in 1983. Since then, it has been adopted by most private payers. The CPT coding system consists of more than 9,000 codes to describe the medical services and procedures, or the "what," provided by the physician or other qualified health care provider for the patient. A new edition of the CPT codebook is released by AMA in late fall of each year to be effective January 1 of the following year. This manual can be purchased online at the AMA bookstore at https://catalog.ama-assn.org or at a variety of other retail providers.

CPT codes are five digits accompanied by narrative descriptions of the procedure and/or service. The CPT codebook begins with an introduction that contains the basics of CPT coding and instructions on use of the codebook. After the introduction, the codes are organized into eight sections according to the types of services or procedures provided. The first six sections pertain to Category I CPT codes. The last two sections pertain to Category II and Category III codes. Each section begins with guidelines that give important coding rules and other information. Billing personnel should be familiar with these sections and what range of codes is included in each one to increase speed and efficiency in finding CPT codes. The first six CPT sections and their associated code ranges are as follows:

- *Evaluation and Management Services (99201–99499).* Codes from this section are used to report office, hospital, consultative, nursing home, and other related services, often called physician "visits."

E/M codes are estimated to be the most frequently reported services for physicians, comprising anywhere from 33 to 40% of all claims paid by payers. For that reason, they are placed in the front of the book for easy referencing.

- *Anesthesia (00100–01999, 99100–99140).* The codes describe anesthesia administered by a physician.
- *Surgery (10021–69990).* The surgery section lists more codes than any other. The procedures range from simple laceration repair to complex surgeries, such as organ transplants. The subsections are organized by organ systems.
- *Radiology (70010–79999).* All radiology services are listed here, with a variety of modalities, such as X ray, ultrasound, and nuclear medicine.
- *Pathology and Laboratory (80047–89398).* Every type of lab test and pathology service is listed here.
- *Medicine (90281–99199, 99500–99607).* Other physician services, such as electrocardiographic, chiropractic, and dialysis codes, are found here.

In addition, supplemental appendices are located in the back of the CPT codebook and include:

- *Appendix A: Modifiers.* Modifiers are located in this appendix; an abbreviated list is located inside the front cover. These two-digit numeric modifiers are added to a CPT code to indicate that a service or procedure has been altered.
- *Appendix B: Summary of Additions, Deletions, and Revisions.* This is a listing of the year's codebook changes. One can use this list to see which CPT codes that apply to a certain specialty have been changed for a particular year.
- *Appendix C: Clinical Examples.* Clinical examples, organized by E/M codes, are listed here. This appendix can be used to further educate physicians on coding.
- *Appendix D: Summary of CPT Add-On Codes.* An add-on code cannot be reported as a stand-alone code and is only used as an addition to an already listed code.
- *Appendix E: Summary of CPT Codes Exempt from Modifier 51.* Procedures on the list of CPT codes that are exempt from modifier 51 are typically performed with another procedure but may stand alone and do not require the attachment of modifier 51.
- *Appendix F: Summary of CPT Codes Exempt from Modifier 63.* Modifier 63 indicates surgery on an infant less than 4 kg and is not needed with the codes in this list.
- *Appendix G: Summary of CPT Codes that Include Moderate (Conscious) Sedation.* When the codes in the summary of CPT

codes that include moderate sedation are reported, no additional code for conscious sedation can be submitted.

- *Appendix H: Alphabetic Index of Performance Measures by Clinical Condition or Topic.* This index is currently only Web-based and lists the performance measures by clinical condition or topic to track performance. Clinical conditions or topics are listed in alphabetical order for quick look-up in the index. (Note: For CPT 2010, this appendix has been removed from the CPT codebook and can be accessed solely on the AMA Website.)
- *Appendix I: Genetic Testing Code Modifiers.* These modifiers allow for diagnostic granularity so that more specific genetic testing information can be tracked.
- *Appendix J: Electrodiagnostic Medicine Listing of Sensory, Motor, and Mixed Nerves.* This is a list of the appropriate nerve conduction study for each nerve.
- *Appendix K: Product Pending FDA Approval.* This appendix lists the vaccines that have been assigned a CPT code in anticipation of future FDA approval.
- *Appendix L: Vascular Families.* This appendix shows branches to first-, second-, third-order, and beyond for help in coding arteriographic procedures.
- *Appendix M: Summary of Crosswalked Deleted CPT Codes.* This is a listing of deleted CPT codes that have been replaced by another code since 2007. In the 2010 CPT codebook, this appendix provides a handy chart showing the crosswalk between the old deleted code and the newly assigned code.
- *Appendix N: Summary of Resequenced CPT Codes.* This is a listing of codes that do not appear in numeric sequence. (Note: This appendix was added for CPT 2010.)

Using the CPT Codebook

The best way to locate a code is to use the index in the CPT codebook. The four primary classes of index entries are:

- procedure or service (eg, endoscopy, amputation, splint);
- organ or other anatomic site (eg, tibia, colon, salivary gland);
- condition (eg, abscess, cyst, Bartholin's gland); and
- synonyms, eponyms (eg, Crohn's disease, Grave's disease, Guillain-Barré virus), and abbreviations (eg, EEG, GGT, GI tract).

Once the best term is found in the index, the next step is to locate the code in the body of the book and read the code description; it is not appropriate to only code from the index. The index in the CPT codebook contains the following guidance: "The alphabetic index is NOT a substitute for the main text of CPT. Even if only one code appears, the user must refer to the main text to ensure that the code selection is accurate."

Selection of the best code requires attention to detail; the distinction between two codes can have a major financial impact. For example, the subsection describing repair of skin wounds (12001–13160) uses the same verbiage multiple times with the only difference being the terms "Simple," "Intermediate," or "Complex." To select the appropriate code, the first step is to read the text at the beginning of the subsection that describes the definitions of simple, intermediate, and complex repair. The appropriate code can then be selected based on the additional criteria of length. The reimbursement for complex repair is quite a bit higher than for simple repair, so accurate coding is imperative.

In addition, notes are found near specific codes in the CPT codebook that give additional information to help in selecting the most appropriate code. For example, code 66220 is described as "Repair of sclera staphyloma, without graft," but the note states "(For scleral procedures in retinal surgery, see 67101 et seq)." These special notes can be critical to improving reimbursement and reducing audit exposure.

Some entries in the CPT codebook are indented. This is done to avoid repeating part of the preceding description in an effort to conserve space. The semicolon is the key to understanding these descriptions; the CPT codebook does not repeat the portion of a description to the left of the semicolon. Instead, it indents subsequent codes to suggest you should look above the code for the first full description and read the missing portion of the current description.

For example,

42215   Palatoplasty for cleft palate; major revision
42220   secondary lengthening procedure

The full reading for 42220 would be "Palatoplasty for cleft palate; secondary lengthening procedure."

CPT Modifiers

Modifiers are two-digit indicators that allow you to report a specific or special circumstance that has altered a service or procedure. Another way to describe a modifier is "we know the rules, but this was an exception." For example, physicians use modifiers to report that (modifier in parenthesis):

- They performed a separate procedure with an E/M visit (25).
- They increased or reduced the service (22, 52).
- They discontinued the service (53).
- They performed the professional portion of the service only (26).

- An unrelated E/M service was provided during a global period (24).
- A bilateral procedure was performed (50).

Modifiers are often confusing because their application varies from payer to payer and they may be added or deleted annually. For compliance purposes, it is important that the information communicated by the modifier is supported in the documentation and not added simply to get the bill paid. (See Appendix A of the CPT codebook for a full explanation of modifiers.)

Evaluation and Management Coding

One of the most important codes for physician practices is the Evaluation and Management (E/M), or "visit," code, yet it can also be the most frustrating. Many physicians find the guidelines ambiguous and vague and end up guessing as to which code to report. To add to the frustration, not only are the documentation guidelines sometimes considered complicated or confusing, the application of the guidelines varies from Medicare carrier to Medicare carrier. Although the CPT codebook does not spell out the specific requirements for each level of E/M, Medicare does, and many private payers have adopted Medicare guidelines. Therefore, it is prudent to use Medicare's documentation guidelines for the practice's standard.

It is tempting for the physician to choose the lower-level E/M code to be safe and avoid the risk of an audit. This has a negative effect on many levels—the practice loses money that it should receive as reimbursement for the service and the third-party payer sees an inaccurate profile of the physician. On the other hand, some specialists will choose the highest-level E/M codes simply because they are specialists, ignoring the documentation requirements and posing a compliance risk. The best way to ensure that physicians are coding correctly is to regularly review their E/M notes with an educational emphasis.

Documentation Guidelines

If the practice decides to follow Medicare's documentation guidelines, the next step is to determine which set of guidelines to follow. The initial documentation guidelines were adopted in 1995, with a second version presented in 1997. The differences are as follows:

- *1995 Guidelines.* These guidelines work better for general practice or when the physician typically examines multiple body areas and/or organ systems. The history of the present illness is documented by four elements. The exam guidelines are vague for the expanded problem-focused and detailed exam. Terms such as "limited," "extended," or "complete" are used, but there are no specifics provided by Medicare on the number of body areas or organs systems that must be examined to meet each level of care. With a lack of specificity, it is often difficult for coders to agree on the level of care documented; likewise, agreement among physicians is also difficult.

- *1997 Guidelines.* The history of the present illness can be documented by four or more elements of the history of the present illness (HPI) or by documenting the presence and status of three or more chronic or inactive conditions. The examination under these guidelines is more objective, and each element is indicated with a "bullet" that is counted to determine the level of service. The criteria are based on 12 specialty exams containing very specific items that a physician may or may not determine appropriate to examine.

Because both sets of guidelines have their advantages and disadvantages, Medicare allows physicians to use the guidelines that are most advantageous to them when documenting or reviewing medical records. Each practice should determine which set of guidelines to use when teaching and auditing their physicians. To date, although there have been many proposals to replace the current guidelines, there has been no consensus to adopt any since 1997. To obtain a copy of the full guidelines for both 1995 and 1997, visit the CMS Website at www.cms.hhs.gov.

E/M Code Components

The following seven components of E/M services are listed in the CPT codebook:

- history,
- examination,
- medical decision making,
- counseling,
- coordination of care,
- nature of presenting problem, and
- time.

Of these seven elements, the first three are considered the key components for selecting the appropriate level of E/M service. Each component is part of the guidelines for both 1995 and 1997.

History. Documentation of the history is comprised of four parts. The *chief complaint (CC)* is a brief description in the patient's words describing why they are being seen that day by the physician and is indicated for all levels of E/M service. The chief complaint should contain enough detail to determine the medical necessity for the patient to be seen by the physician; a brief notation such as "follow up" or "re-check" is not sufficient.

The *history of the present illness (HPI)* is a narrative describing the symptoms of the chief complaint and events that led up to the physician encounter. These symptoms can be described using the following eight elements:

- *Location.* Where the symptom is located on the body (throat, stomach).
- *Quality.* Distinguishing factor (piercing, burning).
- *Severity.* Degree of pain (moderate, improving).
- *Duration.* Frequency (last week, mornings).
- *Timing.* When the symptoms occur (bedtime, when walking, constantly).
- *Context.* The situation associated with the symptom (since beginning antibiotics, after surgery).
- *Modifying factors.* What makes it better or worse (when lying down, after taking aspirin).
- *Associated signs and symptoms.* Other signs or symptoms that appear with the main symptom (wheezing with cough, fever with sore throat).

Although technically CPT only has seven dimensions, it does state that the HPI includes those seven. Medicare specifically lists these eight and includes these eight in their published audit tools. Commercial carriers typically mirror Medicare guidelines.

For an expanded, problem-focused HPI, one to three of these must be in the history documentation; for a detailed or comprehensive history, there must be four or more. Remember that with the 1997 guidelines, the status of three or more chronic conditions can support a detailed or comprehensive HPI.

Part three, the *review of systems (ROS)* asks the patient about other symptoms in pertinent organ systems relating to the chief complaint. This information can be collected by asking the patient pertinent questions or, as a time saver, the patient can record his or her symptoms on a form that asks specific questions before seeing the physician. If the ROS are recorded by ancillary staff or the patient, the physician must document that they reviewed the ROS. The recognized systems for review are as follows:

- constitutional symptoms (weight loss, sleep patterns, fever);
- eyes;
- ears, nose, throat;
- cardiovascular;
- respiratory;
- gastrointestinal;
- genitourinary;
- musculoskeletal;

- integumentary (skin and/or breast);
- neurological;
- psychiatric;
- endocrine;
- hematologic/lymphatic; and
- allergy/immunology.

The ROS consists of three levels: *problem pertinent* includes at least one element documented from the system related to the problem; *extended* requires that 2–9 systems are documented of the positive and pertinent negative responses; and a *complete* ROS requires that 10 or more systems reviewed and documented. Some, but not all, Medicare carriers allow a *complete* ROS with documentation of the pertinent positives and negatives and then a statement of "otherwise ROS is negative."

Part four is the documentation of past family and social history (hospitalizations, surgeries, current medications, etc), family history (as it relates to health and hereditary issues), and social history (marital status, diet, occupation, drinking, smoking, etc), also referred to as "PFSH." These also can be asked of the patient by ancillary staff or recorded on a form filled out by the patient and reviewed by the physician. There are two levels of PFSH: *pertinent* requires only one of the three be documented, and *complete* requires that two or three be documented.

Examination. The second key component in determining the level of care is the examination. There are four levels of exam, but each has different requirements according to the guidelines selected. Figure 4-2 outlines the differences in the general multisystem exam.

Medical Decision Making. The complexity of establishing a diagnosis and the risk of complications to the patient are measured by medical decision making. Three elements are considered: (1) the number of possible diagnoses and management options; (2) the amount and complexity of data ordered or reviewed; and (3) the risk of significant complications associated with the patients presenting problem, tests ordered, and management options selected.

There are four levels of medical decision making:

- *Straightforward.* The problems addressed are straightforward, having minimal decision-making complexity.
- *Low complexity.* The problems are of low severity, low urgency, and low risk of clinical deterioration and complications.
- *Moderate complexity.* Typically, the problems addressed are of moderate severity with low to moderate risk of deterioration. The treatment plan would be expected to be more complicated.
- *High complexity.* The problem is more severe in nature and has a high risk of complications and clinical deterioration.

Exam Level	1995	1997
Problem Focused	Limited exam of the affected body area/organ system	1–5 bulleted items in 1 or more organ systems or body areas
Expanded Problem Focused	Limited exam of affected body area/organ system and additional related systems	6+ bullets items in 1 or more organ systems or body areas
Detailed	Extended exam of affected body area/organ system and additional related systems	2 elements in 6 organ systems or body areas OR 12+ bullets in 2 or more organ systems or body areas
Comprehensive	8+ organ system exam or complete single system exam	9 organ systems or body areas with at least 2 bullets in each

FIGURE 4-2 Levels of Exams by Guidelines.

The three key components of E/M coding, history, examination, and medical decision making form the basis of code selection and, ultimately, reimbursement. The descriptions of the key elements of E/M coding are only meant to be summaries of the documentation required. A more detailed explanation is available at the Medicare Website at www.cms.hhs.gov. Medicare also provides several learning modules for E/M coding on its Website at www.medicare.gov.

Documentation Based on Time

Generally, the key elements of documentation are sufficient to support the service provided by the physician; however, there are times when the visit is dominated by medically appropriate counseling and/or coordination of care. An exception to using the key elements has been provided by CPT using time as the key or controlling factor to support the level of E/M service. Many E/M codes have been assigned a "typical time" in the description in the CPT codebook. To use time as the basis for an office code, the physician should document three facts: (1) the total face-to-face time with the patient; (2) that the counseling/coordination of care dominated >50% of the time; and (3) that the medically appropriate topics were discussed with the patient. For patients in the hospital, the time documented can be a combination of face-to-face time and floor unit time focused on the patient. This rule is helpful for those times when the physician provides such services as discussion of prognosis, treatment options, test results, risk management, and noncompliance issues.

All Medicare updates from local carriers must be reviewed often to ensure compliance with E/M guidelines. The interpretations of various elements of E/M coding vary from carrier to carrier. For example, one carrier may allow for the use of "otherwise review of systems negative" for the documentation of the ROS in the history, but another may not. It is the responsibility of each physician practice to be aware of the specific carrier guidelines and apply them appropriately.

Consultations

One area of E/M coding that is often confusing is when to code a consultation code. Over the years, Medicare has made multiple attempts to better explain the criteria for using consultation codes versus new patient codes, yet much confusion still remains. Effective January 1, 2010, Medicare no longer recognizes consultation codes for physician billing. In the hospital, physicians who are asked for their opinion for patient treatment but are not the admitting physician, will use initial inpatient codes for the first day they see the patient, even if they do not see the patient on the first day of admission. In addition to the E/M code, the admitting physician will use modifier AI to indicate that he or she is the primary physician. In the office or other outpatient setting where an evaluation is performed, physicians and qualified nonphysician practitioners shall use the CPT codes (99201–99215) depending on the complexity of the visit and whether the patient is a new or established patient to that physician. For more direction from CMS, go to www.cms.gov/manuals/downloads/clm104c12.pdf.[6]

A practice should also investigate how its contracted commercial carriers intend to handle consults, because the codes are still listed in the CPT 2010 codebook as valid codes and most third-party payers continue to recognize the CPT consultation codes for non-Medicare reporting. New CPT guidelines for 2010 should also be reviewed for instructions on how to report consultation codes 99241–99255.

The E/M guidelines also include a new definition to preclude reporting the consultation codes for "Transfer of care."

Preventive Services

Also listed in the E/M section of the CPT codebook are services described as "preventive" or wellness. Initially, both Medicare and traditional insurance payers focused on treatment of health problems, such as illness or injury. In recent years, more attention has been placed on treatment to maintain or encourage healthy living. Primary care physician practices often overlook these codes for billing when they may be the most appropriate code for a healthy person seeking health care maintenance. The codes are differentiated by age and whether or not the patient is new to the practice in sections 99381–99387 (new) and 99391–99397 (established). Frequently there is a time component for how often these codes will be paid by payer, such as once a year for adults older than 18. Some health benefit plans cover preventive services without regard to the patient deductible. These are also the codes used to report wellness services provided for children. Be sure to check with the individual payer to determine benefit coverage and what they consider to be part of the preventive visit.

Although Medicare does not pay for these codes as a part of E/M, they do have several preventive services that have been specifically carved out for payment to encourage Medicare recipients to seek proactive medical care. This list of covered preventive services for Medicare changes each year, and, typically, there are details as to when these services are considered covered. The Medicare Website provides a summary table titled "Quick Reference Information: Medicare Preventive Services." This table and other educational products for preventive services provided by Medicare are available at www.cms.hhs.gov/MLNProducts/35_PreventiveServices.asp.

ICD-9-CM Diagnosis Coding

Diagnosis codes are intended to explain the "why" of a patient visit. At this time, coding uses *ICD-9-CM, International Classification of Diseases, Ninth Revision, Clinical Modification*. This codebook is used primarily in the United States to assign codes for diagnoses of the patient's condition, the reason for outpatient and physician office utilization, and procedures associated with inpatient coding. ICD-9-CM codes help to establish the "medical necessity" for various services. In fact, most payers, including Medicare, maintain lists of ICD-9-CM codes that physicians must include on claim forms to receive payment when billing for certain CPT codes. The proper use of ICD-9-CM codes will prevent many problems with denials and help physicians justify the services rendered to patients. But, be careful—the use of a diagnosis code to get a service paid that has not been documented in the physician note could be considered billing fraud or abuse.

The ICD-9-CM codebook is full of information on how to use the codebook and how the text is arranged. Billing staff should familiarize themselves with these directions. To arrive at the most appropriate code, take the following steps:

1. Review the medical record to determine what medical conditions or symptoms are described by the documentation.
2. Look up the disease, sign, symptom, or condition in the front of the ICD-9-CM codebook, volume II, and locate the corresponding code.
3. Find the corresponding code in the volume I tabular list and further analyze the most specific code for the documentation.

Helpful tips to ensure appropriate use of diagnosis codes include the following:

- Use both the alphabetic index (volume II) and the tabular list (volume I). Relying on just one of these sections can lead to errors in code assignment and hinder use of the most specific code.
- Be sure to report the most specific code available. Codes that are not reported to the full number of digits required for that code are considered invalid. The bottom of each page of the tabular list shows the symbol to indicate codes that require a fourth or fifth digit.
- Use signs and symptoms codes when the final diagnosis is not known or has not yet been confirmed in the outpatient setting. This constitutes appropriate billing.
- Only document diagnosis codes that are applicable to that day's visit. If an underlying condition affects the presenting problem, then document both (eg, leg ulcer, diabetes). Some physicians mistakenly believe that listing many problems, even those no longer applicable, increases the level of E/M billed.
- Order the diagnosis codes for billing by priority, with the first code listed to be chiefly responsible for the encounter. Then list co-existing conditions that affect the outcome of the care.

In addition, there are special codes in the ICD-9-CM codebook that are not typically used for a primary diagnosis code but do report additional information for tracking purposes. "Supplementary Classification of External Causes of Injury and Poisoning," or "E," codes (E800-E999) describe the method of injury, including traffic accidents, poisonings, drowning, chemical exposure, environmental exposure, etc. "V" codes, located in the section titled "Supplementary Classification of Factors Influencing Health Status and Contact with Health Services," are used to code circumstances other than a disease or injury as diagnoses or problems. Occasionally a "V" code can be used as the primary diagnosis code for wellness and screening services, but generally a "V" code should not be used as the primary diagnosis when billing. It is important to check billing guidelines for screening exams closely, for both commercial and Medicare carriers.

ICD-10-CM

On January 16, 2009, Medicare published its ICD-10 Final Rule CMS-0013-F, which officially mandated October 1, 2013, as the compliance date for implementation of the ICD-10-CM and ICD-10-PCS code set.

This set of codes will replace the ICD-9-CM and ICD-9-PCS. There will be no impact on CPT or HCPCS codes when the transition takes place. To read the publication in the *Federal Register*, go to http://edocket.access.gpo.gov/2009/pdf/E9-743.pdf.[7]

Why the change? According to Medicare, "The current system, ICD-9-CM, does not provide the necessary detail for patients' medical conditions or the procedures and services performed on hospitalized patients." Medicare also states that ICD-9-CM is 30 years old and contains outdated and obsolete terminology. Therefore, it cannot accurately describe the diagnoses and inpatient procedures of care delivered in the twenty-first century.

Medicare has begun educating physician practices in order to make the transition as smooth as possible. They have created a fact sheet that summarizes the differences and the steps to take to create an implementation plan. That information can be found at www.cms.gov/ICD10/Downloads/ICD10IntroFactSheet20100409.pdf.[8] It is not too soon for every practice to begin planning for ICD-10-CM implementation.

Conclusion

In every medical practice, physicians and those responsible for coding and billing functions must balance capturing revenue appropriately through accurate coding and proper documentation while also following all the billing compliance rules and regulations. Missed steps and errors can spell lost revenue resulting in financial collapse or increased scrutiny for fraud and abuse. This chapter has provided a basic description of coding and documentation along with many resources and guidance for seeking ongoing education. Further, the time for transition to ICD-10 is approaching. Now is the time to prepare.

References

1. American Medical Association. *Current Procedural Terminology (CPT®) Professional Edition 2009*. Chicago: American Medical Association; 2010.
2. *Healthcare Common Procedure Coding System* (HCPCS), National Level II Codes, Salt Lake City, Utah: Contexo Media; 2009.
3. *International Classification of Diseases, 9th Revision, Clinical Modification (ICD-9-CM)*, vols. 1 and 2. Salt Lake City, Utah: Contexo Media; 2009.
4. Jensen PR. A Refresher on Medical Necessity. *Family Practice Management*. Accessed 4/19/2010 at www.aafp.org/fpm/2006/0700/p.28.html.

5. Centers for Medicare and Medicaid Services. Evaluation & Management Services Guide, 2009; 7:4. Accessed 11/1/2009 at www.cms.hhs.gov/MLNProducts/downloads/eval_mgmt_serv_guide.pdf.
6. Medicare Claims Processing Manual, Chapter 12, Physicians/Nonphysician Practitioners, 2010; 12:53. Accessed 5/11/2010 at www.cms.gov/manuals/downloads/clm104c12.pdf.
7. *Federal Register*, 2009; 74:11:3330–3362. Accessed 11/20/2009 at http://edocket.access.gpo.gov/2009/pdf/E9-743.pdf.
8. Centers for Medicare and Medicaid Services. ICD10 Transition: an introduction. Apr 2010. Accessed 5/11/2010 at www.cms.gov/ICD10/Downloads/ICD10IntroFactSheet20100409.pdf.

CHAPTER 5
Revenue Cycle Management
Front-End Processes

OUTLINE

I. Introduction
II. Scheduling Patient Appointments
   A. Capturing Demographic Information
   B. Verifying the Demographic Information
   C. Conducting Authorizations and Pre-Certifications
   D. Confirming the Appointment
   E. Communicating Office Policies
   F. Managing Missed Appointments
III. Registering the Patient
   A. Complying with Identity and Privacy Regulations
      1. Red Flag Rules
      2. The Health Insurance and Portability and Accountability Act
   B. Obtaining Consent for Treatment
   C. Collecting from the Patient at Registration
IV. Checking Out the Patient
   A. Surveying Patient Satisfaction
   B. Creating First Impressions
   C. Using Electronic Records in Patient Visits
V. Completing the End-of-the-Day Processes
   A. Balancing Receipts and Verifying Charges
   B. Contacting No-Show Patients
VI. Conclusion

Introduction

Reimbursement for services rendered in the medical practice is a two-part operation. The first part is "front-office management"; the second is "back-office operations." Although the two components of the revenue cycle differ operationally, the two must have synergy for the practice to succeed. This chapter discusses the specific aspects of front-end office processes involved in revenue cycle management.

Scheduling Patient Appointments

The revenue cycle begins when you schedule the patient. Patient scheduling is more complex than making a telephone call and placing an entry on a calendar. Prior to scheduling, the time needed for each appointment must be determined. The length of an appointment should allow for the time the patient will spend in an exam room or for a procedure requiring the presence and service of the medical providers. The time spent prior to placing the patient in an exam room, ie, triage and check-in processes, should not be part of the time allotted for an appointment. It is customary to allow more time for a new patient or a patient who is being seen for consultative services, because the practitioner must gather more information and possibly perform a more extensive examination. Established patients generally do not require long appointments, because the practitioner is usually aware of the patient's medical history and is focused on the chief complaint for which the patient is being seen.

Capturing Demographic Information

Scheduling is key to reimbursement. If the patient's demographic information at the time of scheduling is inaccurate, the delay in receiving revenue can be significant.

Correct patient and guarantor demographics are critical to timely and accurate payment. Demographics can be obtained either from the referring physician's office or from the patient. The following demographic information should be obtained at the time the patient is scheduled for an appointment, either through direct communication with the patient or from the referring physician:

- name;
- address;

- telephone numbers where the patient can be reached to verify appointments;
- name of the insured;
- insured's date of birth;
- insured's social security number;
- name of insurance company;
- all identifying insurance numbers, such as the group number, the individual insured's number, and insurance company customer service number;
- name of any secondary insurance; and
- if the patient was involved in an accident, information related to workers' compensation or liability coverage.

This information is needed at the time of scheduling or, at the very least, at the time the patient is registered. If the information is received from a referring physician, it is important to verify all information with the patient. Remember that insurance information can change from one day to the next—insurances change, patients move, people change jobs, etc. Also, the referring practice may not have updated its files with information that the patient can provide.

It is also important to get the insurance provider's customer service number so that you can determine whether authorizations or pre-certifications (pre-certs) for services to be rendered are required. If the patient is being referred from a primary care physician and the insurance plan is a health maintenance organization (HMO), an authorization or referral number will be needed; pre-certs are often required for surgeries, out-patient/in-patient admission, and similar procedures. It is usually necessary to get certification or authorization for imaging services, particularly for computed tomography (CT), magnetic resonance imaging (MRI), nuclear studies, and other higher-cost imaging modalities. Frequently these are obtained through radiology benefit management companies, which manage radiology benefits for insurance payers.

After all patient information has been received and entered into your practice management system, the next step is to verify the demographic information.

Verifying the Demographic Information

Using electronic data interchange (EDI), it is possible to verify coverage, the deductible amount, the deductible amount yet to be met, as well as any copayments and co-insurances with the insurance company prior to the patient's visit. This is done using an American National Standards Institute (ANSI) 270 File and the reply, which will return to the practice's system in an ANSI 271 File. These files are processed through an electronic claims clearinghouse that also transmits the practice's electronic claims. This information is critical to the processing of clean claims. In addition, if the patient is scheduled for a procedure or surgery, the appropriate authorizations and pre-certs must be obtained from the patient's insurance.

Conducting Authorizations and Pre-Certifications

Authorizations and pre-certs are usually required by the patient's insurance. The physician must provide the following information to the payer: description of procedure, the procedure codes that are anticipated to be billed, and the diagnosis code. Authorizations and pre-certs should be obtained several days prior to the scheduled procedure; this will allow for a minimum of 24 hours and a maximum of three to four days to receive the authorization from the payer.

Authorizations and pre-certs are also used to inform the patient of payment required for outstanding deductibles or for his or her share of the costs of the procedure. Often this information can be exchanged via the payer's Website. Staff members involved in front-end practice operations should maximize use of the payer's Website to obtain authorizations, pre-certs, and insurance verification and to perform other services that the Website offers in order to ensure accurate demographic information.

Confirming the Appointment

All scheduled appointments should be confirmed at least two days prior to the visit; remind the patient of the scheduled appointment time and the time to arrive and ask the patient to bring an insurance card and a photo identification (ID) card. Also, inform the patient of any copayments or co-insurance due at the time of service. If the appointment is for a procedure, provide instructions regarding food and fluid intake and discuss the need for assistance on the day of the procedure. Because a missed appointment is missed revenue for the practice, it is important to confirm the scheduled appointment, particularly if it is more than three days away. A patient who does not call or advise the practice that they are not coming means an open spot on the schedule and missed revenue.

An appointment can be confirmed by a staff member who calls the patient directly; confirmation can be outsourced to a call center; or appointments can be confirmed electronically. A number of software applications are available that interact with the practice management system and call patients on the schedule book. These systems provide reports on the calling activity so that staff can provide appropriate follow-up for calls not completed due to disconnected or busy numbers.

Communicating Office Policies

It is important to provide patients with clear information regarding your office's policies on how to schedule appointments, how to cancel appointments, and how patients will be notified in case the office has to close for an unforeseen circumstance. Patients should also be advised of how to request prescription refills and the hours and times of day designated for this purpose. In addition, patients should be advised of the practice's financial policies, which should encompass the following:

- when payment is expected on copays;
- when payment is expected on co-insurances;
- what to do if unable to meet financial obligation;
- who to speak to if unable to meet financial obligation; and
- how the practice relates to indigent care.

Office policies and procedures can be sent by letter to the patient prior to his or her first appointment or provided at the time of service. Notice of new policies or policy changes should be sent to every patient, with a notation in the patient's chart stating that he or she was sent a copy of the policies.

Managing Missed Appointments

It is important to track your no-show patients as a percent of the total patient population on any given day. If there are one or two no-shows per day, the schedulers can overbook by one or two patients daily. This provides the physician with a full schedule and prevents dips in revenue due to missed appointments.

Also, it is important to monitor patients and their appointments so that you can inform patients who are chronically late or are chronic "no-shows" of your practice's policies. Policies for these situations are used to modify the behavior of those who have to be rescheduled. For example, you could implement a policy that states that after a third missed appointment, the patient will not get a fixed appointment, rather, the patient will be asked to come in the morning or the afternoon and wait until they can be seen. Another approach is to have a no-show fee. For example, any patient who does not cancel within 24 hours of his or her appointment will be charged a specified amount for the inconvenience and loss of revenue.

Registering the Patient

Registering the patient at the time of the visit is a critical step in the claims and revenue cycle. At registration, it is necessary to confirm the patient's demographics, whether received from the referring physician or from the patient prior to the visit. This includes reconfirming the patient's name and accuracy of spelling, address, date of birth, social security number, insurance number and coverage, and verification of the patient's identity. If the patient is not the person who will be guaranteeing payment, it is necessary to obtain information regarding the responsible party. Figure 5-1 is a checklist of vital information to verify at the time of the appointment.

Although the patient's or guarantor's social security number is no longer used as the identifying number on group insurance cards, the insured's date of birth and social security number are required when filing the electronic claim.

Complying with Identity and Privacy Regulations

Medical practices are required to comply with many federal and government regulations. Two rules that govern the way in which practices interact with patients deal with identity and with privacy—the Red Flag Rules and the Health Insurance Portability and Accountability Act.

Red Flag Rules

On January 1, 2008, The Federal Trade Commission's joint final rules and guidelines, officially known as the Identity Theft Red Flag and Address Discrepancies Under the Fair and Accurate Credit Transactions Act of 2003, became effective.[1] Referred to as "Red Flag Rules," these guidelines were implemented to ensure that identity theft does not occur and that a scheduled patient and his or her insurance information is the patient with insurance who is standing at the registration desk. It is necessary, therefore, to have a picture ID and a state ID (ie, such as a driver's license or a state-issued ID), in addition to the insurance card bearing the patient's or spouse's name. Further, the front desk staff member who is checking in the patient should be able to match the picture ID to the patient, to the insurance card, and to the appointment. Simply, all facets of identification should match. The insurance card should either be scanned electronically into the practice management or electronic medical records system or, if using a paper chart, a copy should be made and stored in the chart for future reference. Also, a copy of the picture ID should be made at this time. Using a modern electronic medical record system, a photo of the patient can be taken using a small computerized camera and attached electronically to the medical record. Not only is this helpful for future identification purposes, the photo can assist the physician in remembering a patient. If he or she cannot recall the patient's name instantly, the photo will often help to link the illness and the patient.

Requirement	Description	Information Obtained
Patient	Patient's name as it appears on his or her insurance verification card	
	Address	
	Telephone numbers	
	• Home	
	• Work	
	• Cell	
	Date of birth	
	Social security number	
Guarantor	Guarantor's correct name	
	Address	
	Telephone numbers	
	• Home	
	• Work	
	• Cell	
	Social security number	
	Other identification information	
Insurance Company	Name of company and plan ID	
	Employer, if this is group coverage through an employer	
	Name of the insured individual (as the insured may not be the patient; it may be the patient's spouse or parent)	
	Insured's date of birth and social security number	
Secondary Insurance Company	Name of company and plan ID	
	Employer, if this is group coverage through an employer	
	Name of the insured individual (as the insured may not be the patient; it may be the patient's spouse or parent)	

FIGURE 5-1 Patient Demographic Requirements at Registration.

Health Insurance Portability and Accountability Act

The Health Insurance Portability and Accountability Act of 1996 (HIPAA) is a multistep approach to improving the health insurance system. Title I of HIPAA protects health insurance coverage for workers and their families when they change or lose their jobs. Title II of HIPAA, known as the Administrative Simplification Provisions, requires national standards for electronic health care transactions and national identifiers for providers, health insurance plans, and employers.

One purpose of the HIPAA regulations is to protect privacy. The HIPAA Privacy Rule provides federal protections for personal health information held by covered entities and gives patients numerous rights with respect to that information. The Privacy Rule also permits the disclosure of personal health information needed for patient care and other important purposes. HIPAA helps to ensure that all medical records, medical billing, and patient accounts meet consistent standards with regard to documentation, handling, and privacy.

The Privacy Rule requires every practice to have a Notice of Privacy Practices. This notice should be presented to every new patient on his or her first visit and to all patients if a change is made to the practice's policy. Simply, every patient must receive an updated copy, and signature verification that the patient was provided a copy of the document must be recorded in the medical record or with patient demographics. The signed verification should be kept either in the paper chart or in the electronic chart for future reference. The Notice of Privacy Practices includes a description of uses and disclosures of protected health information (PHI), the individual's rights as to PHI, and the medical practice's obligations as to PHI.

Obtaining Consent for Treatment

In addition to notices of privacy practices under HIPAA, the practice must obtain the patient's signature on a consent for treatment form for any time the patient receives care in the office. This form can be nonspecific for office visits and should be completed once a year. If the patient will be undergoing a specific procedure, the consent for treatment must indicate the procedure, the process the procedure will follow, and any potential side effects that may result from the procedure. Also, be aware of specific state laws and regulations regarding treatment of minors, especially with regard to drug and alcohol abuse, treatment for venereal disease, HIV testing, birth control and family planning, treatment for sexual assault, and provision of mental health services. Refer to applicable state statutes that include specific requirements regarding consent for treatment; your malpractice insurer may have recommendations on the consent for treatment language.

Collecting from the Patient at Registration

The appropriate copayment should be collected from the patient at registration and reconfirmed at checkout. This should have been discussed with the patient both at the time of scheduling and when the appointment was confirmed. Also, if the patient will be incurring a large expense at this visit or has a large outstanding deductible, it is appropriate to discuss financial arrangements and the office's policies for payments. Usually, outstanding balances are for the amount of an outstanding deductible or co-insurance that was not identified at the time of service and was posted after services were rendered and billed. It may be necessary to discuss large balances with a financial counselor within the practice or a patient advocate who can assist the patient in developing an acceptable payment plan that will clear the balance in an appropriate time frame, in line with the practice's financial policy. The discussion may also include credit cards and other financing options. The practice can implement whatever policies it wishes, providing all policies apply to all patients at all times. Otherwise, the practice could be charged with credit discrimination.

Checking Out the Patient

Several key steps must be completed as the patient leaves the practice. The services rendered by the physician and ancillary personnel should be noted on the encounter, either on the paper form or electronically, and the appropriate diagnosis codes for those services indicated and linked to each procedure that is being charged. In addition, any return appointment for follow-up, additional procedures, or surgeries at the hospital should be discussed with the patient and scheduled as appropriate. The checkout process should include a reconfirmation that any copay had been collected and that any outstanding balances have been discussed. If this was not done at check-in, it can be accomplished at checkout.

Surveying Patient Satisfaction

At checkout, provide the patient with a brief patient satisfaction survey. It can be a short survey with 10 or fewer questions regarding the patient's experience during that day's visit. The survey can be anonymous or the patient can sign or ask to have someone follow up with them. The survey should relate to how the patient was greeted; the office's overall appearance; how medical services were delivered; the accuracy of the explanation of services received, including any instructions related to after-care or prescriptions; ancillary staff courtesy and professionalism; and any other general comments about the day's experience. Patient satisfaction surveys enable the practice to take a reading of their customer service. In addition, the information is extremely helpful and necessary as a basis for explaining to a payer about the quality care that the practice renders.

Creating First Impressions

The front desk and its appearance to patients are critical to the overall office experience. The well-worn cliché, "you never get a second chance to make a first impression," is true regarding your practice's reception desk. The front office *is* the practice—its face and voice. Therefore, front-desk staff members must have the customer service skills needed to handle patients effectively.

Using Electronic Records in Patient Visits

The electronic health record (EHR) is becoming the standard of operation in medical offices, engendering assistance to the practice operations. An EHR

- allows for accurate collection of data;
- allows for accurate documentation of a patient's visit;
- assists in accurate coding of the visit; and
- makes it possible to accurately exchange information with insurance companies and other providers that the patient may need to be referred to for additional services.

The EHR is of such high importance in today's medical office that current governmental assistance with purchasing an EHR is available to practices under the American Reinvestment & Recovery Act, which was passed in 2009. EHRs play an important part in patient visit processes. More and more emphasis is being placed on electronic medical records (EMRs), or EHRs in today's health care environment. As the EHR becomes a standard technology within medical practices, it will significantly change the way in which physicians practice medicine.

Completing the End-of-the-Day Processes

Once patients have been registered, services have been rendered, and patients have been checked out, it is time to process the day's transactions. This involves balancing the day's receipts, verifying the day's charges, and contacting no-show patients for rescheduling.

Balancing Receipts and Verifying Charges

An accounting process must be in place to verify that all copayments, co-insurance, and payments on outstanding balances have been appropriately posted and balanced to the cash received and placed in the cash drawers. This should then be verified by a second party and delivered to the individual responsible for making bank deposits. This verification of charges ensures that all services rendered for the day have been appropriately coded and billed. With today's EMR, this electronic process usually occurs in the billing office when billing staff prepares charges for submission to payers. However, in offices that use paper encounter forms, it is necessary to make sure that all office visits, all labs, and all related charges have been marked and that all charges have been appropriately linked to the diagnosis code for which the services were rendered.

Contacting No-Show Patients

One final end-of-day process is to contact no-show patients. Any patient on the schedule book who did not appear for his or her appointment or contact the practice regarding the appointment should be contacted in an attempt to reschedule. It is important to know why a patient did not show up (eg, transportation issue, availability of a support person). This information can be used to reschedule the patient at a time that is more convenient, preventing future no-shows. Any information the patient provides, such as availability on a specific day of the week, should be noted in the chart for future reference for the scheduling personnel.

Conclusion

Reimbursement for services rendered in the medical practice begins with the front-office operations. The initial step is to schedule appointments. Much more complex than merely filling a date and time slot with a name, scheduling involves obtaining information from the patient about the nature of the visit in order to allot the proper amount of time for the appointment. Scheduling also involves accommodating as many patients in the schedule as possible in order to make the most of the physicians' time.

Once the patient contacts the practice, front-office staff focuses on getting accurate and adequate information in order to achieve reimbursement for services. Every step, from initial call to checking out after services have been rendered, is geared toward achieving reimbursement and protecting the patient and the practice. The final step in revenue cycle management is to account for the revenue billed and collected using adequate checks and balances to protect the practice.

Chapter 6 addresses the back-office operations of the revenue cycle management of the medical practice.

Reference

1. *Federal Register*, Vol. 72, No. 217/Friday, November 9, 2007/Rules and Regulations. Accessed 5/12/2010 at www.ftc.gov/os/fedreg/2007/november/071109redflags.pdf.

CHAPTER 6
Back-Office Processes

OUTLINE

I. Introduction
II. Charge Capture and Entry
    A. In-Office Charges
    B. In-Office Ancillary Charges
    C. Hospital Charges
III. Claims Submission
    A. Claims Scrubbing
    B. Electronic Clearinghouse
    C. Prompt-Pay Laws and Clean-Claim Laws
IV. Remittances and Explanation of Benefits
    A. Lockbox Services
    B. Cash Posting and Contract Monitoring
    C. Balancing
    D. Zero Payments
    E. Denied Claims
    F. Secondary Insurance
    G. Cycle Billing
V. Forms of Payment
VI. Insurance Claims Follow-Up
    A. Contacting Payers
    B. Patient Follow-Up
    C. Bankruptcy
VII. Selecting a Collection Agency
    A. Bad Debt
    B. Right to Cure
    C. Monitoring the Collection Agency
    D. Legal Action
VIII. Conclusion

Introduction

After a patient receives care and checks out, the back-office operations begin. These behind-the-scenes activities involve billing and collections; this is where most of the financial activity occurs. Beyond delivering quality patient care and having satisfied patients, reimbursement is the point where the practice either thrives or collapses. This chapter discusses the workings of back-office operations.

Charge Capture and Entry

Physician practices generally render services in three environments: in the office, through ancillaries in the office, or in the hospital. Reimbursement for these services is captured through coding and documentation of what occurred with the patient, and the revenue is generated by entering the charges into the billing system.

In-Office Charges

Charges can be entered into the practice management system in several ways. Charges incurred for services rendered in the practice can be electronically imported from the practice management system into the billing system using the electronic health record (EHR). If a practice still uses paper charts or prefers to use paper encounter forms, these charges are entered at the time of checkout and verified at that time. If the volume of charges exceeds the front-office staff's ability to input them at checkout, charges should be in the billing office the first thing the next morning for entry into the system, verification, and billing.

In-Office Ancillary Charges

In addition to charges for the office visit, there may be charges for ancillary services, such as electrocardiograms (EKGs), ultrasounds, laboratory work, and other tests performed in order to diagnose the patient. Often these charges are not part of the EHR and exist outside of the system in paper form. These charges must arrive in the billing department the first thing the next day for appropriate processing; they must also be appended to the office visit charges before the claim is forwarded to the insurance payer.

Hospital Charges

In addition, physicians may admit and visit patients at the hospital, provide hospital rounds, and perform procedures at the hospital. The physician is responsible for providing appropriate documentation to the billing office for services rendered, indicating hospital rounds, hospital admits, and hospital consults provided. This information may be captured via a paper or card form that the physician completes or by use of an electronic device. Data are collected and then downloaded to the practice's billing system for posting and claim filing.

If patients receive care in the hospital outpatient or inpatient environment, it is helpful to have an established relationship with the hospital's medical records department so that all procedure notes are provided to the practice in a timely manner in order to account for appropriate billing. Procedures that are scheduled from the office should be tracked and all procedure notes should be received for appropriate billing.

Claims Submission

After charge entry, claims are submitted; this involves claims scrubbing and editing, sending claims to a clearinghouse, making necessary corrections in response to clearinghouse reports, and resubmitting corrected claims to payers. Follow-up to ensure that payers are prompt is the next step in the back-office billing process.

Claims Scrubbing

Once all charges are entered into the billing system, claims are prepared for submission to the various payers. Claims are usually put into batches, and the batches are then scrubbed for edits. This means that the claims are submitted through an electronic process to make certain that the appropriate procedure codes and diagnosis codes are linked, by the payer's definition, to ensure proper reimbursement. The national Correct Coding Initiative (CCI) edits are provided through the Centers for Medicaid and Medicare Services (CMS) for Medicare claims. Also used by commercial payers, these edits identify the Current Procedural Terminology (CPT®) codes that may and may not be billed together. A complete listing of all national and local coverage determination documents is available on the CMS Website at www.cms.hhs.gov/mcd/search.asp?clickon=search. The listing provides the coding, documentation, and diagnosis requirements for procedures covered and payable by Medicare.

Additionally, commercial payers provide their medical policies on their Websites, indicating the procedures and appropriate diagnosis codes for the procedures they have approved for payment. Commercial payers use their own claims editing software and also offer the option of inputting claims in order to determine whether the codes or code combinations are likely to be paid. This information can be included in the practice's practice management system or software from an outside source that allows for this scrubbing of claims.

Once the claims have been scrubbed, an error list is developed. The claims on this list can then be corrected after reviewing the documentation in the medical record and the payer's medical policy.

Electronic Clearinghouse

Once all claims are clean and ready for submission, they are forwarded to an electronic clearinghouse. There are a number of clearinghouses across the country to which electronic claims are submitted. Each day the claims are sorted into batches that are sent to the major payers. For example, Practice A may submit 200 claims that will go to Medicare, BlueCross, United Healthcare, Humana, Cigna, and Aetna. Practice B may submit 700 claims that will go to the same payers, and Practice C may only submit 50 claims that go to the same payer. All claims from Practices A, B, and C that go to Medicare are grouped together and sent to Medicare. The electronic clearinghouse then sends back a report indicating that the claims were successfully transmitted to the payer and also which claims the payer was unable to accept, with the specific error identified. Errors include such things as subscriber's ID not found. This indicates that the identification number for the insurance was not in their system or that the patient's name was not found.

When billing the payer, in particular Medicare, it is important that the name included on the claim is an identical match to the name on the insurance card, even if the name on the insurance card is misspelled. When a name is misspelled, the patient is directed to his or her insurance company or the Social Security Administration for Medicare to correct the spelling.

Claims may be rejected if insurance has terminated. However, if insurance is verified prior to the patient being seen in the office, this rarely occurs. If it does occur, the practice must contact the patient to find out if the patient has new insurance or a new insurance card for his or her group or if the claim needs to be moved from an insurance responsibility to a patient responsibility.

Prompt-Pay Laws and Clean-Claim Laws

After claims are submitted, they are subject to your state's prompt-pay laws and/or regulations regarding timeliness of payment. (Appendix C lists all states' prompt pay laws.) Claims not paid within the required time period may be eligible for additional interest payment from the payer, depending on the reason for the initial denial and whether the health plan is subject to the state law.

Remittances and Explanations of Benefits

Payment from payers comes in the form of electronic remittances and paper explanations of benefits. Electronic payments and remittances are often processed through the same clearinghouse functions that the claims were originally submitted to the payers. Currently, 90% of Medicare remittances are in electronic form. The money is electronically placed in the practice's checking account or bank account; an electronic remittance is available for the practice to post into the patient account system. Many commercial payers, such as Blue Cross, United HealthCare, Humana, Cigna, and Aetna, are moving to electronic payments and electronic remittances. For payers without this electronic feature, payments are mailed to the practice address that is listed in the files, with a paper explanation of benefits and a paper check.

Lockbox Services

Practices with sufficient volume may elect to use bank lockbox services. With this type of service, the bank receives all checks and paperwork addressed to a specific Post Office (PO) box. The bank processes the deposit and puts the funds directly into the practice's account and forwards a copy of the check to the practice, along with any paperwork included with the check. The cash posters in the office are then able to post the payments to the patients' accounts.

Cash Posting and Contract Monitoring

Cash posting is a critical function in the office. It requires extreme accuracy and knowledge of the managed care plans with which the practice participates. If possible, it is helpful to store the fee schedules that have been negotiated in the managed care contracts into the practice management system. If your system lacks this capability, develop a matrix that shows all the procedure codes that the practice bills by payer and what the allowed amount should be. This information should be readily available for the cash posters. Over time, the cash posters will become very familiar with the various reimbursement levels and will be able to ensure that the practice is being paid correctly.

Balancing

Each day, the cash posters' work must be balanced to the deposits received at the bank and all monies appropriately accounted for and posted correctly. This end-of-day balancing function is necessary to confirm that all deposits, either direct deposits or manual deposits, have been recognized and that all postings are accurate and balance to these deposits. Daily balancing makes the month-end closing processes much easier, because it will not be necessary to balance 28 to 31 days individually before the month-end processes are completed.

Zero Payments

Often an explanation of benefits or remittance will indicate zero payment. This type of payment may result when the entire amount is applied to a deductible, the service or procedure performed is not a covered benefit or was not considered to be medically necessary, another payer is responsible for the claim, or a payer states that the procedure is part of another procedure that was also billed on that claim. An assigned insurance follow-up person should review any zero-payment posting to make certain that it is in fact a zero payment and appropriate adjustment is taken. If, after being reviewed against the payer's reimbursement policies, it is determined that the zero payment is an error, the necessary appeal steps are taken, as outlined in the payer's provider manual or managed care contract.

Denied Claims

An explanation of benefits that is returned or an electronic remittance indicating that there are denied claims—denied because the procedure code and the diagnosis code do not match or denied due to medical necessity—should be directed immediately to the insurance follow-up person so that the denial can be reviewed. These denials may need to be reviewed by a coder to determine the correct coding, and an appropriate appeal or corrected claim should be submitted to secure payment. Denied claims should be reviewed and appeals filed within 30 days from the date of the denial. If they are not filed within this time period, the practice may lose the monies due to the timeliness of the appeals process.

Secondary Insurance

After all insurance payments have been posted, any secondary claim must be submitted. Secondary claims are for patients who have a secondary insurance and whose primary insurance did not automatically send a claim to the secondary insurance. The claim should be submitted either electronically through the practice management system or via submission of a paper claim. If submitting electronically, additional information will be needed so that the primary payment can be documented and recognized by the secondary payer. If submitting a paper copy, the primary remittance advice needs to be copied and attached so that the secondary payer receives the information necessary for proper payment of the remaining balance.

Cycle Billing

Patients who do not have a secondary insurance are sent a statement. Statements must be generated regularly. It is recommended that the alphabet be broken into four sections, eg, A-G, H-M, N-S, T-Z, with one section billed each week. This is referred to as cycle billing, which allows for uniform billing and uniform cash flow. Each cycle has approximately the same number of patient statements in it and approximately the same amount of revenue. This method also prevents a large influx of phone calls from patients who have questions regarding their statements. If billing of all accounts is done on a monthly cycle, the entire patient accounts department is likely to be tied up responding to phone calls. To keep things balanced, you can use your modern patient accounts systems to look at the number of statements in a cycle and the total dollar value they represent and move the letters of the alphabet from cycle 1 to cycle 2 if necessary.

Forms of Payment

The practice should be prepared to accept payment in numerous forms. This includes checks, cash, credit cards, and electronic payments from patients' bill-pay checking accounts. Patients' credit card numbers and other identifying information should not be stored in the practice management system. This could create additional exposure in the event of identity theft or "hacking" of the practice's system.

Insurance Claims Follow-Up

Insurance claims that are not paid in a timely manner must be monitored daily with follow-up to the payer regarding the lack of response. The business office may have one person or multiple persons perform all billing and follow-up functions. If multiple persons are involved, follow-up with payers should be split between the various individuals; these individuals will become experts in dealing with a particular payer.

Follow-up should be done on the day that a clean claim should have been paid. If the your state law is 30 days, then insurance follow-up should begin 30 days from the date the claim was filed. For claims that have been paid incorrectly, follow-up should begin the moment (or as soon as practical) the practice becomes aware of an improper payment, with the documentation provided to the insurance follow-up personnel from the payment posters.

Contacting Payers

When calling and contacting payers regarding unpaid claims, make sure the payer is aware of your state's prompt-pay law and/or regulations (if applicable) and understand that the payer has numerous excuses for not paying. If a payer does not pay a claim in a timely manner, most states require that the payer inform the practice in writing that they will not be making payment within the required time frame and the reason why. For example, a payer may look at preexisting conditions or they may look to see if a procedure was related to an accident, in which case it should have been billed to a workers' compensation or liability carrier. If no documentation arrives within the state's prompt-pay time period indicating that the claim is being reviewed, then the prompt-pay laws apply and the payer not only owes the amount noted in the fee schedule, but also the appropriate interest, as reflected by the state's regulations. Because statutes vary, it is essential to become familiar with your state's laws.

Patient Follow-Up

In addition to follow-up with insurance payers, it is also necessary to follow up with patients on outstanding balances. Your practice should have established collection policies that have been shared with staff. This includes the number of statements to be forwarded to patients and the financial policies the practice has in place to assist patients with payment, such as budget payment plans and acceptance of various forms of payment, including credit cards.

All employees who interact with patients in terms of balances and payments must understand the Fair Debt Collections Practices Act, often referred to as FDCPA. This act was originally developed by the federal government and applicable to third-party collectors, such as collection agencies. However, the act now applies to first party attempts to collect and most medical practices. Restrictions include:

- not calling prior to 8 a.m. and after 9 p.m.;
- nondisclosure of the reason for the call to any third party; and
- monitoring or being aware of messages left on any voicemail system asking the patient to return a call.

Therefore, the practice's knowledge of the FDCPA is important in order to prevent violation and potential monetary penalty.

Bankruptcy

It is not uncommon to receive notice of bankruptcy. In these instances, be sure to note the dates the bankruptcy covers and determine how the policy will handle a patient's account going forward. Although a bankruptcy filing stops the statement process for the specific charges, the charges are not removed until the final notice is received from the court discharging the patient in bankruptcy. If the bankruptcy is dismissed, the charges are still the patient's responsibility.

Selecting a Collection Agency

If your practice decides to write off patient balances to bad debt and forward that debt to a third party for collection, a collection agency will be needed. A collection agency should be selected carefully, with sufficient review of the business entity. The collection agency should be a member of the American Collectors Association, thus ensuring the practice that the agency's employees are familiar with the Fair Debt Collections Practices Act and aware of the collection processes they are permitted to use when attempting to collect a debt. Collection agencies commonly charge a percentage of the recovery that they make. That percentage varies by volume and age of the account when it is forwarded to the agency; generally, the percentage ranges from 25 to 35% if no legal action is taken.

If your practice decides to take legal action, such as small claims court or, for larger balances, probate court, the collection agency will usually secure the services of an attorney and the percent charged for recovery will range from 50 to 60%, plus costs incurred.

Bad Debt

Determining when an account is a bad debt is the decision of the practice and should be clearly outlined in the financial policy. In most cases, a debt becomes bad within 90 to 120 days from the date of service or date first billed or after three statements have been sent. Other factors, such as breaking payment arrangements more than three times or not making a payment in three months, will often trigger the bad debt.

Right to Cure

When the collection agency first receives the account, it is required, under the FDCPA, to issue the patient a letter termed the Right to Cure. This gives the patient 30 days to either pay the debt or dispute the debt without the debt being recorded with any national credit bureau. After the 30-day period, the collection agency will place the account on one, if not all, national credit bureau report, thereby showing that the patient has a bad debt that is now affecting his or her credit rating.

Monitoring the Collection Agency

The practice's collection agency should provide several reports on a regular basis. For each group of accounts forwarded to the agency for placement, the practice should receive an acknowledgment report that lists the accounts, the date they were placed with the agency, and the amount. This report should match the report from the practice management system generated at the time the accounts were written off to bad debt and forwarded to the agency.

Collection agencies usually return between 3 and 10% of the gross value of the accounts placed with them. An agency returning more than 10% indicates that the accounts are being forwarded to the agency without appropriate in-house collection activity, ie, an effort has not been made within the practice to effectively collect the accounts. If the issue is volume, it may be possible to make an "early placement or an early out" arrangement with the collection agency. The account will be given to the agency much earlier in the revenue cycle, possibly at 30 days, and will not be in a bad-debt situation. The collection agency will be working for the practice in a self-pay, collections-assistance mode. Services within this type of arrangement are usually at a lower percentage of the collections. After being worked and deemed that the patient is not going to pay the bill, the account is then rolled over into a bad-debt situation. Early-out collections usually have a recovery fee of between 10 and 25%, again depending on the age of the account when it is rolled into that process.

Legal Action

Often the collection agency will inform the practice when it has exhausted all techniques to collect the debt. Based on the value and amount of the debt, the agency may contact the practice to request authorization to proceed to legal action. Prior to recommending legal action, the agency performs an asset check to make sure the patient has assets against which appropriate liens can be placed to secure payment of the account. This usually includes real estate and/or garnishment, if permitted by the state.

Legal action is instituted upon a signed agreement by the practice with the agency to proceed to that level. The agency then files the appropriate paperwork with the small claims or probate court, and the patient is notified that legal action is being taken against them for collection of the debt. Legal action, in addition to increasing the percentage of recovery that will be due to the agency for that service, also imposes liability for the expenses incurred on the practice. Therefore, each case should be reviewed to determine if legal action is appropriate and whether it will secure a payment reasonable for the services rendered.

Conclusion

This chapter describes how the back-office functions in the revenue cycle and defines the responsibilities for capturing reimbursement for the services delivered by the practice. The daily operations are repetitive and multifaceted, with many obstacles and challenges. Nevertheless, with well-trained and highly focused staff doing their jobs the right way every day, a practice can establish a smooth-running and effective business office that affords financial stability for the organization.

CHAPTER 7

Appeals and Reviews

OUTLINE

I. Introduction
II. Managing Appeals and Reviews
III. Know What Payer Contracts Allow
    A. External Resources
    B. Administrative Manuals
    C. Negotiated Reimbursement Rates
    D. Changes to Employer-Sponsored Health Plans
IV. Internal Payer Processes and Timelines for Claim Processing
    A. Clean Claims Criteria
    B. Coding Expert's Role in the Appeals Process
    C. Billing Systems
V. The Appeals Process
    A. Key Components of an Appeals Program
    B. Appealing Claims
VI. Conclusion

Introduction

One important aspect of the revenue cycle that is often neglected and underestimated is the appeals process. Routine acceptance of denials reported by health insurers and writing off charges based on those denials without question is a clear indicator that the terms of the practice's negotiated contract, including the terms that govern the appeals process, are not understood. State managed-care statutes require that health plans administer the appeals and grievance processes under specific processes and rules. Although the process of appealing claims can increase the administrative burden in the short term, ignoring inappropriate denials and allowing continued incorrect payments can create a long-term financial disaster for the medical practice. Development of an effective appeals process and staying diligent in that effort helps to create a more stable claims payment environment by encouraging review and correction of errors in payers' claims-editing software programs. This, is turn, helps to promote more payments that are accurate and reduces the number of errors, which reduces the administrative burden. This reverses the cycle of inefficiency.

This chapter explores the appeals and reviews process as a part of managing reimbursement.

Managing Appeals and Reviews

To manage appeals and reviews effectively, key areas in the practice for reviewing any denials and payment discrepancies must be explored and developed. These areas revolve around understanding the negotiated managed care contract. As discussed in Chapter 2, negotiation of payer contracts requires a clear understanding of the terms of the agreement in order to comply with those terms. The impact these terms will have on the practice, both clinically and financially, must be considered *before* the contract is signed. The negotiated contract is an agreement between the practice and the payer and must be shared with every staff member who can help to enforce the terms appropriately, including but not limited to staff scheduling and checking in patients; clinical staff including nurses, physicians, and providers; the check-out team and referrals coordinators; and most important, the billing office staff who is responsible for reviewing the payments and initiating appeals processes when these agreed-upon terms are not met.

Everyone in the office is responsible for improving revenue to the practice. Of particular importance are the portions of the contract and associated health plan policies and procedures that address the scope of covered services and the negotiated fees; the payers' internal processes for claim payment, review, and denial; and the step-by-step process and timeline for appeal.

Know What Payer Contracts Allow

The most important protection any practice can have to ensure accurate and timely payments is found in the terms of the negotiated contracts. These contracts and the associated references, such as administrative manuals, health plan policies and procedures, and exhibits, must include clear information about the types of services typically covered in a practice of the same specialty, the negotiated rates for payment, the terms for timely payment, and the guidelines for appealing denied or improperly paid claims. Administrative manuals and policies also outline the steps for resolving any discrepancies to those terms. After discrepancies have been resolved, the practice should understand the terms as completely as possible, and take measures to ensure all parties adhere to the contract.

External Resources

Within the body of every managed care contract is reference to external resources that also impact the terms of the agreement. These resources tell the payer and the practice where to look when they are unsure of how to interpret certain sections of the contract. The payer's administrative manual is always listed in this library of references. Without appropriate contract language to clearly identify the prevailing order of documents, the guidelines in the administrative manual could not govern any other reference documents identified. For example, if the contract indicates that the payer must follow standard Current Procedural Terminology (CPT®), Fourth Edition and International Classification of Diseases, 9th Revision (ICDs) coding guidelines but the administrative manual indicates that the payer can make up its own rules for claims payment, it is important to know which statement has greater weight, especially when the two documents contain conflicting information. It is always important to review these manuals and references prior to finalizing the contract because they outline the financial arrangements the practice and patients can expect from the negotiated relationship.

There are also provisions in the contract for making changes to this manual providing appropriate notice is given, which can happen at any time. Larger payers usually announce changes to the administrative manual via newsletters or other communications, which are delivered in print or via electronic notification. The updated administrative manual is always available online; each staff member should have access to the payer site to verify eligibility, covered services, benefit structure, and other specifics. The practice should review all communications from payers, subscribe to all online payer newsletters, and share this information with physicians, providers, and staff. It is very important to stay on top of changes to payer policies and procedures so that claims will be received and paid without rejection.

Administrative Manuals

Administrative manuals (also called policies and procedures manuals) generally include the following: descriptions of health benefit plans offered, credentialing guidelines, claims submission and billing procedures, descriptions of utilization management and case management programs, explanation of coordination of benefits, quality improvement initiatives, and appeals and grievance procedures.

The office staff must be aware of any exclusive contracts or "centers of excellence" programs offered by the health plan. Although the office may be equipped to offer a full range of ancillary services, if the contract prohibits payment to the physician's office because it will conflict with other exclusive arrangements for these services, the practice is required to refer the patient to those preferred providers. Based on the agreement, the practice is also generally required to refer patients to other physicians participating in the patient's plan. The state's department of insurance may require that the network be available within a certain distance for the patient or have certain accessibility requirements. In the specialists' world, this is particularly important for health maintenance organizations (HMOs) and point of service (POS) plans because the plan may require that the referral from the primary care provider (PCP) be documented in order for the specialist's office to be paid. It may be required that documentation of this referral be available before the patient is seen in the office. It is unfair to the patient and to the primary care office to obtain a retroactive referral from a busy primary care office that may be inundated with requests for referrals for services that they may not have recommended. Many insurers will not allow this practice. However, many patients do not understand these restrictions and may have a negative impression of the physician office.

Unfortunately, the medical practice has no control over the plan's terms that the patient accepts. Although patients are responsible for understanding the benefits of their insurance plans, that is not always the case. In the end, the patient's responsibility stops with the copayment or co-insurance, and it is up to the practice to know (before the service is delivered) if it will be paid and the exact amount it will receive from the patient and from the payer. In many cases, patients must be educated about their potential financial liability. In all cases, it is best to collect the patient's portion before he or she leaves the office in order to avoid the cost of back-end billing efforts (eg, administrative time, statement mailing costs, collection agencies). Again, the administrative manual outlines these rules.

Negotiated Reimbursement Rates

The negotiated reimbursement rates are outlined in the contract, usually in the form of an attached fee schedule. If the rates are based on some multiple of Medicare, changes to the allowable may fluctuate annually if Medicare rates are updated annually. Other contracts specify rates for a particular year (eg, 2008 Medicare rates) upon which payments will be made until the contract is renegotiated. These changes can positively or negatively impact the total expected payments. Some payers update their fee schedules with both rates and effective dates to mirror the

Medicare updates. Others decline to update their systems as quickly and establish their own effective dates. Again, the contract terms should outline the update process and offer protection to the practice for appealing any discrepancies to those payments. It is critical to understand the language relating to these rates and to know *exactly* how and when the rates will change. It these terms are not understood, a payer could capitalize financially on the lack of knowledge at the practice level. For example, if the Medicare allowable for a typical office visit (99213) increases by $2.00 and the practice's contract for evaluation and management (E/M) services is based on 150% of the Medicare allowable, the practice would be entitled to an additional $3.00 from that payer every time those services are billed. If the practice has a large population of patients covered by that plan and does not know when the increase goes into effect, it could lose out on $3.00 per patient visit until the correct allowable amount is loaded into the system. Remember, these fee schedules affect all segments of the service line, not just office visits. This can add up quickly.

In most cases, rates remain constant unless the contract language outlines when changes will be made based on some agreed-on event, such as when the contract is renegotiated, at the contract anniversary date, or based on an update to the Medicare fee schedule. It is possible to load multiple fee schedules or payer allowable amounts into most practice management systems. This is a very labor-intensive process that requires constant surveillance and immediate maintenance when the rates change. However, it is an excellent way to identify any variances in the payments received compared to the expected payments based on the contract. Many practice management systems "anticipate" upcoming changes to payments based on contract terms and fee schedules; some systems can even create appeal letters and pull verbatim contract language into the letter. These contract-based programs also require careful planning of the payer infrastructure so that plans are easily identifiable and patients can be matched to the appropriate payer contract and fee schedule.

Many insurance cards reflect multiple plan logos. With the incidence of silent preferred provider organizations (PPOs) (which can be very difficult to handle when they are involved) and discount plans in the market, matching the patient to the correct payer or fee schedule is a challenge for the front-desk staff. Because insurance cards often include conflicting information, it is often impossible for the front-desk staff to know which plan drives the processing and payment of the claim. A decision must be made regarding whether to enter each product line from a particular health plan separately or to enter separate employer groups separately. Staff members with experience in these areas are a definite asset to any practice. If the patient's network affiliation is input incorrectly, the payment will deviate from the expected fee. When this variance is identified, the patient information must be updated immediately to reflect the correct affiliation, so that future payments can be compared to the negotiated fees correctly.

Most errors can be minimized by implementing an effective insurance eligibility and verification program. Many practice management systems include a batch process for verifying the insurance of scheduled patients. For example, the practice management system could be set up to verify every patient appointment two days prior to the scheduled appointment. Typically, this process takes place after office hours, because it ties up the practice phone lines. The following day, a report generated by the eligibility program outlines the insurance status of each patient including the network affiliation (eg, BCBS, UHC, Aetna), the type of plan (eg, PPO, HMO, POS, HSA), the copayment and deductible information, and even an outline of the patient's benefit structure (such as covered preventive services, noncovered services). Additionally, coordination-of-benefits information (other primary or secondary insurance), which alerts the practice to request an update of the information when the patient comes into the office, can be outlined in the process.

The front-desk staff is also responsible for ensuring compliance with the terms of the payer agreement by capturing the correct patient demographic information and collecting copayments at each and every visit. Errors in collecting this information can impact accounts receivables in several ways: eligibility and benefits cannot be verified, statements can be sent to wrong addresses, and copayments and co-insurance can be loaded incorrectly. Depending on the specialty, this can be a very costly mistake. In a surgical practice where expensive procedures are scheduled, failure to verify patient insurance information could result in expensive delays and denials that could significantly damage the cash-flow process. In a primary care practice, failure to keep current with changes to employer-sponsored plans can result in large groups of claims going to the wrong payer or being submitted with the incorrect group number, which greatly affects the revenue that sustains the practice.

Loading the correct patient copayment or co-insurance information into the billing system and collecting this at each visit is also a contractual requirement. The only way to collect 100% of the payer's allowable is by collecting the appropriate patient portion, ideally at the time of service. Estimates of the coinsurance and deductible can be obtained during the verification of insurance process, which is frequently done through the payer's Website. For example, Blue Cross Blue Shield of Alabama providers verify all contract benefits online through the provider access portal. Providers are able to pull up the patient summary plan description, choose a category grouping such as physician benefits (in-office), and see exactly what the co-insurance and/or copayment will be. The practice can contact the payer directly for clarification, if necessary. The same process is used to determine a patient's benefits for outpatient surgery.

Many practices see a dramatic effect on their bottom line by simply asking for the copayment at the time of service with a simple question, such as "Will that be cash, check, or credit card?" The importance of the staff assigned to these front-end positions can make or break a practice (see Chapter 5). Again, it is a part of the contractual agreement to collect the patient's portion at each visit.

Changes to Employer-Sponsored Health Plans

Another important aspect of the revenue cycle involves keeping informed about changes to employer-sponsored health plans. Because of the competitive nature of the insurance industry, the negotiations to secure large pools of employees escalates just before the open enrollment period, which is usually September and October. The current economic climate can dramatically impact the insurance options available to the work force. As employers try to improve their bottom line by taking better control of expenses, changes to the employer-sponsored health benefits can affect a large group of employees and patients, which can in turn dramatically affect the practice's bottom line. Depending on the plan options offered, an employee could go from paying a $15 copayment at each visit to paying 100% out-of-pocket based on a negotiated fee schedule. If staff is not aware of the local changes to employer plans, the changes can dramatically impact the practice's bottom line. When multiple plan options are available, it is the patient's responsibility to know his or her benefits, but the practice will have an advantage if it keeps abreast of local changes. Again, an effective eligibility process can alleviate some of the problems associated with changes to coverage options.

Understanding the terms of all negotiated contracts and knowing how to translate contract terms into systems and processes in the physician offices is necessary in order to capture revenue and avoid unnecessary denials. Educating staff and keeping them updated on changes to payer contracts is the best way to defend the practice's claims submission processes and support appeal efforts. After all, the payer agreed to the rules, too.

Internal Payer Processes and Timelines for Claim Processing

As the saying goes, "the devil is in the details," and it is very true when it comes to following the letter of the law with payer processes and timelines. Again, the contract between the practice and the payer outlines the requirements (on both sides) to ensure that claims are submitted and paid as quickly as possible. If the billing staff knows the rules, revenue can be optimized. If the rules are ignored, revenue cannot be captured effectively.

Clean Claims Criteria

Every negotiated managed care contract has clauses that outline the requirements and timelines for submitting claims and for processing and paying those claims. Because of these requirements, the American Medical Association (AMA), along with several other health care industry sector representatives, have conducted a nationwide initiative to educate health care providers, managers, and staff about the steps required to process charges efficiently.[1] The electronic transmittal of insurance claims cannot be completed at the practice level or at the payer level if incomplete or inaccurate patient information is submitted or if basic coding guidelines are not followed. The foundation of the rules rests on the submission of a clean claim within the time period outlined in the contract. The definition of a clean claim is usually identified in the contract and can vary by type of payer. For example, Medicare defines a clean claim as one that "has no defect, impropriety or special circumstance, including incomplete documentation that delays timely payment."[2] A claim is considered clean if all the required data elements along with any required attachments are provided within the time limits established by the claims processor. An omission of a single data element can cause the claim to be rejected or denied. For the HCFA 1500, these required data elements typically include:

- subscriber's information (name, date of birth, gender, plan ID, policy number, address);
- patient's information (name, date of birth, gender, plan ID, address, relationship to the subscriber);
- insurance provider's information (name, disclosure of any other insurance);
- information about the service provided (date, place of service, rendering provider name/National Provider Identifier [NPI]/billing address, referring provider name and NPI, referral authorization);
- appropriate coding according to AMA standards (CPT-4, ICD-9, Healthcare Common Procedure Coding System [HCPCS]);
- charges per service, total charges; and
- signature of the provider (or signature on file) and assignment of the benefits by the patient to the provider.

The clean claim provisions were originally designed by the health plans to dispute allegations that payers were deliberately delaying the payment of claims in an attempt to hold on to their money for as long as possible. From the payer's standpoint, they could not process claims that were incomplete or contained erroneous information. In reality, these requirements put much greater responsibility on the physician's office to submit claims with all the information necessary for the payer to identify the patient, provider, and service provided. This in turn requires greater accountability for collecting information accurately at each and every visit. Ultimately, the prompt-pay laws led to a greater emphasis on the payer requirements to pay claims according to the terms of the agreement or according to state laws that require the payers to either pay the claim immediately according to the contracted rates or provide a valid reason why the claim was denied.

In most states, a physician's office can apply timely payment principles to its private payers because of the prompt-payment laws designed to protect health care providers by requiring payment of claims within certain reasonable time periods for health care services. To take advantage of the protection afforded by these laws, providers need to be aware of prompt-payment statutes, which can be affected by several factors—the states in which they provide care, the states in which their patients live, and the states in which their payers are located. The prompt-payment statute of the state in which the provider is located may not apply to an out-of-state payer or it could apply only to state-regulated health insurers and not to self-insured employers. By being aware of their rights and obligations under these laws, physicians can use the prompt-payment regulations proactively to avoid payment backlogs without resorting to litigation.

A quick glance at Appendix C identifies many differences between the prompt-payment laws in the 50 states. Because the rights afforded under these statutes vary widely from state to state, the mere existence of a prompt-payment law should not be taken as a guarantee that payment will be made quickly. In order to take full advantage of the laws, providers and their staff must become educated about their rights under their applicable state laws and be proactive in asserting them. For example, Georgia law requires clean claims to be paid within 15 days. If this does not occur, the payer is penalized and the provider is entitled to the additional payment of 18% per annum. If the claim is judged to be unclean and not paid, the payer is required to notify the practice within that same 15 days why the claim was denied. Reviewing the denials and reworking claims is a practice expense that can be avoided if the appropriate claim processes that help ensure that the claim is clean before it leaves the practice are in place on the front end.

Timing is everything, because most prompt-payment statutes mark the payer's obligation to pay a claim from the time the payer receives a clean claim. To ensure that the claims submitted are complete, providers should review the submission protocols established by their payers, review them with their staff, and document their compliance with those requirements. As contracts are renegotiated or terms change (such as when the fee schedule changes), re-educating the staff is the key to continuity of a solid claims submission program. Failure to keep the staff updated results in a higher denial rate, a sluggish cash flow, and greater practice expense. A clear understanding of the payer's internal processes is key to understanding where the claims-processing bottlenecks are and how to overcome them. Have processes in place that will overcome any objection the payer may have to paying the claim quickly and accurately. Know the answers to the following questions in order to respond to denials and rejections:

- Who has to comply with the timely payment laws? (They may only apply to HMOs, preferred provider benefit plans, and indemnity plans issued by insurers. They do not apply to self-funded Employee Retirement Income Security Act [ERISA] plans, workers' compensation claims, Medicare, Medicaid, Medicare supplements, TRICARE, or the Children's Health Insurance Program [CHIP], to name a few.)
- What are the claim filing deadlines? How many days from the date of service? Are days expressed in terms of business days or calendar days? What is the deadline for submitting the secondary claim after receipt of primary payment?
- How are notices about denials and other communications sent? When will they be sent out? Will they be sent electronically or by mail?
- What is this payer's definition of a clean claim and how quickly are clean claims paid?
- What are the coordination of benefits policies and how do they affect the allowable amount?
- How are refunds or recoupments identified and what is the process for resolving the situation—refund check or automatic recoupment?
- What is the deadline for requesting refunds for overpayment (or underpayment) of claims? Can the payer come back to the practice in five years and request a refund for services that were paid incorrectly?
- What are the late-payment penalties, how are they calculated, and how will they be paid?

Understanding these claim-payment basics offers insight into the payer billing processes and provides information needed to appeal improperly paid claims objectively. An appeals expert armed with this information can speak with confidence and authority when challenging a suspected payment impropriety.

Coding Expert's Role in the Appeals Process

A valuable addition to any billing department is a trained coding professional who has claims and appeals experience. This individual can help increase the chances that a clean claim will be submitted, which means it has a greater likelihood of being paid correctly. By understanding the coding and documentation guidelines, the coder can more easily recognize deviations from standard coding logic. Most payers have their own payment "logic" built into their claims editing system. Some of these bundling edits may be based on industry standards, even though they may deviate from coding standards. The coding and bundling edits the payer uses to process claims are usually outlined in the administrative or online manuals with the payer's explanation of why codes may be combined or denied. Because the contract refers to the administrative manual as the resource for understanding coding and bundling edits, it is already agreed that the practice will accept these terms. It is important to regularly review the explanations of benefits (EOBs) to verify that services have been paid according to the terms and rates in the agreement. If the billing office staff does not have the name of an individual (or several individuals) in the claims processing department of every major payer, they are not challenging enough claims.

Billing Systems

An excellent billing system can be worth its weight in gold if it is set up correctly. Setting up a knowledge base to complement the practice and designing systems that will take care of the practice today and also prepare the practice for the future is a massive undertaking that requires a great deal of forethought and planning. The process should not be rushed or taken lightly, because this foundation will ultimately affect the profitability and stability of the practice, possibly for years. A program that does not fulfill the needs of the practice can be costly to correct. The setup standards should be developed as a collaborative effort with input from staff members from multiple areas of the practice so that different perspectives are included in the system design. This also fosters better acceptance of the system. By effectively eliminating the claims that might have been submitted with incomplete or erroneous information and might require rework on the back end, practice expense is decreased and cash flow is positively affected. Examples of the types of rule-building that help to make a practice more profitable include the following:

- Front-end edits can be set up in most practice management systems to ensure that the basic data elements (identified above) are in place and in the right format to be accepted by the payer.
- Rules can be built to make sure that the elements submitted make sense (ie, hospital service CPT codes have been submitted for a hospital place of service; billing an injectable drug also requires billing for the actual administration of the drug; a hysterectomy can only be submitted for a female patient).
- National and local coverage determinations can be uploaded into the system to make sure that services (eg, lab, imaging, diagnostic) meet medical necessity based on diagnosis coding.
- Procedures that require referral or pre-authorization can be held until the appropriate information is received and put into the system.

- If the system is linked to an eligibility program, errors in subscriber or patient identifying information can be corrected before the claim is submitted electronically.
- If fee schedules are set up by a contracted payer, the system can send an alert when the approved payment amount does not match the contracted amount and automatically generate a letter to the payer (and can even cut and paste the exact verbiage from the contract in the appeal letter).
- Appeal letters can be set up to be generated automatically if a claim is paid incorrectly.

The tracking of denials and rejections is another bonus of using an automated billing system. Although each carrier may have its own rejection codes, most codes can be categorized into several major denial categories, which will provide excellent reporting information for the future. By understanding the reasons for denials, effective measures can be taken to educate the providers and staff so that claims are not delayed in the future. Outlining coding and billing errors for your providers offers an opportunity to educate them for the future. Correlating the revenue impact associated with these errors usually makes an even greater impact on the providers.

Tracking the detail of a claims submission program provides an audit trail, which is particularly important with the advent of the electronic claims submission process. Every step in the submission process, from input into the billing system to receipt at the clearinghouse to payment by the payer, can be tracked and reproduced electronically. This is a great tool when assessing where the "ball dropped." The standard claim submission response, "claim not on file," can be challenged with the audit logs from the billing system.

Additionally, tracking denials by payer provides excellent information that can be used to renegotiate contracts. Quantifying the detail of revenue written off because of payer administrative rules or bundling edits is very effective at the negotiating table and offers the practice the leverage of accurate information. Rest assured that payers come armed with this information and know exactly where the practice weaknesses lie. This is the payer's opportunity to capitalize on ignorance or misuse of available information.

The Appeals Process

Understanding the payer rules and knowing how to identify improperly paid claims requires streamlining the claims submission processes and internal auditing practices. Watching collections reports to identify payment delays and gaps is a quick way to recognize potential problems. In states with prompt-payment laws, the accounts receivable report can identify any outstanding claims that then can be investigated to determine why it has not been paid.

Collection reports often highlight other problems. For example, the identification of a particular payer who has a growing accounts receivable balance could indicate that something is wrong with the electronic submission process, signal that a physician has a credentialing problem, or reveal that payments are being sent to the wrong address. Information can be used to reduce the administrative burden of the appeals process, reduce the administrative cost of the process, and enable greater financial return on behalf of the practice.

Failing to appeal and recoup the monies due for services rendered disables a necessary segment of the revenue cycle and enables payers to hold on to funds that are due and payable to contracted providers. Having processes in place that identify these errors quickly and efficiently reduces overhead expenses by reducing administrative staff time spent correcting and refiling claims. It also sends a clear message to payers that payment errors are not acceptable and enables them to correct errors in their claims payment system, which can initiate positive changes to the payment protocol for other practices as well.

Key Components of an Appeals Program

The key components of an effective appeals program include:

- a knowledgeable claims appeal expert;
- access to and understanding all payer resources (eg, contracts, administrative manuals, coding resources such as CPT-4, ICD-9, HCPCS);
- a clear understanding of the state claim-processing payment laws and regulations;
- a clear understanding of the payers' explanations of benefits and the reasons for denial or rejection;
- effective claims appeal letters;
- effective follow-up; and
- education for providers and staff to prevent future errors.

The practice's appeal expert should be knowledgeable in all of these areas and should have the following qualifications:

- be knowledgeable in coding and billing;
- be able to interpret payer contracts and payment processes and develop effective relationships with payer representatives;

- be able to interpret messages on the explanations of benefits and respond quickly to those messages;
- be able to develop and maintain a library of standard appeals letters that can be used for multiple purposes (see Appendix G, Library of Sample Appeals Letters);
- be organized and able to develop a claims and denials follow-up system; and
- be able to translate this information and educate providers and staff about maneuvering through the claims adjudication process using specific examples of denials and payments.

If mistakes are being repeated but there is no education on how to prevent the errors, the process is being perpetuated rather than alleviated. The appeal expert should be allowed time to focus on this activity without interruption. If the system design includes a thorough review of this part of the claims process, the financial return on these efforts should be trackable and measurable.

It is imperative the appeals specialist has access to and an understanding of all resources necessary to correct a claim and resubmit it quickly. By having access to the contract so that the exact language in the contract can be quoted in an appeals letter, your practice can effectively show the payer that the rules are understood and the challenge is validated. Knowledge of how to use coding resources, such as the CPT-4, ICD-9, and HCPCS manuals, is valuable in many parts of the practice. However, the appeals expert must understand the standards, especially if the contract indicates that these resources are the basis for the payer claims editing program.

Understanding resources that are specific to the payer, such as fee schedules, administrative manuals, and claims payment policies, allows the appeal expert to speak intelligently when challenging the denial. It is important to have immediate access to the current negotiated fee schedule so that payment inconsistencies can be identified quickly in the billing system. It is also important to track this information so that patterns with particular payers can be recognized quickly. For example, if Payer A always bundles the office visit with the injection administration code and the logic is outlined (and justified) in its administrative guidelines, then there is no reason for appeal (because this was accepted in the contract). If such a process is not specifically addressed and the denial conflicts with standard coding guidelines, then there may be grounds to question the denial. Recognizing that an E/M code level is reduced, ie, a service is downcoded (paid at a lower level), requires knowledge of the schedules, as well as an understanding of how to interpret documentation to support the charge, which could help to justify reversal of the downcoded charge. It is essential to know the applicable state payment laws and regulations and to know how (and if) they apply to the denial being reviewed. Many claims will not be covered by prompt-payment laws if they are processed by Medicare, Medicaid, workers' compensation, or any self-funded ERISA plans.

Skill, practice, and determination are required to understand the explanation of benefits and the patient's benefits and then interpret what the payer is requesting requires. Although all payers may use the same general categories (eg, charge, approved amount, patient responsibility, payer responsibility), each payer can have its own internal denial codes and code descriptions. These descriptions can be confusing. A standardized set of denial codes could be used across the managed care continuum, which would make reporting on denials of a particular category much easier. Universal code sets are being implemented, slowly but surely. Once the reason for denial is understood, swift action is required to appeal the claim if warranted. It is essential to respond to requests for additional information quickly and to document this in the denial tracking system carefully. This process requires patience and determination. Keeping accurate records of phone calls, e-mails, faxes, letters, and other communication sent to the payer can be useful if claims need to be escalated within the managed care organization.

Be aware that discounts are routinely taken by physician network rentals, sometimes referred to as "silent PPOs," that may not have been identified on the patient's insurance card.[3] Learn to identify these in order to know when to appeal an inappropriate discount. The patient's benefit structure is a valuable tool and can be accessed at the point of eligibility verification. This information should be printed out and kept current and available before services are rendered to the patient. Though it is the patient's responsibility to understand his or her benefits, the practice will bear the brunt of the financial risk if services are that are not payable are delivered. Having a copy of the patient's benefit structure can be very helpful if the patient is unsure if a service is covered. For example, most patients believe they have benefits that cover an annual physical. If this has not been verified or if the patient does not remember when the last physical was performed, this service could be denied if it has not been at least 12 months since the last physical. If not recognized before the patient leaves the office, delivery of services that the insurer will not cover results in higher patient financial responsibility and may lead to increased collections efforts.

Appealing Claims

The first step in appealing a claim should be done verbally. If this does not provide the resolution expected, develop effective appeals letters that include pertinent claim information (eg, name, date of service, CPT code, ICD-9 code, total charge). If possible, direct the letter to a specific person (perhaps the person talked to on the telephone) to expedite the review. Document the justification for denial with supporting, objective data (eg, copy of the documentation, newsletters, and coding resources).

If possible, have the physician or provider review sign the appeal letter. (Sample appeal letter templates are included in Appendix G.)

Maintain effective follow-up of all claim appeal efforts and track those efforts in case an appeal goes to the next level with the payer. Sometimes multiple communications (verbal and written) are required to get the claim paid properly. By following the payer's appeal protocol and timelines you are letting the payer know that the practice understands their process and is taking the proper steps to comply. When doing follow-up, refer to the exact dates, times, and person communicated with in order to substantiate the validity of the appeal; the payer will recognize that this claim cannot be ignored. If attempts to resolve the disputed claim do not achieve the result as expected, be prepared to escalate the appeal through the grievance process outlined in the contract.

Regardless of the outcome (hopefully, it is positive), meet regularly with physicians, providers, and other staff to update them on recognized patterns with particular payers and educate them on ways to eliminate denials in the future. If there are services that will never be paid for, providers need to know that if they continue providing these services, zero revenue from the payer will be the result and the service will be payable by the patient. To be able to bill the patient, the patient should be informed of the situation before the service is provided. If there is a team of appeals experts, have them share information regarding the tools for appealing claims that have been effective.

If all verbal and written attempts to reconcile a claim with the payer fail, the state may have a formal process—one that involves the insurance commissioner—for filing complaints. This is where well-documented attempts to appeal improperly paid claims will help most. It is critical to follow the outlined process and completed all necessary paperwork. Clear documentation of the charges, denials, and specific contact information (including date/time, contact name, further instructions to affect reconsideration) should be submitted. In the absence of an outlined protocol, include a letter that clearly outlines the payer error and attempts to reach a resolution. (See Appendix G, Sample Letter to State Insurance Commissioner or Other Entity that Regulates Various Health Payers Regarding Late Payment.)

In most states, the insurance commissioner's office can be an advocate for the physician's office and carries much more authority than a single physician's office. Additionally, if the office sees repeated patterns and offenses by particular payers, it can contact the state medical society and request that action be taken on behalf of all physician practices. This could include fines, penalties, and lawsuits to institute positive change on behalf of the practices within the state. This also helps to establish precedent for other states that may be seeing similar violations of state laws and contracts.

The insurance commissioner's office may even be available to meet with office staff to discuss effective appeals resources and outline how the office staff can help to recoup appropriate reimbursement for services rendered to managed care patients. Keep in mind that this office typically has no control over self-funded ERISA plans, workers' compensation claims, Medicare, Medicaid, Medicare supplements, TRICARE, or Children's Health Insurance Program (CHIP). However, even though they cannot force these payers to make changes, they usually have a network of contacts with all agencies and can gently suggest that they review and reconsider processing claims. Check with your state insurance commissioner's office to verify how they might be able to help in this effort.

Conclusion

Understanding the terms of negotiated contracts is the first step in optimizing revenue for submitted claims. Even a "perfect" billing process can result in claims that are inappropriately denied, delayed, or reduced by the payer. Neglecting and underestimating the appeals process can create instability in the revenue cycle. By implementing effective processes for reviewing these denials and appealing with appropriate documentation and justification, collections can improve on charges that may have otherwise been written off.

Claims appeals require diligent efforts and constant attention in order to stabilize the claims payment environment in the practice. The ability to identify inappropriate denials and opportunities for appeal requires a clear understanding of contract terms, timelines, and processes. It is necessary to keep a current library of all contracts and knowing the effective dates of changes to the contract is required so that the billing system can be updated to include the most current information. Routine acceptance of denials reported by health insurers and writing off charges based on those denials without question is a clear indicator that the terms of the practice's negotiated contract, including the terms that govern the appeals process, are not understood. Remember that the payer is struggling to make a profit for their shareholders and would like to hold on to the provider's money for as long as possible. Although the process of appealing claims can increase the administrative burden in the short term, ignoring inappropriate denials and allowing continued incorrect payments can create a long-term financial disaster for the practice. Development of an effective appeals process and staying diligent in that effort helps to create a more stable claims payment environment by encouraging review and correction of errors in payers' claims-editing software programs. This, is turn, helps to promote payments that are more accurate, reduces the number of errors, which reduces the administrative burden, and in term reverses the cycle of inefficiency.

Remember that cycle improvement is not limited to the billing staff. It is the responsibility of every person in the practice to support initiatives to reduce costs and increase revenue. An effective process for informing the staff about the contents of managed care contracts, an understanding the payers' internal processes and timelines, and an effective appeals program will lead to increased revenue for the practice.

References

1. Accessed 4/22/2010 at www.ama-assn.org/ama1/pub/upload/mm/31/stakeholders-to-obama.pdf.
2. Accessed 3/1/2010 at www.cms.hhs.gov/ManagedCareMarketing/Downloads/2008-21686_PI.pdf, pages 37–38.
3. Berry, E. Model law banning silent PPOs could serve as draft for state legislatures, *AMNews*, December 29, 2009. Accessed 3/1/2010 at www.ama-assn.org/amednews/2008/12/29/bisa1229.htm.

CHAPTER 8
Benchmarking and Monitoring Reimbursement

OUTLINE

I. Introduction

II. Financial Measures of Tracking Reimbursement and Efficiency
   A. Benchmarks
      1. Benchmarking Sources
      2. Essential Components
   B. Budgeting
      1. Revenue
         a. Gross Revenue
         b. Net Collections
         c. Forecasting Patient Volume
      2. Expenses
         a. Fixed Expenses
         b. Variable Expenses
         c. Period Expenses
      3. Final Steps
         a. Physician Buy-In
         b. Calculating the Percentages
         c. Reality Check

III. Monitoring and Trending
   A. Importance of Constant Review
   B. Monitoring Key Statistics
      1. Aging Report
      2. Collection Percentages
      3. Days in Accounts Receivable
      4. Payer Mix
   C. Dashboard Reports

IV. Conclusion

Introduction

Benchmarking is a highly effective method for improving a practice's collection and reimbursement performance. By setting objectives and developing action programs, it is possible to understand current positions and future trends in order to achieve positive outcomes. Benchmark ratios are inherently measurable and comparable. They provide an objective standard by which to measure performance. The tracking of key measurements at regular intervals points to key factors that affect performance. Further, benchmark results can and should be communicated regularly to an organization's leaders.

Likewise, budgeting is an exercise in setting parameters for practice financial performance and creating stability. A budget is a financial plan that is used to estimate the results of future operations and it is frequently used to help control future operations.

This chapter provides a roadmap for benchmarking and budgeting. It includes practical applications for keeping reimbursement measures on the right track through observation of trends.

Financial Measures of Tracking Reimbursement and Efficiency

Two metrics are used widely for evaluating the effectiveness and efficiency of a practice's collection efforts: (1) the gross collection rate and (2) the net collection rate. Both are easy to calculate and understand.

Gross collection rate measures the percentage of total charges collected. It is calculated by dividing total payments collected by total gross charges (without consideration of contractual allowance and discounts). The payments and gross charges information can be obtained easily from the practice management system. The formula for gross collection rate is as follows:

$$\text{Gross Collection Rate} = \text{Collections/Gross Charges}$$

For example, a practice charges $100 for an office visit. It receives $15 from the patient and $35 from the patient's insurer. In this case, the gross collection rate for this service is 50%.

Gross collection rate is very straightforward to communicate and is used frequently by practices to assess billing performance. However, because it is highly reliant on the practice's fee schedule, in most cases, this ratio varies from practice to practice.

In the same example, if another practice charges $80 for the same service and is paid $50, the result is a 62.5% gross collection rate, 125 basis points higher than for the other practice.

Because gross collection rate is highly reliant on a practice's fee schedule, it will result in meaningless conclusions for practices with fee schedules that are set differently. Although the gross collection ratio is not always applicable to direct benchmarking, it can be a useful ratio to consider because it gives a relative comparison of what was billed with what was actually collected. Gross collection ratio should not be an end-all analysis but rather as a component of analysis. This is especially useful when considered over a time period, ie, measuring from quarter to quarter or from year to year, especially if the practice knows how much its fee schedule has changed and can make adjustments for these changes. If significant changes occur from period to period, then layers can start being peeled back to determine the reason for the changes.

Net collection rate is derived by dividing payments (collections) received by the net charges (also referred to as gross collections). Net charges are charges that are adjusted by contractual allowance and discounts. Different from gross collection rate, this ratio measures collection as a percent of what is available to collect. The formula for net collection rate is as follows:

Net Collection Rate = Collections/Net Charges (Gross Collections)

As in the previous example, the practice charges $100 for the service and the contractual allowance is $50. The practice receives $50 total from the patient and the insurance company; this makes the net collection rate 100%.

Different from the gross collection rate, which can vary from practice to practice, the net collection rate should be close to 100%. The difference? Net collection rate is a better measurement for external benchmarking purposes than gross collection rate because it evaluates the amount of reimbursement the practice receives for every dollar of collectible charges. It is less subjective to fee schedule and payer mix.

The net collection rate is also a good measure of a central billing office's ability to collect. Theoretically, after all contractual adjustments have been made, 100% of that figure should be "collectible." Thus, the net collection rate should be as close to 100% as possible; however, this is not always the case due to such issues as inefficiencies in the billing office and bad debt. An acceptable rate typically runs between 97 and 99%; this will differ based on payer mix, amount of self-pay, and other factors that affect bad debt. Again, another way to evaluate this figure is to compare it to internal numbers over set periods of time to see the fluctuations.

Benchmarks

A benchmark is a statistical comparison that forms economic standards upon which to compare the actual performance results of a practice against some set of standards (usually independent, market-driven standards). They are important standards upon which to measure the practice's performance. When used within reason, benchmarks provide a good comparative analysis. Benchmarking is a way to establish targeted performance and is a good business/management tool to monitor results. Benchmarking allows for objective, measurable performance standards to be compared with actual performance as a way to pinpoint trends and receive early warning signals that may be indications of either strengths or weakness.

A key point to note is that benchmarking is the use of "external" sources to compare "internal" performance. Although it is important to measure performance against internal standards, such as the budget and the previous year's performance, it is also beneficial to use external standards. For benchmarking to be credible, the data must be comparative, which is usually the greatest challenge in terms of benchmarking comparisons within the medical practice. For example, when using benchmarking comparisons for productivity within the medical practice, productivity should be defined comparatively, as in comparing "apples to apples."

Every industry, including health care, uses benchmarks to define economic standards for that industry. Businesses gauge themselves against these benchmarks to determine if they are operating at or near average for their industry.

In medical practice, benchmarks often vary by specialty and by geographic region. For example,

- The average operating cost for a family practice in the Southeast may be 56% of gross revenue while in the Northeast, 58% may be the average or benchmark.
- Average office operating costs for a family practice may be 56%, while operating cost for a surgical specialty may be 48%. This is due to the fact that most of the surgeon's income is generated in the hospital, not in his or her office.

Different ratios can be considered as important measurement tools to use to determine the outcomes and ongoing performance of various practice components. For example,

- Ratios that are related to the performance of accounts receivable correspond to the activities and general productivity of the billing department.
- Ratios that relate to overhead correspond to administration and operations and the proficiency of this area of the practice's management.
- Ratios pertaining to revenue respond to the performance of the providers relative to their individual practices.

It is essential to define benchmarking comparisons and to use them consistently. Some data for benchmarking are less complex to compare. For example, relative value units (RVUs) are a standard measurement. Therefore, when they are defined and consistently applied, they provide a good comparative analysis (eg, work only versus the entire RVU). Other standards for benchmarking comparisons are more viable when data such as number of full-time equivalent employees and costs are used. It also helps to break the data into smaller components such as total support staff cost and even accounts receivable, eg, total accounts receivable dollars over a certain number of days or aging.

Listed below are several key ratios that practices should consider (this is not a complete list). Some of these ratios may be evaluated in greater detail or separated on a departmental basis (ie, the same ratio that is reviewed for the whole practice may be used to determine performance within an individual department or division within the practice):

- collection ratio,
- days of revenue and accounts receivable,
- visits per provider per day,
- collections per provider,
- nonmedical staff members per provider,
- total staffing per provider,
- practice overhead percentage,
- occupancy expenses per provider,
- average revenue per patient,
- average cost per patient,
- no-shows versus scheduled appointments,
- physician cancellation rate,
- collection agency and rate of charges,
- payer mix ratios,
- marketing costs per new patient, and
- departmental expense ratios.

Benchmarks must be applied appropriately. If they are not, the outcomes could be adverse. For example, a practice may think it is in line with benchmarks, when it is far outside the boundaries and vice versa.

The following questions illustrate the problems that result when using benchmarking comparisons:

- Does the external source define productivity as gross charges, net charges, gross or net collections, or a combination of some of these things?
- If using gross charges, what about the variances in fee schedules that occur from one practice to another?
- If using net charges, what about the variance in contractual allowances?

- What is incorporated within revenue?
- Does revenue include ancillary services that may or may not be a direct part of the practice's professional fees?

The same problems arise when comparing expenses:

- Are the expenses inclusive of any physician benefits or salaries?
- What about employed physicians? Is their expense included in overhead?

Benchmarking Sources

Several organizations publish regional and national benchmarks for the medical practice, including the Medical Group Management Association (MGMA), American Medical Group Association (AMGA), and Sullivan Cotter and Associates (SCA). In addition, there are numerous resources, including benchmarks that are available from professional organizations. A benchmarking source is likely to be available for most specialties and organization types, depending on what information is needed.

Essential Components

Regardless of the type of benchmark used, it must have two components: (1) clean data and (2) a significant number of results from which the data were drawn. The clean data aspect is simple and follows the garbage in/garbage out system; that is, if the data used to determine the benchmarks are faulty, then the benchmarks themselves will be useless. To ensure clean data, use a reputable source that has experience in benchmarking. Gathering and disseminating data for benchmark purposes is not easy, especially in the medical field where data can be suspect. However, if the benchmarking agency has good processes and policies to scrub data and validate that it is accurate, then this should not be a problem.

A critical step in the process is to ensure there are enough responses in the benchmarking data to provide a reasonable representation of the market. If only a few results are used to generate the benchmarks, then the information may be suspect. If there are 10,000 results for family practitioners in the Northeast and only 10 in the Southeast, then the "national" benchmarks may not be reflective of the Southeast.

When some things appear to be outside of the norm, people will question the validity of the data, even if the benchmarking was performed by a well-known benchmarking agency. Even if you are using the most accepted benchmarking tool, keep in mind that every organization is different and outliers exist, some good and some bad. Benchmarks should be used but they also should be used with caution.

Internal benchmarks are helpful for established organizations that can source good historical data in order to measure their practice. It is possible to choose a self-imposed benchmark. For example, a practice may commit to holding its overhead below 35%. This goal does not have to come from a standard benchmark; management may say that in order to return X, the practice must generate or do Y. Those become the practice's benchmarks.

Budgeting

A budget is the foundation for all financial activities of the medical practice. Budgeting includes the coordination, control, and reporting of variances between budgeted results and actual results. The budget provides and coordinates the controls needed to manage the practice effectively. It relates to all policies and procedures needed to accomplish a practice's objectives.

A budget is generally prepared for a short period of time (compared to long-range and strategic plans) and is expressed using basic financial terminology. It should be simple enough for the nonaccounting professional to understand and use. Simply stated, a budget measures actual financial performance against standards. A parallel example is to set a personal or professional goal and direct all activities to reach it.

From a practical standpoint, a budget can be used to gain an understanding of the productivity and expense levels that are required to keep the practice financially healthy. By comparing the actual results with the budget throughout the year, the practice administrator is made aware of trends that facilitate better control of future costs. Preparing and monitoring a budget throughout the year (ie, actual performance versus budgeting standards) provides early warning signs of negative trends within the practice.

Budgeting is as much a cognitive process as an accounting process. The physician(s) and staff must seriously reflect upon changes in the health care industry and how those changes relate to the practice. Plans for expansion, operational changes concerning services and payer mix, and the physicians' future goals and plans must be considered in the process.

To summarize, a budget accomplishes the following:

- provides an accurate, timely tool to review anticipated versus actual results;
- helps control current performance;
- helps predict future performance and anticipated problem areas;
- determines where resources should be allocated;
- provides an early warning device of budget variations;
- highlights early signs of future opportunities;
- provides the physician(s), office personnel, and practice administrator a practice management tool; and
- provides a concise financial summary in an understandable format.

The budgeting process begins with gathering the information that will be used when formulating the initial budget. The information needed includes:

- year-end financial statements for the prior three fiscal periods, preferably broken down by month or, at the very least, by quarter (depending on the legal structure of the practice, tax returns may also be beneficial);
- all legal documents supporting contractual agreements, including real estate leases, equipment leases, contracts for cleaning maintenance, landscaping, and similar documents;
- a list of major equipment purchases anticipated for the coming year, including the estimated cost and suggested method of payment for each (consider all possible acquisitions regardless of the cost impact on the practice [ie, a "wish list" of items]); and
- fee schedules.

Once this information has been collected, plan on an extended session, or sessions, for incorporating the necessary analysis and discussion processes. Budgeting consists of many steps. The following information will help participants complete the process systematically by using various inputs to develop the fundamentals of the budget.

Revenue

Two components drive revenue in the medical practice: (1) patient volume and (2) revenue per unit (or patient). Relative to budgeting, revenue is viewed as gross revenue and as net collections. These drivers are considered in the scope of the following budgeting process.

Gross Revenue. Gross revenue generally refers to all production placed "on the books" by the physician for services rendered. This includes office visits, consultations, hospital visits and procedures, ancillary procedures, nursing home work, and outpatient procedures. Gross revenue can be the starting point for budgeting revenue in the process of making changes to the fee schedule, potential contractual changes by payers, and other changes that will affect revenue.

Another step in forecasting revenue is to determine if the practice is planning to make an increase in the fee schedule and how much that increase will be. At a minimum, a practice should adjust its fees at the beginning of each year. This can be accomplished using one of two simple methods:

- Apply a percent of increase to every fee based upon inflation, an inflation index, or a cost-of-living change or specific factors in the individual practice that ultimately dictate an adjustment.

Also, reflect any adjustments to Medicare's fee schedule in this analysis.

- Review each fee and increase those fees that have increased in cost to deliver. Knowing costs is a significant component of successfully negotiating and securing a managed care contract. A fee schedule can be based upon such contracting. Although fee schedules may vary by payer type (eg, indemnity insurance, Medicare, health maintenance organization [HMO], or preferred provider organization [PPO] managed care), it is best to have a consistent fee schedule that does not change to accommodate different types of payers. However, practice management software allows the user to input different fee schedules for each managed care plan. The software enters the proper fee initially, eliminating the need for adjustments.

Competition is another factor to consider when making a change in the fee schedule. It is helpful to know what the competition is charging for comparable services. Remember, it may be acceptable to "shop" competitive prices (on a limited basis, informally), but it is illegal for practices to agree to uniform pricing schedules.

Although it may be difficult to anticipate the effect of a fee schedule change in the budget planning process, a safe approach is to apply a 2 to 3% cost-of-living adjustment for inflation. Budgeting is primarily for internal use and requires a realistic approach. If a fee schedule is certain to increase by more than a simple cost-of-living adjustment, reflect that in the budget. However, if it is not a certainty, particularly when completing the budget planning worksheet, then a simple increase may be justified. On the other hand, if managed care contracting will result in lowering the fee schedule, then this should be realistically reflected in the projections.

Net Collections. Because most practices use the "cash basis" of accounting, the number representing net collections is the "actual revenue" referred to for the budget planning process. It represents the actual receipts of the practice, net of all contractual agreements, and is a result of the actual collections of accounts receivable from all sources of professional services performed by the physician. The net collections total, therefore, is the most critical item on the revenue side of the budget planning process upon which decisions are to be based.

If the practice has projected an increase in its fee schedule or other gross charge-related items, then it will probably not realize a 1:1 growth ratio for net collections. It is likely that the gross collection rate will fall. However, one's objective should be to achieve a net increase in net collections even when the gross collection rate goes down. Making this estimation will likely be the most difficult aspect of revenue projection for the budgeting process.

Forecasting Patient Volume. Once the average revenue per patient per unit is determined, patient volume must be projected. To establish a basis to forecast patient volume, answer the following questions:

- What patient volume trends have developed over the past three years? Is the average percent of change in patient volume for the past two years expected to continue?
- Will there be any significant changes in managed care contracting that will result in an increase, decrease, or discontinuation of contracts that result in less volume?
- Will the practice add a mid-level provider?

Many factors affect the number of patients seen. The practice cannot assume that patient volume will increase every year. Remember that the example used actually assumed no increase before considering other new factors (ie, the new managed care contract and the new practice). The more aware the practice is of what is going on in its market area and the industry in general, the more accurately it can forecast changes.

The real benefit of a well-planned practice budget comes from careful consideration of changes and the ability to accurately reflect or forecast these upon the practice operations.

As noted, determining patient volume is the first step in forecasting revenue. This example considered both internal and external changes anticipated within the practice to develop a logical projection of patient visits for the coming year.

Expenses

Budgeting considers the following types of expenses:

- fixed expenses,
- variable expenses, and
- period expenses.

Fixed Expenses. Fixed expenses are those expenses not affected by patient volume. Examples are rent, salaries (excluding commissions), interest payments on fixed debt, insurance, property taxes, and utilities. Fixed costs are relatively easy to project because they are fixed in nature and generally do not change without some forewarning (eg, rent payments should not change unless stipulated in the rent agreement).

Variable Expenses. Variable expenses are those expenses that change in direct proportion to some number such as the number of patients seen or the number of procedures performed. Examples are medical supplies, office supplies, laboratory costs, medications, and interest on an operating working capital line of credit. In order to forecast variable expenses, one must first find out what the "driver" is; that is, what makes the expenses move. Is it the number of patients seen, number of vaccines given, number of scans performed? This knowledge will also allow the practice administrator to project costs. Because most costs are driven by patient volume, which has already been projected when forecasting revenue (see above), it is possible to address two issues at one time.

Period Expenses. Period expenses are costs incurred over time, as opposed to level of activity. As an example, salaries are quoted as an annual amount but paid over a period of time during the year.

Final Steps

The budgeting process calls for cooperation and support from the physicians before it can become a viable tool for practice management, as described in the following paragraphs.

Physician Buy-In. Calculations and input completed for the budget forms a good start toward the final budget figure. Before proceeding, consider all other factors within the practice that will influence the final budget total. These factors include a realistic overview of what is going on within the practice and the knowledge of an external or internal factor that will significantly change the initial budgeted total to the final budgeted total entry. The key decision makers should review each line entry to formulate the final budget. Remember, regardless of how thoroughly a budget has been analyzed, it requires buy-in by the physician(s) and/or other owners of the practice to be taken seriously and to be used as the management tool it is intended to be.

Calculating the Percentages. Once a realistic budget figure for each projected expense and the operating revenues have been determined, the final step is to calculate the percent of each expense to total revenue projected. It is important to interpret all budgeted data, especially expense entries, on a line-by-line basis. Also, it is essential to convert expenses as a percent of total net collections. For example, a practice that operates at a 50% or less expense factor (ie, 50% of net collections for total expenses, excluding physician compensation) is generally viewed as having a fairly efficient structure. Conversely, a budget that results in an expense total in excess of 50% requires further research to ascertain if this is acceptable. Historically, if a practice has operated on an expense factor of 55 to 60% of net collections, the physician(s) and/or other owners of the practice may find this acceptable. If the owners do not object, the final budget may reflect a higher-than-standard (industry) expense total.

Expense-to-earnings percentages vary with geographical locations, the specialty, and the type of practice, such as solo versus group. The benchmark figures for a specialty are available from several sources (eg, AMGA, MGMA, and local consulting firms). In addition, *Medical Economics Magazine* publishes these expense averages each year in a November issue. Thus, the final step of calculating the percentages of each expense item to total net collections is a process that brings the budgeted figures into perspective.

Reality Check. Completion of a budget planning worksheet is an internal assessment, or reality check, for the practice. After the budget is set and complete with final entries, the practice administrator and physician(s) should look at the totals as a whole. As previously noted, determining the percentages of expense items to net collections is an ongoing process of budget development and should not be delayed until the budget is complete. On the other hand, after the numbers have been entered and the calculations made with the totals set for the budget, it is logical to take a broad view of the outcome in relation to the reality of running the practice.

During the reality check, ask the following questions for each entry:

- Is this entry realistic?
- Can the practice afford the increases or decreases?
- Will the increases maintain the practice at a competitive level and result in efficient operation compared to prior years?
- What does management (usually the physicia[s]) really want?

Another part of the reality check is to determine if the expenses are reasonable in light of where the practice is going and what has traditionally been acceptable performance. Physicians are sometimes more concerned with maintaining a certain level of quality or prestige in their practice than with the costs to maintain these items. For example, certain practice commodities, such as providing a coffee service or bottled water, are not necessary. Logically, a practice that is under pressure to cut expenses would cut nonessentials first. Before cutting or eliminating these expenses, however, the physician(s) must be consulted and agree to the change.

Monitoring and Trending

Benchmarking and budgeting are worthwhile activities only if they are used and continually monitored. The exercises of benchmarking and budgeting and then leaving the information on the shelf until next year are useless. It is as helpful as not going through the exercise at all.

Importance of Constant Review

Continually comparing actual performance to projected performance, benchmarks, and budgets is the best method of detecting early warning signs that something may be wrong. Consider this: if the net collection rate is consistently monitored against the budget and the rate is declining a bit each month, collections will be directly impacted. The reasons may be due to changes in coding patterns for one of the physicians, increased claim denials by one or more payers, or claims not being submitted in a timely manner. There are infinite scenarios where trending and budgeting will help identify potentially big problems.

Monitoring Key Statistics

Dashboard reports that are monitored on a daily or weekly basis offer a quick view of trends that may identify problems. Dashboards provide key diagnostic indicators of how things are going within a very short time frame. The key is to choose three or four statistics that are most applicable to the practice; avoid the tendency to over analyze by trying to capture every statistic, as this defeats the purpose. The goal is to watch the dashboards on a regular basis and, in the event they move outside of a predetermined range, delve in and gather more information or do additional analysis and determine why they have changed.

Benchmarking the practice's revenue is extremely important in order to monitor trends in payment and reimbursement. Who in the practice needs to know about payment and reimbursement performance? The chief executive officer, chief financial officer, chief operating officer, practice administrator, patient accounts manager, physicians, and physician board need to know how the practice compares to itself and to similar practices. Knowing the numbers helps to take the pulse of the health of the revenue cycle. Numbers, such as collection percentages, total accounts receivable (A/R), and days in A/R, should be trended and watched. Any significant change indicates a potential problem.

Aging Report

The aging report indicates the amount of practice revenue that has been billed and the length of time without payment. Common categories, often referred to as buckets, are the current column or the 0–30 days column, 31–60 days, 61–90 days, 91–120 days, and 120+ days, which can be broken down to 121–150 days. Ideally, the largest figures are in the current or 0–30 days column, with decreases as the buckets age out. Aging dollars are noncollectible dollars. Once an account reaches approximately 180 days, or six months, it is worth about 56 or 57 cents of what it was worth when the services were rendered. If an account ages beyond a year, the value may be as low as 25 to 30 cents on the dollar.

Collection Percentages

As discussed earlier in the budgeting section, collections are measured in two ways: (1) gross collection percentage and (2) net collection percentage. Gross collections are a simple calculation of the gross dollars received divided by total dollars received, which equals the gross collection percentage. In most practices, the number is approximately 35 to 45%, depending on the fee schedule. The net collection percentage is the revenue received divided by the total charges less contractual and other adjustments. This number usually falls into the 90% category if the collection function is running superbly. Using national benchmarks, a practice should measure itself against other practices in the same geographic area as well as across the country. In addition, a practice can use its own performance to monitor trends against past performance. Any significant change in these percentages should be easily explained, such as additional effort to collect past-due balances or reduction in aging through bad-debt write offs.

Days in Accounts Receivable

Accounts receivable (A/R) and the phrase *days in A/R* are frequent points of discussion in practice management. This is a calculation of the average revenue charges for the last 30 days divided into the total A/R, equaling the number of days of outstanding billings. The lower this number is the better, with an excellent number being around 30 days in A/R.

Payer Mix

Payer mix refers to the percentage of the A/R that is billed to each payer. For example, the practice submits claims to Medicare, Medicaid, Blue Cross Blue Shield, various managed care payers, commercial payers, workers' compensation carriers, and liability insurers. The total charges billed to each payer divided by the total charges equals a percentage that, when added together, equals 100 and represents the practice's payer mix. The payer mix is another factor to monitor. Any significant shift from one payer to another, depending on the payer's contracted reimbursement rates, could result in a significant change in practice revenue.

Dashboard Reports

Practice benchmarking and monitoring are ongoing processes, and the numbers that result from these processes should be reviewed on a monthly basis, after the month's accounting is closed. The practice should establish a financial dashboard or an A/R dashboard report. This brief, one-page report presents all of the financial data in a format that is easy to review and analyze. The data can be benchmarked against national benchmarks or compared to one's own practice. By making comparisons to one's own practice allows, trends can be monitored and identified and analyses of the causes shown. A financial dashboard should; at a minimum, reflect charges for the month; charges for the year to date; current year versus the same period a year prior; the same revenue categories for the current year and the prior year, and adjustment for those years. In addition, the dashboard should show the total accounts receivable, preferably in their individual categories or buckets, and the amount that is related to insurance as well as the amount related to each patient's responsibility. The dashboard can also include number of patient visits; a breakdown between office visits and procedures; and the RVUs generated for office visits and procedures. Depending on the practice's structure and the desire to monitor physician productivity, these numbers can also show a physician's productivity when compared to his or her peers and also to him/herself for the same period of time a year prior.

In some cases, dashboard reports are color coded for easy evaluation at a glance. Colors often used include "green" when the actual results are better or within benchmarks; "yellow" when actual figures have become progressively worse against benchmarks, or are at the point where they need attention; and finally, "red" when actual results have fallen to critical levels compared to benchmarks.

Tables 8-1 through 8-4 show example dashboard reports that can be beneficial for monitoring trends. The reports are for gross collections, work RVUs (wRVUs), days in A/R, and budget, respectively.

TABLE 8-1 Gross Collection Dashboard Report

Period: June, 20XX

Provider	Current Month %	Year-to-Date %	Benchmark %
Smith	45.25	46.10	45.30
Jones	47.62	47.50	45.30
Wilson	46.22	46.55	45.30
Young	35.15	45.33	45.30

Legend
Light Gray: Within or better than benchmarks
Dark Gray: Trending below benchmarks
Black: Fallen to critical levels.

TABLE 8-2 wRVU Dashboard Report

Period: June, 20XX

Provider	Current Month	Current Benchmark	Year-to-Date	Year-to-Date Benchmark
Smith	687.67	710.58	4,255.20	4,263.50
Jones	759.25	710.58	4,703.58	4,263.50
Wilson	728.08	710.58	4,300.29	4,263.50
Young	654.50	710.58	4,441.19	4,263.50

Legend

Light Gray: Within or better than benchmarks
Dark Gray: Trending below benchmarks
Black: Fallen to critical levels.

TABLE 8-3 Days A/R Dashboard Report

Period: June, 20XX

Provider	Year-to-Date	Benchmark
Smith	42.00	42.50
Jones	40.25	42.50
Wilson	41.10	42.50
Young	43.00	42.50

Legend

Light Gray: Within or better than benchmarks
Dark Gray: Trending below benchmarks
Black: Fallen to critical levels.

TABLE 8-4 Budget Dashboard Report

Period: June, 20XX

	Period		Budget		Variance			
	Current $	YTD $	Current $	YTD $	Current $	Current %	YTD $	YTD %
Revenue	2,158,982	13,458,798	2,200,000	13,300,000	(41,018)	−1.86%	158,798.00	1.19
Personnel	1,089,256	8,523,457	1,150,000	8,620,000	(60,744)	−5.28%	(96,543.00)	−1.12
Supplies	75,892	890,256	82,000	910,000	(6,108)	−7.45%	(19,744.00)	−2.17
Net Income	252,777	1,255,585	205,000	1,245,000	47,777	23.31%	10,585.00	0.85%
Net Income % of Revenue	11.71	9.33	9.32	9.36		2.39		−0.03

Legend
Light Gray: Within or better than benchmarks
Dark Gray: Trending below benchmarks
Black: Fallen to critical levels.

Conclusion

Benchmarks can be used to gauge and measure the practice's standing. However, one must determine what is right for the specific practice and the standards that will apply. The same is true for the budgeting process, which is nothing more than developing the practice's own internal benchmark to follow over time. Regardless of what is used as a guide, just like a good map, it can only help if it is used on a regular basis. It is important to follow the established plan and determine that the practice is still on the path.

Benchmarking and budgeting are worthwhile activities only if they are used and continually monitored. The exercise of benchmarking and budgeting and then leaving the information on the shelf until next year is useless. It is as helpful as not going through the exercise at all.

CHAPTER 9
Billing and Reimbursement for Ancillary Services

OUTLINE

I. Introduction
II. What Are Ancillary Services?
III. When to Provide Services and Who Provides Services
IV. Be Aware (or Beware) of Stark
V. Negotiate Separately Within the Managed Care Contracts for Services Normally Provided by Physician
VI. Monitor Usage, Cost to Deliver, and Revenue Generated
VII. Conclusion

Introduction

As physician groups and hospitals continue to evaluate their financial viability, a common theme continues to emerge—the practice is doing more work for less revenue. This underlying factor compels organizations to think of creative ways to increase the bottom line. One approach is to initiate new services that are beyond the scope of seeing patients for office visits. When well planned and aptly administered, ancillary services allow physicians to enhance their net incomes significantly. This chapter provides a current perspective on ancillary services and addresses measures necessary to ensure that reimbursement is received for the work. Topics covered in other chapters, such as managed care contracting and compliance with Stark regulations, are presented here as they relate to ancillary services.

What Are Ancillary Services?

Ancillary services are those services offered by a hospital or physician practice other than room, board, and professional services. Ancillary services can assist the physician in his or her ultimate goal of providing quality medical care, often in the practice setting, while producing additional revenue. Some examples of ancillary services include:

- X ray, computerized tomography, and ultrasound services;
- laboratory services;
- physical therapy;
- diagnostic testing;
- diabetes and weight management programs;
- wellness center;
- retail products (eg, eye glasses, hearing aids);
- free-standing ambulatory surgery center (ASC);
- dialysis center;
- infusion therapy center;
- catheterization laboratory;
- sleep center;
- anti-aging center;
- skin care center and skin care products;
- anti-addiction center; and
- urgent treatment center.

Within the walls of the practice, a group can offer any product or service that fits its specialty area and is provided to its patient base. Normal regulatory compliance is required depending on the rules and guidelines of each state. This includes a possible certificate of need, business licenses, and accreditation standards. It is advantageous for the patient to receive these types of ancillary services within the practice, because of the convenience of having the service performed at one location and at one time. It is likely that the cost for the service will be less or no more costly than having the service provided in a different setting. The quality of care is as good and often better and correlates with better continuity of care based on the service location. Because quality of care remains a priority for most physicians, economic ramifications are still secondary to quality of care and continue to be a major part of the decision-making process for ancillary services. Most physicians will not consider an ancillary service unless it maintains or improves quality of care.

When to Provide Services and Who Provides Services

Physicians and hospitals consider ancillary services as part of their organizations for several reasons. Due to a long-standing trend of declining reimbursement, physicians' core revenue source of seeing patients in an office setting is often not enough to generate the revenue needed to keep the practice profitable. The ability to diversify services increases revenue, especially if someone other than the physician can perform these services. Stark regulations have also broadened the ability to offer ancillary services. Of course, there are important things to know before you start offering these services. (Stark regulations are discussed later in this chapter and also in Chapter 10 regarding compliance.)

Another reason ancillary services are becoming more popular is the increased sense of control over all aspects of patient care. These types of services often improve the delivery of care in terms of both efficiency and quality.

Practices that are thinking of providing ancillary services should ask the following questions as part of the decision-making process:

- Will the ancillary service be reimbursed by third-party payers?
- Will it need to be a cash-only service?
- What are the revenue possibilities?
- What does the return on investment look like? When will a profit be realized?
- Does the service add to the quality of care for the patient?
- Does addition of this service increase patient compliance?
- Can the service be supervised easily by the physician on an ongoing basis?

Ensure the ancillary service chosen is feasible for the practice and confirm that the service will complement the existing practice. Track the referrals and tests referred to other providers to determine if they can be performed in house.

Once the decision has been made to expand the practice and offer ancillary services, several steps must be completed. First, and foremost, perform the necessary due diligence. This covers management of the ancillary service and regulatory, compliance, and legal matters. Start with a well-thought-out business plan and create a budget for the service(s) you want to offer. Review the referral patterns, develop a marketing plan, and look within the practice's patient base. Determine if the service will only enhance the practice with its current patient base or actually bring new business into the practice. Review the service need in the practice area and have a good understanding of the targeted population area and identify other practices that are offering the same services. Determine the feasibility of offering the same services as others within the targeted service area.

Next, bring together an experienced team to help with implementation. This may include outside consultants and vendors to structure and develop the business. Hire competent legal counsel who are well versed in health care law and regulatory compliance. Develop an implementation timeline that clearly outlines the responsibility of each team member and dates for completion of tasks.

Ancillary services are offered by physician offices, hospitals, private investors, and private companies. Each entity faces different challenges when looking at implementing ancillary services. Hospitals have faced this challenge for years because they have been forced to look at new ways to deliver care. Traditional thinking has changed as hospitals continue to look at ways of delivering quality care while reducing costs. Historically, hospitals have been slow in making major changes to the delivery of care due to the enormous capital outlay for equipment and personnel. However, the sense of urgency to improve bottom-line performance has required hospitals to forge ahead in developing new programs for ancillary services.

Physicians have been at the forefront of implementing ancillary services within their practices. Technology and equipment advancements have made it possible for physicians to expand their services. The skill of performing these services is part of the physicians' training and is seen as part of the continuity of care for their patients. However, one driving force is economics, and many physicians rely on the additional income brought in by ancillary services to augment their bottom-line profits.

Private companies and independent investors have also been a major player in the ancillary services arena. Many companies build and manage the ancillary center or service and partner with hospitals and physicians or contract for services. One major concern with involving private companies in ancillary services is quality of care. However, in most cases, these companies deliver the highest quality of care that is often better than that performed solely by physicians. These companies bring expertise and a solid plan for the business to succeed. Although the motivation is bottom-line profits, reimbursement is based on the care delivered; therefore, quality is their first priority.

Billing for ancillary services can vary by payer, especially for commercial and managed care payers. In most cases, the physician and/or group practice bills for the service or for supervising the service under its own billing number or company, which is wholly owned by the group. A third-party billing company can also bill the service. In all cases, determining how to bill and the requirements for getting these services authorized should be researched before the services are implemented. In many cases, not only the reimbursement for the service but also the process for billing can be negotiated directly with the payer. In addition, certain ancillary services may require a separate contract and fee schedule and may be subject to a credentialing process by the health plan. Services such as computed tomography (CT) and sleep studies may also be subject to specified preauthorization requirements. The one exception is government payers, which have set rules regarding billing and reimbursement for ancillary services. Knowing the practice's payer mix is imperative when considering implementing these types of services.

Be Aware (or Beware) of Stark

Stark regulations provide specific guidelines on how to provide ancillary services. Section 1128B(b) of the Social Security Act (42U.S.C.1320a 7b(b)) provides criminal penalties for individuals or entities that knowingly or willfully offer, pay, solicit, or receive remuneration in order to induce business that is reimbursable under federal or state health care programs. This regulation now prevents physician groups from compensating an individual physician based on the amount of revenue he or she generates from ancillary services. However, revenue from ancillary services can be distributed equally to each physician in the group regardless of how much revenue he or she individually generated from the service.

Stark rules have evolved over the past several years. Named after the author of the original statute, California Representative Pete Stark, Phase III changes are currently in effect. This is the final phase of the Stark rules and seeks to further clarify the Stark II statute. Basically, the Stark rules apply if a physician refers Medicare beneficiaries and Medicaid recipients to an entity for the following ancillary services:

- clinical laboratory service;
- inpatient and outpatient hospital services;
- outpatient prescription drugs payable under Medicare Part B;
- physical therapy, occupational therapy, speech and language services;
- home health services;
- prosthetics, orthotics, prosthetic devices;
- radiation therapy;
- durable medical equipment; and
- nutritional supplies.

Ask the following questions when determining if your practice needs to beware of Stark regulations: Is there a direct or indirect financial relationship between the physician referring the ancillary service and the entity providing the service? Is there a referral from the physician to the entity providing the ancillary service? If the answer is yes to either question, then the Stark regulations apply unless there is an exception to the specific situation.

A financial relationship is defined as a direct or indirect ownership or a compensation arrangement for an entity that provides these types of ancillary services. However, a physician can have a financial arrangement with an entity that provides ancillary services if the financial arrangement is unrelated to the ancillary service. An example would be a physician who holds equity or a membership interest in a limited liability company that owns and operates an ambulatory surgery center.

A compensation arrangement is basically any arrangement that involves remuneration of any kind between a physician and an entity providing the service. This includes payments or other benefits given directly or indirectly to the physician. A compensation arrangement can include:

- cash,
- space,
- equipment leases,
- physician professional services,
- medical director services, and
- management services.

The Stark regulations are written in very broad terms in regard to limitations on financial and referral relationships that can exist. However, there are exceptions if they comply with the current regulations; these exceptions should be researched before implementing ancillary services. The Stark regulations have established exceptions for both ownership interests and financial/compensation arrangements. Yet, in order to meet the exception criteria, documented compliance with the regulation generally needs to exist and financial arrangements must be at fair market value.

There will always be a financial consideration and ownership aspect in a physician's office that offers ancillary services. Within a group practice, there are exceptions for referral and financial compensation when the ancillary services are provided personally or under the supervision of another physician within the group. The Stark regulations for a group practice are complex when it comes to compensation and referral arrangements.

Also, Stark exceptions apply to certain employment agreements. These exceptions are for compensation and are met when employment is for an identifiable service; the amount of compensation is based on current fair market value and is not determined based on referrals or volume of referrals for the service. Also, compensation is in accordance with an agreement that would be considered "reasonable" even if no referrals were made to the employer.

Physician practices and ancillary service entities are required to understand Stark regulations and adapt quickly to law changes, otherwise serious consequences could result. These types of Stark violations can carry penalties of up to $15,000 per violation plus reimbursement of refunds back to the Centers for Medicaid and Medicare Services (CMS).

Negotiate Separately Within the Managed Care Contracts for Services Normally Provided by Physician

Physicians and other ancillary providers have seen many changes in reimbursement and referral guidelines for the delivery of ancillary services. Because of the shift from high-cost inpatient service to lower-cost outpatient service, physicians and ancillary entities have increased opportunities to provide these services. However, discounting services and aggressive cuts in reimbursement make it necessary to look at these services separately as "carve outs" when negotiating managed care contracts.

Many physician offices negotiate reasonable managed care contracts, and savvy administrators (and even some physicians) ensure that all the basic elements are covered. However, even the most savvy practice can sign an agreement that should have been reviewed more judiciously or that has provisions that become a problem later. This includes not ensuring that reimbursements for ancillary services are provided for in a cost-effective and profitable way.

It is wise to get good contracting advice or to outsource this process. Managed care agreements tend to be long and complicated. Often the language and terms are unfamiliar to most physicians and office administrators. Remember, managed care agreements are written by managed care plans and offer terms that are not always in the physician's or practice's best interest. (Chapter 2 addresses managed care contracts comprehensively.) It is not unusual for managed care plans to show willingness to discuss and negotiate specific reimbursement for only certain areas of the practice or specific procedures. This is referred to as carving out selected portions of the negotiated agreement. The principles outlined in Chapter 2 also apply to negotiations for carve-outs for ancillary services.

Physicians should not be afraid to pass on a bad contract or one that does not allow the ancillary business a cost-effective way to be managed or to be profitable. It is wise to gain insight into how other physicians deal with managed care plans. Physicians who already have contracts in place can be a great source of information. The managed care plan's provider directory lists the names and phone numbers of other physicians who are currently working with the plan. Call a few, particularly those within the same practice specialty. Ask about the administrative burden of managing the plan. This is often an area that is overlooked and can cause a huge hardship after the agreement has been signed.

In further exploring negotiating agreements indicated in Chapter 2, carve-outs should be addressed specifically. Because of the potential pitfalls in negotiating or, more important, not negotiating with managed care plans, the best way to ensure successful patient management is to develop a solid strategy. Look at the market realistically and plan accordingly. What (if any) leverage is there? Are other physicians offering the service or are many physicians offering the service? If the latter, carve-out services may not be realistic. Specific to carve-outs, the contract should include explicit information regarding patient's eligibility for all services and how referrals for service work. Overutilization of a service based on inappropriate referrals can make carve-outs for specific services difficult. Develop a plan on how this process will be managed and inform the managed care company. Use this in your negotiations with the payer and set a positive tone for the relationship.

Monitor Usage, Cost to Deliver, and Revenue Generated

Once an ancillary service(s) is implemented, it must be managed and monitored in terms of its clinical and business operations. This often starts with appropriate usage and productivity training for both clinical and nonclinical staff. It is also necessary to monitor coding and claims collection. Although some of these items need to be managed and monitored on a monthly basis, others such as training and compliance with regulatory bodies can be monitored quarterly or semi-annually depending on the type of service offered.

It is important to run monthly financial reports and compare them to the original numbers in the business plan to ensure that the practice is staying on track with initial projections. Look at the performance and then benchmark against others in the industry. Do not forget to plan strategically throughout the process and each year. Is there room to expand services? Should the management of the service be outsourced? Is the practice getting the expected results? These questions should be part of a yearly examination of all services the practice is providing. Again, continually look for changes in Stark regulations and applicable CMS laws and rules ensure compliance. Look at equipment needs and future outlay of capital and evaluate staff and how they are contributing (or not) to the success of the venture.

Other areas to assess on a regular basis include:

- coding,
- variance between revenue goals and actual revenue,
- expenses and costs per procedure,

- ongoing training needs,
- return on investment, and
- ability to provide adequate access to the service.

Additional Resources on Billing and Reimbursement for Ancillary Services

Many factors affect the potential for reimbursement of ancillary services. Among those are the current legislation as well as managed care contracts that cover the reimbursement fees and arrangements. Managed care contracting is complex and multifaceted, as noted in this chapter and in Chapter 2. The following resources provide helpful information for understanding the concepts of billing and reimbursement for ancillary services:

1. Zingarelli, T. Creating outpatient clinics for ancillary services, *Physician's News Digest*, January 2000. Accessed 12/18/2009 at www.physiciansnews.com/business/100.html.
2. Walpert, B. Negotiating a doctor friendly contract, *ACPInternist*, June 1999. Accessed 12/18/2009 at www.acpinternist.org/archives/1999/06/docfriend.htm.
3. Hursh, D. Negotiating a managed care contract, *Physician's News Digest*, February 2004. Accessed 12/18/2009 at www.physiciansnews.com/law/204.html.
4. Tinsley, R. Tips for negotiating managed care contracts, *Physician's News Digest*, March 5, 2009. Accessed 12/18/2009 at www.physiciansnews.com/2009/03/05/tips-for-negotiating-managed-care-contracts.

Conclusion

Ancillary services can be offered to increase a practice's bottom-line revenue through its existing business. This is one reason why these services are so attractive to physicians. Most ancillary services can be accommodated within the current practice structure, and most specialty practices can offer some type of ancillary service while maintaining or even improving their patients' quality of care. In many cases, access to these types of services is more convenient for patients and reduces their out-of-pocket expenses. The finalized Stark regulations provide more opportunity to offer ancillary services. With the right support, ancillary services can be very profitable. However, ancillary service business ventures should not be entered into lightly, and a solid plan of action is necessary for success. Always start with a clear business plan and bring in the most experienced team to help with implementation and continued management of any service offered.

CHAPTER 10
Compliance Programs

OUTLINE

I. Introduction
II. Sanction Authorities
   A. False Claims Act
   B. The Anti-Kickback Statute
   C. Physician Self-Referral (Stark Laws) Regulations
      1. Exceptions
   D. Health Insurance Portability and Accountability Act
      1. Security Rule Enforcement
      2. Enforcement and Penalties for Noncompliance
   E. Red Flags Rule
   F. Commercial Insurer Fraud and Abuse Programs
      1. Penalties for Fraud and Abuse
      2. Practice Protection
III. Who Else Is Watching?
   A. Medicare Claims Review Programs
      1. Recovery Audit Contractors
      2. Comprehensive Error Rate Testing
      3. Medicaid Integrity Program
      4. Office of Inspector General
IV. Developing an Effective Plan
   A. Designating a Compliance Officer
   B. Implementing Written Policies, Procedures, and Standards of Conduct
   C. Conducting Effective Training and Education
   D. Developing Effective Lines of Communication
V. Enforcing Standards Through Well-Publicized Disciplinary Guidelines

A. Responding Promptly to Detected Offenses and Developing Corrective Action
   1. Refunding Overpayments
   2. Disclosure
B. Conducting Internal Monitoring and Auditing
   1. Warning Lights and Monitors
      a. Business Relationships
      b. "Incident To" Services
      c. Other Areas to Review
VI. Conclusion

Introduction

The term *compliance*, the act of adhering to a law, regulation, or guideline, is a common concern of health care providers and health care billing organizations. When compliance is mentioned, most in the medical field think of correct Medicare and Medicaid billing or conducting business within the Stark guidelines. Compliance touches many aspects of the physician practice, including referrals, ownership issues, patient privacy, treatment of emergencies, occupational health and safety, and identity theft.

Many are confused as to what needs to be done to become or remain compliant, and there is a certain "fear factor" associated with compliance or the lack of it. It is little wonder. Compliance violations can cost organizations huge sums of money and, in some cases, can result in criminal penalties including incarceration of key staff members.

For the first half of fiscal year (FY) 2009, the Department of Health and Human Services (HHS) Office of Inspector General (OIG) reported expected recoveries of more than $274.8 million in audit receivables, including $551.7 million in non-HHS receivables resulting from OIG work (eg, the states' share of Medicaid restitution). These amounts include all OIG investigations of pharmaceutical companies, hospitals, nursing homes, and similar organizations. For that same reporting period, the OIG reported exclusions from participation of 1,415 individuals and entities for fraud or abuse involving federal programs. The report also shows 293 criminal actions against individuals or entities and 243 civil actions.[1]

This information indicates that compliance is not something to be taken lightly. But with whom or what are we to be in compliance?

Although the list of laws and regulations grows daily, most regulations have their roots in one of four major pieces of legislation: the False Claims Act Amendments of 1986 (FCA) 31 USC §§3729–3733 (1986) and the Fraud Enforcement and Recovery Act of 2009 (FERA); the Medicare and Medicaid Patient Protection Act of 1987, as amended,

42 U.S.C. §1320a-7b (the Anti-Kickback Statute); the Omnibus Budget Reconciliation Act of 1989 (OBRA 1989; the Stark Referral Law and Regulations); and the Emergency Medical Treatment and Labor Act (Section 1867 of the Social Security Act [rw USC §1395 dd]). These four pieces of legislation and associated laws and regulations focus almost exclusively on Medicare compliance. Other laws and regulations also apply to reimbursement, such as the Health Insurance Portability and Accountability Act (HIPAA) (both for transactions and privacy), red flags rule, and commercial insurer fraud and abuse programs.

Sanction Authorities

In the struggle to remain or become compliant, it is beneficial to understand what statutes and regulations require compliance. The following sections describe health care laws and their sanctioning authorities.[2]

False Claims Act

The False Claims Act (FCA) was enacted in 1863, with significant updates in 1986 and 2009. It states that those who knowingly submit, or cause another person or entity to submit, false claims for payment of government funds are liable for three times the government's damages plus civil penalties of $5,500 to $11,000 per false claim.

In 2009, the act was amended to expand the scope of potential FCA liability, redefined the definition of "claim," and enacted other changes to strengthen the law. The FCA contains the qui tam provision (31 USC 3730 b), which allows citizens to bring action on behalf of the United States. Citizens may share in up to 25% of the proceeds from an action or settlement.[3]

Examples of false claims include:

- *Billing for services or supplies that were not provided.* A common false claim is billing for services or supplies that either were not provided or were provided but not documented in the patient record.

- *Billing twice for the same service.* Duplicate billing can result from sloppy claims filing or it can be deliberate. Submitting claims to Medicare and another payer as though both were the primary payer or billing Medicare for tests that another provider has billed (eg, billing for the global fee when only the technical or professional component should have been billed) are examples of duplicate billing.

- *Misrepresenting the diagnosis to justify the service.* Physician offices sometimes use "cheat sheets," or lists of covered diagnoses from the Medicare carrier's Local Medical Review

Policy or National Coverage Determinations. With more aggressive policies in place to reduce the number of inappropriate tests, the tendency is to select a diagnosis from the covered list. If the diagnosis selected is not reflected in the patient's chart, the provider may be suspected of committing fraud. Another example of misrepresentation is to code a rule-out or suspected condition as a confirmed diagnosis.

- *Altering claims in any form to obtain a higher reimbursement.* Adding modifiers, changing dates of service, or revising the Current Procedural Terminology (CPT®) code or reason for a test to obtain coverage or a higher reimbursement will result in the submission of a false claim.[4]

- *Inappropriate balance billing of patient accounts.* Providers have the option of being participating or nonparticipating providers with Medicare. A participating provider accepts Medicare assignment. This means that Medicare will pay the provider directly for 80% of the Medicare allowable charges, and the patient is responsible for the remaining 20% of the Medicare allowable charges. Billing the patient for more than 20% is inappropriate balance billing. Similarly, a nonparticipating provider may bill a patient up to the "limiting charge," as defined by Medicare. The patient pays the physician directly, and the Medicare payment is sent to the patient. It is also a violation to bill the patient for more than the limiting charge.

- *Poor resolution of overpayments.* Tempting as it may be to let a Medicare overpayment sit on the books to make up for the money you believe Medicare owes the practice, it is not advisable. Resolution of overpayments is one of OIG's targeted areas to watch. Practices should have a written policy in place outlining how overpayments will be handled and requiring that refunds be made within 30 days.

- *Willful misuse of provider identification numbers.* Submitting any claims for services that were not actually provided by the indicated physician is a misuse of the provider number. Allowing new providers to share a billing number, billing incorrectly for mid-level providers under the "incident to" rule, and billing for work that medical students performed are ways that physicians can misuse their provider numbers.

The Anti-Kickback Statute

The Medicare and Medicaid Patient Protection Act of 1987, or the anti-kickback statute, is another law that affects health care entities. Originally enacted in 1972, the statute forbids making or receiving kickbacks for items or services covered by Medicare, Medicaid, and other federal health care programs.

Kickbacks can distort medical decision making, cause overutilization, increase costs, and result in unfair competition by freezing out competitors who are unwilling to pay kickbacks. Kickbacks also can adversely affect the quality of patient care by encouraging physicians to order services or recommend supplies based on profit rather than on the patients' best medical interests.

Section 1128B(b) of the Social Security Act, 42 USC §1320a-7b(b), prohibits knowingly and willfully soliciting, receiving, offering, or paying anything of value to induce referrals of items or services payable by a federal health care program. Both parties to an impermissible kickback transaction are liable. Violation of the statute constitutes a felony punishable by a maximum fine of $25,000, imprisonment for up to five years, or both. The OIG also may initiate administrative proceedings to exclude persons from federal health care programs or to impose civil monetary penalties for fraud, kickbacks, and other prohibited activities under sections 1128(b)(7) and 1128(a)(7) of the act.[5]

In 1987, the OIG was given the power to exclude practitioners who violate the statute from being Medicare providers. In addition, Public Law 105-33, the Balanced Budget Act of 1997, increased the OIG's power by allowing it to seek civil money penalties rather than criminal penalties for violation of the law. Thus, the OIG no longer had to prove intent when charging an organization with violations of the statute.

Examples of violations of the anti-kickback statute include:

- *Giving cash for patient referrals.* Giving cash in exchange for patient referrals is one of the most common forms of kickback.
- *Conducting contests and giveaways.* Any prize, gift, cash payment, coupon, or bonus in exchange for prescribing or purchasing specific products is subject to investigation.
- *Waiving copayments and deductibles.* Routine waiver of Medicare Part B copayments and deductibles is a violation of the statute.
- *Providing remuneration to induce referrals.* Fees given to providers to induce referrals are improper.
- *Creating below-fair-market agreements between providers and suppliers.* This includes rental space as well as services rendered. To be in compliance, all agreements must be in writing, for at least a year, and of fair-market value.
- *Providing compensation for minimal services.*
- *Creating cross-referral arrangements.* These arrangements typically involve two providers, where one is given the opportunity to make money in exchange for referrals to the other.
- *Offering any prize, gift, or cash payment in exchange for prescribing or purchasing specific products.*
- *Accepting free employee health services provided by a supplier.*
- *Accepting free computers, fax machines, or other equipment provided by a supplier.*

Personnel in many physicians' practices inadvertently find themselves violating this statute because they were not aware of the far-reaching arm of this regulation. Penalties can be great—fines of up to $25,000 and imprisonment—if a vendor is found guilty of a criminal action. With the implementation of the Balanced Budget Act of 1997, the government no longer has to show intent to defraud the government (which evokes a criminal action) but can seek damages under the civil monetary penalties clause. This allows the OIG to seek action for noncriminal causes, for which no intent has to be shown. Therefore, a physician who is inadvertently doing something that he or she is not even aware is illegal could still be subject to fines of up to $50,000 for each violation.

Under the Civil Monetary Penalties section 1128A of the Social Security Act (42 USC §1320a-7a), a person is subject to penalties, assessments, and exclusion from participating in federal health care programs for engaging in certain activities. For example, a person who submits or causes to be submitted to a federal health care program a claim for items and services that the person knows or should know are false or fraudulent is subject to a penalty of up to $10,000 for each item or service falsely or fraudulently claimed. For the purpose of this law, *should know* is defined to mean that the person acted in reckless disregard or deliberate ignorance of the truth or falsity of the claim.[6]

Physician Self-Referral (Stark Laws) Regulations

The Omnibus Budget Reconciliation Act of 1989 (OBRA 1989), which bars self-referrals for clinical laboratory services under the Medicare program, became effective January 1, 1992. This provision is known as Stark I. In 1993, Congress expanded the law to apply to 10 additional health services in Stark II, which became effective in 1995. The Stark Law, which actually incorporates three separate regulations, governs physician self-referral for Medicare and Medicaid patients. The law is named for U.S. Congressman Pete Stark, who sponsored the initial bill.

The 11 designated health services from which physicians are barred from self-referring include:

- clinical laboratory services;
- physical therapy services;
- occupational therapy services;
- radiology services;
- radiation therapy services;
- durable medical equipment and supplies;
- parenteral and enteral nutrients, equipment, and supplies;
- prosthetics, orthotics, prosthetic devices, and supplies;
- home health services;

- outpatient prescription drugs; and
- inpatient and outpatient hospital services.

Penalties for violation of Stark I and II regulations include denial of payment for the designated health services, refund of amounts collected in violation of the provision, and civil monetary penalties up to $15,000 for each service. Physicians and entities entering into an arrangement to circumvent the referral restriction law are subject to civil monetary penalties of up to $100,000 per occurrence.[7]

Phase III of Stark II, the final rule, was published in 2007. It did not change the designated health services but it does clarify some provisions for office space and equipment lease arrangements, eliminated the safe harbor for "fair market value," modified the definition of "physician in a group practice," and made other changes.

Other proposed statutes and regulations may impact Stark in the near future. These include the 2008 Medicare proposed physician fee schedule limits "per-click" (or per unit of service) compensation that applies when a physician leases space or equipment to an entity that performs designated health services (DHS) and then refers patients to that DHS entity. CMS believes these arrangements give physicians the incentive to make unnecessary DHS referrals. The agency has requested comments on other arrangements in which an entity performing DHS pays the owners of space and/or equipment per unit of time or per unit of service and in which the units reflect referrals from the space and/or equipment owners. The proposed limit on per-click compensation was not included in the final rule. However, this provision was included in the Medicare hospital inpatient prospective payment system (IPPS) rulemaking for FY 2009 and went into effect October 1, 2009.

Exceptions

As with the anti-kickback statute, there are exceptions to the general Stark Rule prohibiting a physician from making a referral for certain designated health services payable by Medicare to an entity with which the physician or an immediate family member has a financial relationship, unless an exception applies. Some exceptions are similar to the safe harbors listed for the anti-kickback statute. The exceptions fall into three categories:

- *Those based on compensation, investments, and ownership.* These exceptions apply to physician services personally provided by the physician, ancillary services provided by the ordering physician or another member of the group or supervised by the ordering physician, services furnished to enrollees of risk-based Medicare health maintenance organizations, and services furnished in ambulatory surgery centers or end-stage renal disease facilities.

- *Those based on both ownership and investment.* These exceptions include ownership or investment in publicly traded securities and mutual funds and certain hospital exceptions.
- *Those based on compensation only.* These exceptions deal with office rental, equipment rental, employee relationships, group practice arrangements within hospitals, and group purchasing arrangements.

The Stark Law, however, is based on fact rather than intent. Whether or not people intended to violate these laws, if they are in violation—well, they are in violation! Unlike the anti-kickback statute, which can apply to any health care provider, this law currently pertains only to physicians, defined as doctors of medicine, osteopathic physicians, dentists or doctors of dental surgery, podiatrists, optometrists, and chiropractors. Recently, questions have been raised pertaining to Stark laws and mid-level providers. This applicability is still being tested.

Health Insurance Portability and Accountability Act

The Health Insurance Portability and Accountability Act of 1996 (HIPAA) required the secretary of HHS to develop regulations to protect the privacy and security of certain health information. To fulfill this requirement, HHS published what are commonly known as the HIPAA Privacy Rule and the HIPAA Security Rule. The Privacy Rule, or Standards for Privacy of Individually Identifiable Health Information, establishes national standards for the protection of certain health information. The Security Standards for the Protection of Electronic Protected Health Information (the Security Rule) establish a national set of security standards for protecting certain health information that is held or transferred in electronic form. The Security Rule operationalizes the protections contained in the Privacy Rule by addressing the technical and nontechnical safeguards that organizations known as "covered entities" must put in place to secure individuals' electronic protected health information (e-PHI). Within HHS, the Office for Civil Rights (OCR) has responsibility for enforcing the Privacy and Security Rules with voluntary compliance activities and civil monetary penalties.

Security Rule Enforcement

The Security Rule is a set of federal security standards that protect the confidentiality, integrity, and availability of e-PHI. The secretary of HHS delegated authority for administration and enforcement of the Security Rule to the OCR on July 27, 2009. Before that date, CMS was responsible for enforcing the Security Rule, including investigating complaints and conducting compliance reviews.

Enforcement and Penalties for Noncompliance

Enforcement and penalties for noncompliance are described in the following paragraphs.

- *Compliance.* The Security Rule establishes a set of national standards for confidentiality, integrity, and availability of e-PHI. The HHS OCR is responsible for administering and enforcing these standards, in concert with its enforcement of the Privacy Rule, and may conduct complaint investigations and compliance reviews.
  Consistent with the principles for achieving compliance provided in the rule, HHS will seek the cooperation of covered entities and may provide technical assistance to help them comply voluntarily with the rule. The rule provides processes for persons to file complaints with HHS and describes the responsibilities of covered entities to provide records and compliance reports and to cooperate with, and permit access to information for, investigations and compliance reviews.

- *Civil Monetary Penalties.* HHS may impose civil monetary penalties on a covered entity of $100 per failure to comply with a Privacy Rule requirement. That penalty may not exceed $25,000 for multiple violations of the identical Privacy Rule requirement in a calendar year. HHS may not impose a civil monetary penalty under specific circumstances, such as when a violation is due to reasonable cause and did not involve willful neglect and the covered entity corrected the violations within 30 days of when it knew or should have known of the violation.

Red Flags Rule

The Red Flags Rule is a set of regulations issued in November 2007 by the Federal Trade Commission (FTC) that require any institution considered a "creditor" to develop and implement written identity theft prevention and detection programs to protect consumers from identity theft. Although the American Medical Association (AMA) has expressed its concerns about whether physician practices are subject to the Red Flags requirements and has successfully delayed implementation of the rule until December 31, 2010, the AMA has prepared guidance and sample policies for physicians.[8] This simple identity theft prevention and detection program can be incorporated into existing compliance and HIPAA security and privacy policies.

A "red flag" is a pattern, practice, or specific account activity that indicates the possibility of identity theft. The FTC identifies the following as red flags:

- alerts, notifications, or warnings from a consumer reporting agency;
- suspicious documents and/or personal identifying information, such as an inconsistent address or nonexistent Social Security number;

- unusual use of, or suspicious activity relating to, a patient account; and
- notices of possible identity theft from patients, victims of identity theft, or law enforcement authorities.

The Red Flags Rule requires organizations to have "reasonable policies and procedures in place" to identify, detect, and respond to identity theft red flags. The definition of "reasonable" depends on a practice's specific circumstances or specific experience with medical identity theft, as well as the degree of risk for identity theft in the practice. These policies and procedures should complement a practice's existing HIPAA privacy and security policies and procedures, which outline the administrative, technical, and physical safeguards the practice uses to ensure the security of patients' PHI.[9]

A guidance document and sample policies for physicians are available at www.ama-assn.org/ama1/pub/upload/mm/368/red-flags-rule-edu.pdf.

Commercial Insurer Fraud and Abuse Programs

Because of the escalating pace of legislative and administrative health care reform activities, a practice is likely to be in technical violation of at least one billing regulation at any given time, no matter how scrupulous and thorough its billing procedures. In addition, commercial insurance programs, or "private payers," have their own rules for proper billing that must be followed for payment to ensue. Commercial insurers monitor claims to detect and review possible cases of fraud and abuse. Thus, it is becoming more important for physicians to have compliance plans in place to prevent fraud and abuse and to protect the practice in the event it falls under scrutiny for billing practices. In addition, health care fraud is under increased scrutiny at the state level through state insurance regulators and at the federal level with penalties prosecuted under the U.S. Code.

Penalties for Fraud and Abuse

Violators of health care fraud can be prosecuted under 18 U.S.C. 1347 Health Care Fraud, as described here:

> Whoever knowingly and willfully executes, or attempts to execute, a scheme or artifice— (1) to defraud any health care benefit program; or (2) to obtain, by means of false or fraudulent pretenses, representations, or promises, any of the money or property owned by, or under the custody or control of, any health care benefit program, in connection with the delivery of or payment for health care benefits, items, or services, shall be fined under this title or imprisoned not

more than 10 years, or both. If the violation results in serious bodily injury (as defined in section 1365 of this title), such person shall be fined under this title or imprisoned not more than 20 years, or both; and if the violation results in death, such person shall be fined under this title, or imprisoned for any term of years or for life, or both (Title 18, Part I, Chapter 63, §1347).

Practice Protection

A practice is obligated to report suspected fraud and abuse by calling the insurer. Most commercial companies have a hotline to call or an online form to complete. Additional practice protection includes the following:

- Have a process in place to keep up with benefit and policy changes released by the company through written and online publications.
- Do not waive deductibles and/or coinsurance.
- Keep provider numbers confidential and do not allow other providers to bill for their services with another physician's provider number.
- If someone else is authorized to bill for the physician's services, have a process in place to ensure accurate billing that reflects the services provided.
- Maintain a treatment record for each patient and document all services, orders, and prescriptions.
- Have internal audits in place to detect billing inaccuracies promptly.
- Make copies of each patient's insurance card and driver's license.
- Do not advertise "free" services that are subsequently billed to an insurer.
- Do not bill an insurance company for services provided to a relative who is related by blood or marriage or who lives in the provider's household.

Who Else Is Watching?

In addition to these sanctioning authorities, CMS, state Medicaid agencies, and private payers have increased their incidence of claims reviews and audits in an effort to prevent reimbursement for false or invalid claims.

Medicare Claims Review Programs

CMS provides complete information about its five claim review programs in a booklet titled, *Medicare Claim Review Programs: MR, NCCI Edits, MUEs, CERT, and RAC.*[10] Table 10-1 shows a division of the programs based on performance of prepayment or postpayment reviews.

The information in this section considers recovery audit contractors (RACs), the Comprehensive Error Rate Testing (CERT) Program, the Medicaid Integrity Program (MIP), and the Office of Inspector General (OIG).

Recovery Audit Contractors

The Medicare Prescription Drug, Improvement and Modernization Act (MMA) 2003 SEC. 306 required the three-year RAC demonstration project. The Tax Relief and Health Care Act of 2006 (H.R. 6111) required that a permanent and nationwide RAC program be implemented no later than 2010. Both statutes gave CMS the authority to pay the RACs on a contingency fee basis.

RACs are tasked with detecting and correcting improper payments on Medicare claims (ie, collecting overpayments and paying back underpayments). RACs review claims on a postpayment basis and use the same Medicare policies as do carriers, fiscal intermediaries (FIs), and Medicare administrative contractors (MACs) (see Table 10-1). RACs can look back three years from the date the claim was paid. Any organization that bills Medicare claims can be subject to a RAC review. In an effort to minimize the burden reviews place on billers, RACs limit the number of records they request from a provider. The following information gives the number-of-records limit per entity:

- Inpatient hospital, inpatient rehabilitation facility, skilled nursing facility, hospice:
    10% of the average monthly Medicare claims (maximum 200) per 45 days per national provider identifier (NPI)
- Other Part A billers—home health (HH):
    1% of the average monthly Medicare episodes of care (maximum 200) per 45 days per NPI
- Physicians (including podiatrists, chiropractors):
    Sole practitioner: 10 medical records per 45 days per NPI
    Partnership (2 to 5 individuals): 20 medical records per 45 days per NPI
    Group (6 to 15 individuals): 30 medical records per 45 days per NPI
    Large group (16+ individuals): 50 medical records per 45 days per NPI

TABLE 10-1 Medicare Prepayment and Postpayment Claim Review Programs

Prepayment Claim Review Programs	Postpayment Claim Review Programs
National Correct Coding Initiatives edits	Comprehensive Error Rate Testing Program
Medically unlikely edits	Recovery audit contractor
Carrier/FI/MAC medical review	Carrier/FI/MAC medical review

FI: fiscal intermediary; MAC: Medicare administrative contractor

- Other Part B billers (durable medical equipment [DME], laboratory, outpatient hospital):

    1% of the average monthly Medicare claim lines (maximum 200) per 45 days per NPI

When the RAC identifies something that was paid in error, it will issue a demand letter to the provider. If the provider agrees with the RAC's determination, it has the option of paying by check or allowing recoupment from future payments or requesting and applying for an extended payment plan.

If the provider disagrees with the determination, the provider has an opportunity to appeal the decision. The provider is given an opportunity to discuss the improper payment determination directly with the RAC. The review determination follows Medicare's outlined normal appeal process. Additional information on the appeals process is available at www.cms.hhs.gov/RAC/Downloads/AppealUpdatethrough83108ofRACEvalReport.pdf.

When the RAC identifies an issue, the determination must be approved by CMS before it is open for widespread review. The approved issues are posted on the RAC Website. Because CMS holds the same determination for other RACs, it is beneficial for practices to view posted determinations on all RAC Websites. The RAC contact information is available at www.cms.hhs.gov/RAC/Downloads/RAC%20contact%20information.pdf.

Comprehensive Error Rate Testing

CMS developed the CERT program to produce a national Medicare fee-for-service error rate as required by the Improper Payments Information Act of 2002 (Public Law No: 107–300). The CERT review contractor and the CERT documentation contractor conduct CERT reviews. CERT randomly selects a small sample of Medicare fee-for-service claims and reviews the claims and records for compliance with Medicare coverage, coding, and billing rules.

CERT contractors generate a number of measurements and statistics for review and analysis by CMS. There are four categories for which Medicare contractors are responsible:

- paid claims error rate including documentation,
- paid claims error rate excluding documentation,
- processed claims error rate, and
- provider compliance error rate.

To better measure the performance of the Medicare claims processing contractors and to gain insight into the causes of errors, CMS decided to calculate a national Medicare fee-for-service paid claims error rate that measures the percentage of total dollars that Medicare contractors paid erroneously. Medicare also measures a provider compliance error rate, which measures how accurately providers paid claims for submission.[11]

Medicaid Integrity Program

In February 2006, the Deficit Reduction Act of 2005 was signed into law and created the Medicaid Integrity Program (MIP) under section 1936 of the Social Security Act. CMS has two broad responsibilities under the MIP:

- to hire contractors to review Medicaid provider activities, audit claims, identify overpayments, and educate providers and others on Medicaid program integrity issues; and
- to provide effective support and assistance to states in their efforts to combat Medicaid provider fraud and abuse.

The Social Security Act required CMS to develop a five-year comprehensive MIP and to report to Congress on the effectiveness of the plan. The plan will be fully funded and operational in 2010. The stated purpose of the MIP is to review the actions of entities or individuals furnishing items or services for which payment is made under the state plan to determine whether fraud and abuse have occurred or are likely to occur, to identify overpayments to individuals or entities, and to educate providers of services, managed care plans, and beneficiaries with respect to integrity and quality of care.[12] Additional information on comprehensive MIP is available at www.cms.hhs.gov/DeficitReductionAct/Downloads/CMIP2006.pdf.

Office of Inspector General

The purpose of the Office of Inspector General (OIG) is to protect the integrity of HHS programs as well as the health and welfare of the beneficiaries of those programs. OIG duties are carried out through a nationwide network of audits, investigations, inspections, and other mission-related functions performed by OIG components. Among other initiatives, the OIG:

- issues advisory opinions on the application of the anti-kickback statute;
- publishes fraud alerts and bulletins;
- negotiates compliance obligations in the form of corporate integrity agreements as part of the settlement of federal health care program investigations;
- establishes and oversees the exclusions program and maintains a list of excluded providers; and
- provides for compliance plan guidance for health care entities.

The OIG also publishes an annual work plan outlining the areas it has identified as being susceptible to fraud and abuse. In recent years, the following areas are among those that have been included in the OIG work plan:

- provider-based status for outpatient facilities,
- hospital ownership of physician practices,
- Medicare secondary payer,
- place-of-service errors,
- "incident to" services,
- evaluation and management (E/M) services during a global period,
- unbundling of laboratory tests,
- high use of ultrasound services in identified areas,
- physician reassignment of benefits,
- unbundling of hospital outpatient services,
- billing service companies, and
- payment for initial preventive physical examinations.

Despite the increased oversight by government agencies, compliance remains a confusing arena for many health care managers and providers. This is primarily because of confusing directives, lack of clarity in the regulations, and an abundance of misinformation and individual interpretation.

To take a proactive approach to compliance and minimize damages if there are unintentional infringements, many organizations are adopting compliance plans. In an effort to reduce the number of erroneous claims or prevent providers from engaging in unlawful conduct, the OIG has developed compliance plan guidance for selected areas of the health care industry, including hospitals, clinical laboratories, nursing facilities, ambulance services, physician group practices, and third-party billing companies.

What are the advantages of implementing a plan? The internal benefits include the submission of more accurate claims, improved documentation to support the services that were rendered, and better internal communications. In addition, the OIG considers the existence of an effective compliance program that predated any government investigation when addressing the appropriateness of administrative sanctions.[13] However, these benefits will apply only if the organization has implemented what the OIG considers an "effective compliance program." Following the published compliance plan guidance can help organizations develop effective programs.

Developing an Effective Plan

Depending on the size and nature of your organization, you may want to refer to specific compliance plan guidance (eg, for physician practice, hospital, home health agency) in addition to the compliance plan guidance for third-party medical billing companies. These guidance documents can be found on the OIG Website at http://oig.hhs.gov/fraud/complianceguidance.asp.

Each guidance plan outlines the following seven steps, which should be included in any effective program:

1. Designate a compliance officer and compliance committee.
2. Implement written policies, procedures, and standards of conduct.
3. Conduct effective training and education.
4. Develop effective lines of communication.
5. Enforce standards through well-publicized disciplinary guidelines.
6. Respond promptly to detected offenses and develop corrective action.
7. Conduct internal monitoring and auditing.

Adjustments and allowances have been made for the physician compliance plans, because the OIG realizes that physician practices may not have the resources to implement plans to the extent that larger entities do. However, it is recommended that these seven key steps be taken.

Designating a Compliance Officer

The first step in developing a program is to select a compliance officer and committee to oversee the program. The guidelines for a compliance officer for physician practices suggest the following possibilities:

- An existing employee can be appointed to oversee the plan.
- Several employees can share the responsibility.

- The practice may join other entities, such as hospitals or billing companies, and become part of their plan.
- The practice may choose a legal or consulting firm.
- The practice may share an officer with another practice.

Responsibilities include:
- overseeing and monitoring the implementation of the program;
- establishing methods, such as periodic audits, to improve the organization's efficiency and quality of services and to reduce vulnerability to fraud and abuse;
- periodically revising and updating the program to address changes in the needs of the organization or to reflect changes in law and standards;
- developing, coordinating, and participating in compliance plan education and training; and
- investigating and reporting any allegations concerning possible unethical or improper billing or business practices.

When choosing a candidate to oversee compliance, ask the following questions:
- Does the candidate have sufficient professional experience working with health care regulations, medical billing requirements, clinical records, and documentation to perform the assigned duties successfully?
- Does the candidate have sufficient authority to effect change?

Figure 10-1 can be used to in the selection of an effective compliance officer.

Implementing Written Policies, Procedures, and Standards of Conduct

Once a compliance officer/committee is designated, the organization can begin developing its standards of conduct. These standards, which outline the tenets of the organization, will vary depending on the size and nature of the organization. Typically, they will address such issues as:
- employee hiring and retention;
- general marketing and marketing arrangements;
- business arrangements, referral patterns, and compensation agreements;
- quality of patient care;
- compliance with laws and regulations for health care entities;

1. What can we afford to pay for this position?
2. If a physician or existing employee assumes this responsibility, will he or she be compensated extra? _____ If yes, how much? _____
3. Of all the options for fulfilling the compliance director responsibilities, which would we prefer if money were no object?
   - Have the employees share the responsibility
   - Be part of a hospital or billing firm's plan
   - Share a compliance officer with other offices
   - Use a consulting firm or legal firm
   - Appoint one person in-house
   - Hire a full-time compliance director
4. If an employee (eg, office manager) assumes the role, which physician will oversee the employee and assist with disciplinary issues?
5. What role do we see this individual performing, and how will it be performed?
   - Performing the audit or arranging for outside audits
   - Performing the training or arranging and overseeing the training
   - Writing the compliance plan or fulfilling the plan once written by outside counsel
   - Disciplining wrongdoers or reporting wrongdoing to physicians to discipline
6. Who will be able to override this individual's decisions?
7. How much of this individual's time will be spent on compliance issues?
8. Will he or she be required to do other work and perform compliance tasks only a few hours a week?
9. What is the education budget for this position?
10. What is the biggest fear on the appointment to this position?
11. If we use another firm or organization, who is going to handle compliance tasks in-house and be the contact person?
12. Are all the partners committed to compliance and the appointment of a director?
13. Is this position a figurehead only?

FIGURE 10-1 Compliance Officer Evaluation.

- conflicts of interest for owners, providers, and staff members; and
- billing, coding, and records integrity.

For example, some standards of conduct for a practice may be similar to the following:

- We will take steps to ensure that an individual is not on an excluded or sanctioned OIG list before extending an offer of employment.
- We will not engage in marketing initiatives that involve cross-referral arrangements, exchanging goods or money in return for patient referrals, or offering free services such as "insurance only" billing.
- We will provide high-quality care and related services to patients in a responsible, reliable, appropriate, and cost-effective manner.
- We will operate this business in accordance with high moral and ethical standards and in full compliance with applicable laws, rules, and regulations.
- We will refrain from and avoid conflicts of interest, or the appearance of conflicts, between the private interests of any employee and his or her official responsibilities and duties performed on behalf of the practice.
- We will protect patient information from improper disclosure in compliance with Health Insurance Portability and Accountability Act guidelines.
- We will maintain timely and accurate patient records and bill only for services actually rendered as documented in the patient record.
- We will take care to accurately submit all claims to third-party payers with regard to patient information, services rendered, and the reason for those services.
- We will take steps to ensure that all claims are submitted with the appropriate rendering physician's provider number.
- We will implement internal guidelines to ensure adherence to "incident to" guidelines.

Written policies of "how we do things" can reinforce the standards of conduct. They may cover such issues as:

Billing

- how charges are to be entered,
- who is responsible for assigning the procedure and diagnosis codes,
- bill only under appropriate provider's number,
- rules to follow when assigning modifiers,

- importance of checking National Correct Coding Initiative (NCCI) edits before submitting claims,
- appropriate posting of explanations of benefits, and
- how to handle overpayments.

Documentation

- to reflect work actually performed,
- to meet official guidelines,
- the reason for tests or referrals,
- when a patient cancels an appointment,
- telephone calls with patients,
- billing and coding directives from payers,
- national or local coverage determinations: how the practice is to advise patients that a test or service may not be covered and how to obtain the signed advance beneficiary notice,
- how to check the assigned diagnosis code to determine whether it meets medical necessity, and
- avoiding assignment of a diagnosis code simply because it is on the approved list.

These written policies will be a work-in-progress and will change to reflect payer guidelines. For this reason, it is important to review the written instructions periodically to ensure that they reflect the most current requirements.

Conducting Effective Training and Education

The next step to effective compliance is to educate staff members on the existence of a plan, what the plan means, and how it will affect them.

The OIG recognizes that there are many forms of training but it has publicly favored training programs that are delivered in person. The initial compliance plan training typically includes:

- reviewing the seven elements of a plan,
- introducing the person overseeing the plan,
- providing an overview of fraud and abuse issues that are pertinent to the organization,
- outlining the standards of conduct the organization expects staff members to achieve, and
- outlining the lines of communication to use in the event of a lapse in compliance or a suspected lapse in compliance.

A typical training agenda is shown in Figure 10-2.

9:00 am to 9:10 am	Sign in and welcome

9:10 am to 10:00 am	Overview of compliance program

Reinforce the mission, vision, and values

1. Emphasize the organization's commitment to good compliance practices at all levels
2. Encourage employees to resolve any problems/concerns through the chain-of-command
3. Describe the structure and operation of the compliance program
4. Explain the hotline operation and underscore employee rights to anonymity and confidentiality
5. Review policies and the code and their application to workplace scenarios
6. Review what fraud and abuse are
7. Review compliance plan
8. Identify who is responsible for overseeing program in the office
9. Discuss the job responsibility of that person
10. Explain employees' duty to report suspected misconduct or seek clarification on issues they are unclear about
11. Assure employees that there will be no retaliation for reporting
12. Describe review and audit procedures the plan calls for

10:00 am to 10:30 am	Discussion of scenarios, questions and answers

10:30 am to 10:45 am	Post-training quiz

10:45 am to 11:00 am	Closing comments

Wrap up

A sign-in sheet should provide evidence that participants:

1. Have received a copy of the practice's code of conduct
2. Have been trained in compliance
3. Have learned how to apply the code to recognizable work situations
4. Understand the reporting mechanism
5. Understand the lines of communication

FIGURE 10-2 Training Program Agenda.

Interactive training that gives attendees the opportunity to ask question works well and is favored by the OIG. In addition to providing training, organizations must be able to provide evidence that the written guidance was effectively communicated to all employees. For that reason, some form of post-training quiz in which attendees can demonstrate their understanding will support the effectiveness of the training.

During the training program, it is important to inform employees that they have a duty to report anything they believe is questionable conduct as it relates to fraud and abuse issues. This duty to report puts responsibility on every staff member and provides clear direction to an employee who may be aware of inappropriate practices but not know how to handle the information.

In addition to knowing about this duty to report, staff members must be assured that there will be no retaliation for reporting or for questioning the organization's policies or actions.

Once the initial training is given, it is advisable to review the requirements annually in order to address any new issues. Additionally, an annual review will refresh compliance in staff members' minds.

Figure 10-3 provides an evaluation tool for assessing the effectiveness of your compliance training.

- Are employees trained on compliance within first 60 days of employment?
- Have you provided for annual training of all personnel?
- Can your employees pass the post-training test?
- Does your training program adequately summarize fraud and abuse laws?
- Are your trainers qualified to train?
- Can employees identify risk areas?
- Do employees know the procedure for reporting an incident?
- Have you developed a method to track employee training in the compliance plan?
- Do you have a training budget?
- How do you determine who needs training?
- How do you determine where training dollars are spent?

FIGURE 10-3 Have You Developed an Effective Training Program?

A second type of education and training is ongoing training pertinent to individual jobs. This may be the most difficult step because it involves assessing the educational needs of staff members, finding the resources to meet those needs, budgeting for those educational sessions, and setting aside the time to implement the education.

Needs assessments can include the following:

- reviewing chart documentation to determine whether physicians need additional training in documentation guidelines,
- reviewing explanations of benefits to identify where the mistakes and lapses occurred,
- asking in-depth questions of staff members to assess their knowledge levels, and
- observing staff members as they complete their work.

Establishing an education and training budget each year will help the practice meet the staff's training needs.

Fortunately, many educational opportunities are offered by CMS, carriers/MACs, and specialty societies. Most CMS online modules are free of charge, as are many of the carrier/MAC programs. Ongoing training for the compliance officer as well as staff members is essential to functioning within regulatory guidelines.

Developing Effective Lines of Communication

Ask almost any health care organization today what it believes needs to be improved, and you will probably hear, "We need better communication." In this age of information overload, we continue to struggle to get the right information to the right people at the right time.

Communications, as it pertains to compliance plans, primarily focus on reporting methods. What happens when a staff member believes there is improper billing, inappropriate activities, or a violation of one of the fraud and abuse laws? There must be an outlined reporting method so that an individual knows where to go with the concern or information.

A major concern for staff members who want to question or report an action is, "What will happen to me if I report this?" In order to protect employees who have concerns, the OIG recommendation for large organizations is to have a 24-hour hotline or other method of providing anonymous reporting. The hotline number should be posted for access by all employees. Several agencies offer this hotline service.

Other methods that organizations might consider include having a post office box number where inquiries can be sent, a voice mail system where staff members can leave a message, a reporting box where employees can provide their concerns, as well as the open-door method in which they can come in and talk. For each method, there must be documentation of what was reported, the time and date of the report, and what actions were taken. Figure 10-4 is a sample form for report documentation.

In addition to guidelines on how to report incidents, organizations should review how other information is communicated by asking these questions:

- Who is responsible for distributing payer guidelines and changes in payer requirements?
- Which staff members need that information?
- If a payment poster notices services that are regularly denied, how does that information reach the provider?
- If patients call to report that they received a bill that they have already paid or they have given updated insurance information at check-in several times and it is still incorrect, what steps are taken to ensure that these lapses in service will be eliminated?

The answers to these and other important questions could be answered in an intra-office newsletter or postings on a staff bulletin board. Figure 10-5 provides a checklist to ensure that the organization has developed effective channels of communication.

Enforcing Standards Through Well-Publicized Disciplinary Guidelines

Some organizations are reluctant to discuss or establish disciplinary procedures as they develop their plans. It is not uncommon to see generic phrases that refer to "appropriate disciplinary procedures" and "in the event of misconduct" tiptoeing across the pages of compliance plans. Every person hopes he or she will never have to use disciplinary action and do not want to risk creating trouble by outlining disciplinary measures that could be interpreted as too lenient or too severe.

However, generalizations in compliance plans can be dangerous. An effective compliance plan will "have teeth" in it in order to indicate that the organization takes compliance seriously. Although somewhat unpleasant to address, the written plan must include a section on the specific procedures the organization intends to use for enforcement. The discipline must be consistent for all levels of personnel and carry appropriate sanctions for violations, misconduct, and repeat offenses. This is much easier to do before actions are necessary.

Disciplinary actions may include the following:

- oral warnings,
- written reprimands,

Description of possible violation:
_____
_____

When did it occur? Provide exact dates, if possible.
_____
_____

Who was involved?
_____
_____

How did you come to learn of this incident?
_____
_____

Do you have any evidence?
_____
_____

Would you be willing to discuss further?
_____
_____

Have you discussed this with anyone else?
_____
_____

Are you aware of anyone else who might have information?
_____
_____

Date: _____
Name (optional): _____
Signature (optional): _____

We will take all possible steps to investigate each report of suspected violation. Be aware that if we cannot contact you for additional information, we may not be able to carry out a thorough investigation.

FIGURE 10-4 Report of Suspected Violation.

> - Have one or two reporting methods been established?
> - Are the reporting methods designed to protect confidentiality?
> - Does your employee handbook clearly state that it is the employee's responsibility to report suspected misconduct?
> - Does your employee handbook clearly state that employees who report will not suffer retaliation?
> - Do you communicate an open-door policy in your practice?
> - Do your bulletin boards and office correspondence carry messages to promote compliance?
> - Have you clearly stated to employees the intent of the plan and their roles in making the plan successful?
> - Would an entry-level person be able to explain:
>   — Why you have a plan
>   — When it was effective
>   — What the plan is supposed to do
> - Could an entry-level person talk to the compliance officer if he or she had to?

FIGURE 10-5 Compliance Communication Checklist.

- probation,
- demotion,
- temporary suspension,
- termination, and
- restitution of damages.

It is advisable to have legal counsel review the disciplinary measures before they are fully enacted.

Responding Promptly to Detected Offenses and Developing Corrective Action

Offenses are like skeletons in the closet. Once you find them, you have to deal with them. Regardless of the scope or the method by which the misconduct or suspected misconduct is discovered, all investigations must be handled systematically and with a cool head. Overreacting, becoming extremely angry, assuming someone is guilty before a thorough investigation because the person has always been suspected of inappropriate billing, or bringing a physician in front of the group can result in embarrassment and a loss of faith in the program. If a possible violation is detected, all reports and investigations should be held in strictest confidence, and any evidence that is discovered should be carefully documented. Although the discovery of evidence may be detrimental to the practice, it is extremely important that the investigators resist any temptation to bury, cover up, or alter evidence. Figure 10-6 can be used to document a discovered lapse in compliance.

Once the report has been filed, the compliance officer should keep facts and circumstances confidential and limit discussion of the findings to those parties who need to know. Centralizing reporting and oversight of investigations with a compliance officer and having a physician oversee the investigation enables the practice to consistently apply standards. Feedback on how the investigation is proceeding and findings regarding the possible need for policy or procedure changes can be given to physicians. Although it may be tempting to change some part of the compliance policy, all investigators should consider any changes to the plan as the result of investigations. A key consideration before making any changes is whether the changes are actually good for the plan or whether they are being recommended because the investigations were too unpleasant.

Refunding Overpayments

When a billing error occurs—whether or not it is intentional—any overpayment from Medicare must be refunded. Making the refund is simple to do, providing that the overpayment was for one service—that is, that it was an isolated incident. Overpayments are the result of an incorrect billing practice that has been in place for months (or even years). In this situation, determining the amount of overpayment and making the refund can be hazardous. For this reason, it is best to obtain legal counsel before proceeding.

Disclosure

Although the practice does have an obligation to refund money due Medicare or Medicaid, there is currently no legal responsibility to self-disclose. However, the OIG has given life to the belief that a practice has a legal duty to self-report incidents of misconduct. The OIG announced that compliance plans should include a policy of self-reporting and has published instructions regarding how, when, and to whom to report.[14] In its Provider Self-Disclosure Protocol, the OIG encourages providers to self-report in a prescribed manner.[15]

Providers who are interested in disclosing information concerning irregularities are asked to submit the disclosure in writing to the OIG and to do the following: (1) include information identifying the providers and entities involved; (2) indicate whether the provider has

Date report initiated: _____

Person(s) conducting investigation: _____
_____
_____

Description of incident: _____
_____
_____

How was the incident discovered? _____
_____
_____

Describe investigations performed: _____
_____
_____

People Interviewed			
Date	Name	Interviewer	Subject

Findings: _____
_____

Results of investigation: _____
_____

Disciplinary action taken: _____
_____

Corrective action implemented: _____
_____

Date incident closed: _____

Signed: _____

FIGURE 10-6 Billing Error/Misconduct Investigation.

knowledge of a current government or contractor inquiry into the matter; (3) provide a full description of the matter, including the type of claim, transaction, or conduct involved; (4) identify the type of provider and the provider's billing numbers; (5) set forth the reasons that the provider believes there may have been a violation of a criminal, civil, or administrative law; and (6) certify that the information submitted to the OIG is truthful and based on a good-faith effort to notify the government to resolve potential liabilities.

The protocol states that a disclosure report include a written narrative that, among other things, identifies the potential causes of the incident or practice, such as "intentional conduct" or "circumvention of corporate Government regulations." It also states that a disclosure report identify "corporate officials, employees, or agents who knew of, encouraged, or participated in" the incident of practice. Further, according to the protocol, the report should identify the "corporate officials, employee, or agents who should have known of, but failed to detect" the incident or practice at issue.[16]

Although a practice has no legal obligations to self-disclose, if serious overbilling is detected and no self-disclosure is made, the OIG could interpret this as the practice not having an effective compliance program in place. However, the following points should be taken into account when considering the terms of the OIG self-disclosure protocol:

- There are no assurances regarding the government's consideration and actions taken as a result of the voluntary disclosure protocol, although the OIG has indicated it will work in a cooperative fashion with the provider in discussing the disclosure to law enforcement agencies.
- No allowance is made for anonymous or hypothetical disclosure that will meet the standard of this protocol. The protocol calls for the furnishing of basic information that identifies the provider, the nature of the conduct, the type of matter being disclosed, and the health care provider numbers of those reporting.
- There are risks involved because the disclosure protocol requires multiple certifications by the provider as to the truthfulness and completeness of the information provided to the government and the provider's willingness to engage in a good-faith effort to assist the OIG in its inquiry and in the verification of the disclosed matter. These certifications carry substantial risks of further legal liability for the entity and for the person making such certifications.
- The protocol also seeks the names of the culpable individuals—those individuals who knew, or should have known and failed to detect, the practice.
- With the voluntary disclosure protocol, attorney-client privilege is waived.

Self-disclosures should never be decided on, for or against, without the assistance of legal counsel.

Conducting Internal Monitoring and Auditing

The OIG compliance plan guidance recommends that an audit be conducted within 90 days of establishing the compliance plan. This audit can act as a baseline, or "snapshot," to be used as part of the benchmarking analysis, which enables the practice to judge its progress in reducing or eliminating areas of potential vulnerability. These self-audits can be used to determine whether:

- bills are accurately coded and reflect the services provided,
- services and items are reasonable and necessary,
- any incentives to provide unnecessary services are in place, and
- medical records contain sufficient documentation to support the codes that are billed.

The audit should establish a consistent methodology for selecting the examining records to determine whether improvements are made during the life of the plan.

The compliance guidance further recommends that audits be conducted at least once a year. No set formula currently exists regarding how many records should be reviewed. A basic guide is 2 to 5 medical records per payer or 5 to 10 medical records per physician.

The guidance states:

> There are many ways to identify the claims or services from which to draw the random sample of claims to be audited. One methodology is to choose a random sample of claims/services from either all of the claims/services a physician has received reimbursement for or all claims/services from a particular payer. Another method is to identify risk areas or potential billing vulnerabilities. The codes associated with these risk areas may become the universe of claims or services from which to select the sample. The OIG recommends that the physician practice evaluate claims or services selected to determine if the codes billed and reimbursed were accurately ordered, performed, and reasonable and necessary for the treatment of the patient.[17]

One way to select records is to find where the physician's E/M code utilization varies significantly from the national distribution and focus on reviewing those codes. A comparison of utilization is shown in Figure 10-7.

In this example, Dr. A's utilization graph shows that he uses code 99213 much more than the national distribution. There is a high probability that some of his services coded 99213 were actually 99212, which means that they were overcoded and could pose a compliance risk. Conversely, some of those 99213 codes may have supported a higher code (with proper documentation) that represents a loss of revenue.

Dr. B, on the other hand, falls within line of the national distribution. A review of all levels of his code would verify that the documentation supports the level assigned.

Comparison of Provider Utilization

Computer-generated reports can reveal coding patterns and utilization for each code, broken down by procedure. Provider utilization can then be compared among the physicians in the practice or benchmarking standards. Presenting a graph (such as the one below) can clearly show the provider how his or her utilization compares with that of the other providers in the practice.

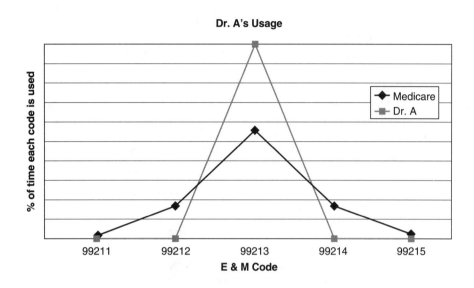

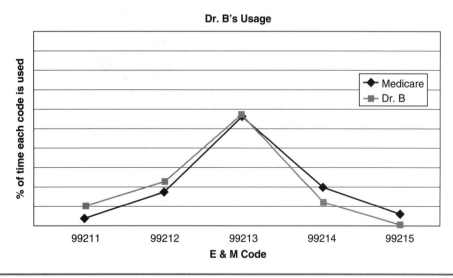

FIGURE 10-7 Comparison of Provider Utilization.

Once the audit has been completed, the results can be shared with the provider on a form such as a coding audit checklist. This feedback will assist the physician in learning where the lapses are.

Using a pie chart such as the one shown in Figure 10-8 is an excellent method to give feedback to providers regarding their accuracy in coding and documentation.

Warning Lights and Monitors

In developing the compliance plan, a practice may want to establish safeguards to detect problems before they become overwhelming issues. For example, the practice may want to monitor claim rejections or reductions of payment amounts. Figure 10-9 provides a sample of an explanation of benefits review form.

Monitoring can be accomplished by using various methods. In determining which method to use, the practice should select a monitoring plan that will work best for it. For example, if one person posts insurance payments, monitoring may be simple. The poster may review

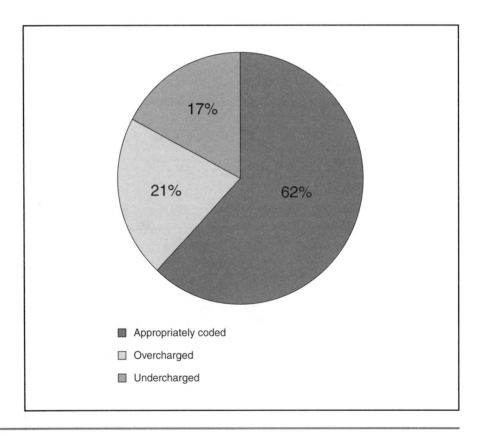

FIGURE 10-8 Overall Department Performance.

Period Ending: _____

Payer: _____

	Yes	No
Are contractual write-offs according to contract?	☐	☐
Are there any balance billing issues?	☐	☐
Are any services denied?	☐	☐

If yes, list:

Patient ID	Provider ID	CPT Code	Diagnosis Code	Reason

	Yes	No
Were there requests for additional information?	☐	☐
Where there any overpayment issues?	☐	☐

Findings: _____

Corrective action taken: _____

_____

_____

Review conducted by: _____ Date: _____

Abbreviations: Current Procedural Terminology (CPT); Explanation of Benefits (EOB); Identification (ID)

FIGURE 10-9 Sample Explanation of Benefits Review.

explanations of benefits on a weekly basis and report to the manager findings that summarize the following:

- the number of denials received,
- the reasons for the denials,
- corrective actions taken, and
- whether this is a pattern or a one-time incident.

Another way to measure how accurately the organization is submitting claims is by reviewing claims scrubber rejections. Often, only a limited number of staff members have access to these rejections, and the errors are typically corrected on the spot and the claims resubmitted. There is valuable information in these rejections that can tell an organization important information such as whether:

- the patient insurance information was entered correctly,
- the diagnosis code supports the service rendered,
- the diagnosis code is valid, and
- the NPI number associated with the claim is correct.

Monitoring these rejections closely will show a practice where its errors are. Monitoring should also include the following:

- periodic (such as quarterly) utilization review that examines coding patterns of E/M services, procedures, and diagnoses;
- monitoring of referral patterns—both referrals going out of the practice as well as those coming in;
- notation and review of large-dollar charge amounts as well as high payment adjustments from carriers. A periodic review of these areas may help a practice to correct irregularities before they become big problems.

Chart audits usually come to mind when we think of performing due diligence; however, practices can look in a variety of places to see whether they are in violation of any compliance issues. These areas are covered in the following discussion, which includes examples of actual discoveries.

Business Relationships. The first place to look is at the business relationships that the physicians and the organization have with other entities. All existing agreements or contracts should be reviewed to make sure that there are no violations. Although this process seems straightforward, and providers are accustomed to complying with the Stark Law and anti-kickback regulations, often organizations are engaged in contracts that are in clear violation of various statutes.

As an example, it was discovered that XYZ Pharmaceutical Company paid for a physician and his staff to attend a large, elegant banquet as a thank-you for prescribing the company's drugs. At the end of the evening, the Physician stood up and said, "Remember folks, be sure to sell XYZ Pharmaceuticals." The pharmaceutical company, in effect, was giving cash for patient referrals.

"Incident To" Services. Investigations into "incident to" services continue to appear on the OIG work plan. It is important to determine which nonphysician providers can bill E/M codes. Only four classifications of nonphysician providers can render E/M services at a level higher than CPT code 99211. They are

- certified clinical nurse specialists,
- certified nurse midwives,
- physician assistants, and
- nurse practitioners.

"Incident to" guidelines require that the physician be present in the office suite when the service is rendered in order for the procedure to be eligible for "incident to" billing. Additionally, the physician must have seen the patient initially and established a plan of care in order for the services to be "incident to." Guidelines also require that the physician have an active part in the patient's ongoing care.

Some practices make the mistake of applying "incident to" guidelines to all services that the support staff furnishes. Diagnostic and therapeutic procedures do not fall under the "incident to" guidelines but have their own set of guidelines under the supervisory requirements of testing. The supervision requirements for each test can be found by CPT code on the CMS Website Physician Fee Lookup Tool at www.cms.hhs.gov/PFSLookup/.

Some nonphysician providers, such as nutritionists, geneticists, and diabetes educators from a certified American Diabetes Association training program, have no technical codes to bill. Because they are not permitted to use the E/M codes, these practitioners have no way to bill directly for their services. To avoid this problem, many offices incorporate some very ingenious—yet questionable—ways to attempt to gain reimbursement. Although some may use code 99211, which is "non-MD visit," or code 99499, the "unlisted procedure" code, these practitioners cannot be separately reimbursed for their services.

Even providers who are entitled to bill for E/M services must take care that those services are adequately provided and that the services are documented according to guidelines. Moreover, these providers must follow the guidelines that physicians must follow and they must bill either under the physician's provider number, which calls for following "incident to" guidelines, or under their own provider numbers and receive less reimbursement from Medicare.

Other Areas to Review. Other areas to review for possible compliance violations include the following:

- If practicing at more than one location (eg, a satellite office), physicians need separate provider numbers for each location. If a satellite location should close, the physician must advise Medicare that he or she is no longer using that provider number. Stealing practitioners' provider numbers and using them to bill is a form of intentional Medicare fraud that unscrupulous providers are using. As a result, physicians' provider numbers should be guarded as carefully as Drug Enforcement Administration numbers or Social Security numbers.

- Violations may occur due to lack of awareness. Therefore, it is important to educate employees about important issues. For instance, staff must understand that they are not allowed to accept gifts in return for referrals, nor can they accept gifts of cash. Also, they cannot engage in arrangements to purchase goods for a referral stream, such as with a relative who sells equipment and says, "You know, I have lots of contacts—I could send you lots of patients if you buy your office supplies from me." Employees who enter into such agreements, written or not, leave the practice vulnerable.

- Review explanations of benefits rejections, denials, and requests for additional information—this is often a good way to find out where billing problems are occurring. Also, look at how services are being billed. Billing clerks and collectors may be adding a modifier to get a claim paid, but that modifier may or may not be appropriate to coding guidelines.

- Monitor front-desk and billing functions to make sure that protocols are being followed. Often, when employees are questioned, they can repeat the rules and protocols verbatim. Nevertheless, if they do not understand the importance of those protocols, these employees may not perform their job functions as the protocols stipulate.

- Education and training can be a big problem if you have a high rate of staff turnover. Processes that were reviewed and working well six months ago may not work well now because of new staff members who have not yet been trained. Therefore, ongoing evaluation and assessment of training is of the utmost importance. Likewise, offices with little or no staff turnover might have a longtime employee who is reluctant to modify routines or feels loyal by supporting the doctor in his or her reluctance to change. Assessing the personalities and working relationships in the office is also beneficial. Chart audits, of course, are central to due diligence, and it is advisable to establish a baseline passing grade or compliance performance. A good consulting firm should then help the organization establish a follow-up plan that the organization can easily use.

- What happens to Medicare newsletters and directives? If these are not being kept in a central location, it is likely that some of the information is getting lost and not being implemented. Ask the people in charge of billing and coding, "Who do you go to when you have a coding question?" If they do not have a ready resource, chances are they are doing a lot of guesswork if something new comes up. Ask to see the office's coding resources. At the minimum, there should be current *Current Procedural Terminology (CPT®)*; *International Classification of Diseases, 9th Edition*; and *Healthcare Common Procedure Coding System* manuals published by reliable sources.[18,19] Other resources to have on hand are specialty coding books, information from seminars the employees have attended, publications by your specialty society, Medicare newsletters and directives, and a *National Correct Coding Initiative Coding Policy Manual for Medicare Services* (coding policy manual).[20]

Conclusion

The goal of compliance is to reduce the likelihood of risk and exposure to penalties that infractions would bring upon the practice. However, experience shows that compliance plans are difficult—if not impossible—to enact if the practice's motives are different from this goal. Compliance plans will fail if the objective is anything less than adherence to the legislation in place. Moreover, for a practice's plan to remain an effective tool against violations of fraud and abuse statutes, compliance programs require repetitive training of employees.

When the OIG looks at a plan to determine its effectiveness, it considers a number of factors. Among them is management's commitment to compliance measured by funding and the legitimate support and involvement of its high-ranking members.

References

1. U.S. Department of Health and Human Services, Office of Inspector General. Semiannual Report to Congress, October 1, 2008–March 31, 2009. Accessed 9/30/2009 at http://oig.hhs.gov/publications/docs/semiannual/2009/semiannual_spring2009.pdf. Page v.

2. *Ibid*, pp. 74–75.
3. U.S. Department of Justice. *False Claims Act Cases: Government Intervention in Qui Tam (Whistleblower) Suits*. Accessed 6/11/2010 at www.justice.gov/usao/pae/Documents/fcaprocess2.pdf.: 1.
4. American Medical Association. *Current Procedural Terminology (CPT®) Professional Edition 2009*. Chicago, IL: American Medical Association; 2008.
5. U.S. Department of Health and Human Services, Office of Inspector General. Semiannual Report to Congress, October 1, 2008–March 31, 2009, p. 74. Accessed 9/30/2009 at http://oig.hhs.gov/publications/docs/semiannual/2009/semiannual_spring2009.pdf.
6. U.S. Department of Health and Human Services, Office of Inspector General. Semiannual Report to Congress, October 1, 2008–March 31, 2009, p. 74. Accessed 6/11/2010 at http://oig.hhs.gov/publications/docs/semiannual/2009/semiannual_spring2009.pdf.
7. U.S. Department of Health and Human Services, Centers for Medicare and Medicaid Services. *42 CFR Parts 411 and 424, Medicare Program; Physicians' Referrals to Health Care Entities With Which They Have Financial Relationships (Phase III); Final Rule*. Accessed 9/5/2007 at http://edocket.access.gpo.gov/2007/pdf/07-4252.pdf.
8. Since the Federal Trade Commission (FTC) first issued the set of regulations referred to as "Red Flags Rule" in November 2007, there has been a controversy regarding application of the Rule to physicians and medical billing services. At the end of May 2010, the American Medical Association successfully obtained yet another delay from the FTC regarding the Red Flags Rule until December 31, 2010.

    The AMA continues to work to convince the FTC that physicians should be exempt from the rule. It should be noted AMA has held this position for the past two years. The Rule applies to an institution which operates as a "creditor". It has been FTC's stand that physicians fall into the creditor status because they provide services on credit awaiting insurance payment or in some instances enters into payment arrangements with patients for their medical billing services. http://ezinearticles.com/?Red-Flags-Rule—Facts-For-Physicians&id=4435826. June 11, 2010.
9. Practice Management Center, American Medical Association. Protect your patients, protect your practice: What you need to know about the Red Flags Rule. Accessed 4/26/2010 at www.ama-assn.org/ama1/pub/upload/mm/368/red-flags-rule-edu.pdf.
10. U.S. Department of Health and Human Services, Centers for Medicare and Medicaid Services. *Medicare Claim Review Programs: MR, MCCI Edits, MUEs, CERT, and RAC*. October, 2008; p. 1. Accessed 10/1/2009 at www.cms.hhs.gov/MLNProducts/downloads/MCRP_Booklet.pdf.
11. TrailBlazer Health Enterprises. *Part B Provider Compliance Error Rate (PCER)*. August, 2009; p. 1. Accessed 10/30/2009 at www.trailblazerhealth.com/Publications/Job%20Aid/PCERjobaid.pdf.
12. U.S. Department of Health and Human Services, Centers for Medicare and Medicaid Services, Center for Medicaid and State Operations, Medicaid Integrity Group. *Comprehensive Medicaid Integrity Plan of the Medicaid Integrity Program, FY 2006 – 2010*. July, 2006. Accessed 10/1/2009 at www.cms.hhs.gov/DeficitReductionAct/Downloads/CMIP2006.pdf.

13. U.S. Department of Health and Human Services, OIG Compliance Program. *Guidance for third party medical billing companies. Fed Reg.* 1998;63(243):70138. Accessed 6/11/2010 at http://oig.hhs.gov/fraud/docs/complianceguidance/nhsolicit.pdf.
14. Luce GM. Falling on your sword doesn't have to be deadly. *J Health Care Compliance.* 1999;March/April, 1(2):35–39.
15. U.S. Department of Health and Human Services, *OIG's provider self-disclosure protocol. Fed. Reg.* 1998;63(210):58399. Accessed 6/11/2010 at http://frwebgate.access.gpo.gov/cgi-bin/getdoc.cgi?dbname=1998_register&docid=98-29111-filed.pdf.
16. Wackler AP, Avery PA. OIG issues new voluntary government investigations. *J Med Pract Manage.* 1999;15(3):147–149.
17. U.S. Department of Health and Human Services. *OIG Compliance Program for Individual and Small Group Physician Practices. Fed. Reg.* 2000;65(194):59438. Accessed 6/11/2010 at www.umsl.edu/~garziar/OIG_compprog.pdf.
18. Coding is the process of assigning a procedure code (CPT® or HCPCS code) and a diagnosis code (ICD-9 DM) to a physician service that accurately describes what the physician did for or to the patient and the patient's condition or the reason for the service. It includes rules for the use of modifiers and description of multiple procedures.
19. HCPCS codes are standard code sets used by health care providers and health insurance payers to report and pay claims. Level one HCPCS codes are CPT® codes developed, maintained, and copyrighted by the American Medical Association. The level two codes are developed and maintained by CMS to describe services not defined by CPT® codes.
20. *National Correct Coding Initiative Coding Policy Manual for Medicare Services* (Coding Policy Manual). Accessed 12/11/2009 at www.cms.hhs.gov/NationalCorrectCodInitEd/Downloads/NCCI_Policy_Manual.zip.

CHAPTER 11
Information Technology and Reimbursement

The Role of Information Systems in the Revenue Cycle

OUTLINE

I. Introduction
II. Revenue-Enhancing Features
    A. Electronic Health Records Charge Capture
    B. Portability Devices for Providers
    C. Patient Portal Access and Kiosks
    D. Real-Time Insurance Verification
    E. Reporting Tools
    F. Telephone and E-mail Reminder Systems
    G. Automated Advanced Beneficiary Notice Checking
    H. Simplification of Documentation
III. Best of Breed versus One Throat to Choke
IV. Managing a Conversion Successfully
    A. Assembling an Implementation Team
        1. Clinical Support
        2. Technical Resources
    B. Establishing Buy-In
    C. The Implementation Plan
    D. EHR Implementation Strategy
        1. Set Expectations
        2. EHR "Roll-Out" Timing
        3. EHR Specialist Role
        4. Training

E. Transforming Workflow
   1. Why, When, and How to Improve Workflow
   2. What Needs to Change
V. Conclusion

Introduction

Modern information systems that are properly deployed and implemented can shorten the revenue cycle and, in turn, improve cash flow. Many new features are available that enhance a practice's income, including automated charge capture and portable devices that enable charge capture at the point of service from remote locations such as hospitals, patient portals, and real-time insurance verification. The return on investment (ROI) for upgrading or purchasing a new information system can definitely justify the expenditure. If the proper expectations are set at the beginning and implementation is intentional, the ROI is significant. If the practice management (PM) system does not support real-time claims monitoring through electronic submission and remittance, direct patient-entered demographic and insurance information, automated payment posting, and user-friendly reporting tools, it is time to consider replacing this legacy system with a new one.

This chapter addresses the revenue-enhancing features of information technology, the pros and cons of integrated systems and single systems, successful management of conversion from paper to electronic applications, and essential changes in workflow with the adoption of an electronic process.

Revenue-Enhancing Features

Among the applicable features of information technology available to augment the revenue cycle are electronic health records (EHR) charge capture, portability devices for providers, patient portal access and kiosks, real-time insurance verification, reporting tools, telephone and e-mail reminder systems, automated advanced beneficiary notice (ABN) checking, and simplification of documentation.

Electronic Health Records Charge Capture

Fully integrated EHRs and practice management systems advance the revenue cycle by improving coding at the point of care, ensuring more accurate claims by providing decision support that links proper

International Classification of Diseases, Ninth Revision (ICD-9) codes with procedures, decreasing the time frame from charges incurred to claim submission, and improving documentation to support higher visit codes. Using an EHR to document a patient visit can improve profits by reducing costs. Documenting an office encounter electronically can save on transcription time and services, file storage, and costs associated with chart distribution. A fully implemented EHR can assist a provider in proper coding, adding 3 to 15%, on average, to the visit. Additionally, a practice can realize a 1.5 to 5% increase in billing by ensuring all charges are captured.[1]

Full integration, which is having a practice management system that is capable of applying accurate demographic, insurance, and clinical information to every encounter and charge, is a key feature. Full integration ensures charges are passed from the point of the encounter to the PM system and through the clearinghouse with minimal effort and with great reliability and accuracy. Full integration also guarantees that the practice management and EHR systems are always in sync and functioning as a single system to seamlessly support both the business and clinical aspects of the practice.

Portability Devices for Providers

With devices such as iPhones, BlackBerrys, and other mobile tools, providers can capture their charges at the point of service and transmit them directly to the practice management system for submission to the clearinghouse. Gone are the crumpled papers containing provider's rounds charges, which may or may not get returned on a timely basis. This technology makes it possible to send information more efficiently with the net result of a shortened revenue cycle and improved cash flow.

Patient Portal Access and Kiosks

The best way to improve the accuracy of patient demographics and insurance information is to have the patients enter this information themselves. Patient portals allow patients to use the Internet to access their personal information. Through a secure log-in, patients can view their accounts, pay outstanding balances online, and ensure demographic information is accurate and up-to-date. Similar to airport self check-in, kiosks allow patients to check in at appointment time and verify the accuracy of demographic and insurance information. The benefit to the patient is minimal waiting and accurate claims management. The benefit to the practice is improved accuracy, which minimizes denials for inaccurate patient demographics and require fewer staff to handle the registration process. Many practices use patient portals to allow patients to schedule appointments and to invite patients in for preventive and health maintenance visits.

Additional cost savings are realized when patients request prescription refills and check lab and test results through the portal. The revenue cycle improvements are transparent. The benefit to the patient is improved patient convenience and response times. The benefit to the practice is improved patient satisfaction and patient compliance. Additionally, patients are engaged in their health care, which is rewarded through pay for performance. Portals also support asynchronous communication, which improves the efficiency of patient communication for the practice; patients' needs can be addressed at the convenience of the staff, and phone interruptions are minimized.

Real-Time Insurance Verification

Most modern PM information systems allow the practice to send an inquiry to the patient's insurance company and request verification of coverage in real time when the patient presents for an appointment. The insurance company response alerts the practice if the patient is not eligible for services. The insurance company can also send additional relevant information regarding the patient payment due at the time of the office visit, such as co-payments and needs for prior authorization. At the time of service, the practice knows if it has the right insurance, holding down rejections downstream in the revenue cycle. This feature is continually improving as more practices use the function, thus encouraging payers to deliver better real-time information.

Reporting Tools

Information accessibility through reports and digital dashboards is improving and creating strong decision tools. User-friendly reporting allows access to real-time information for improved and quicker decision making; decentralizes access to data to individual managers; and provides for robust analysis of business data. It allows management to identify and focus on areas that will have the greatest impact on the organization. As a result, the practice is more apt to solve problems at their source. Data entered into these systems can be easily queried and reported on with more sophisticated tools than ever before. The key is to select a system with robust reporting tools that enable the practice to create its own reports as needed in addition to prewritten reports included in the system.

Telephone and E-mail Reminder Systems

Patients and providers often forget to talk about preventive and health maintenance services. Reminder systems have a two-fold solution to this problem. First, they are set up to automatically call patients and remind them of appointments. Although this type of system has been a part of most medical practices for some time, modern systems allow for rules to be formulated to support population-based care. Second, the practice can query and contact patients who are due or overdue for routine health screenings, disease prevention procedures, and health maintenance activities and invite them in for care. Sophisticated telephone and e-mail reminder systems empower practices to improve ancillary and provider productivity, therefore, improving revenue.

Automated Advanced Beneficiary Notice Checking

Some systems offer automated advance beneficiary notice (ABN) checking that is integrated with the practice management and EHR systems. At the point of care this software provides decision support to the provider that an ABN will be required, suggests existing problems on the patient's problem list that would support the test being ordered, and decreases the number of denials for not obtaining and including the ABN with the claim.

Simplification of Documentation

Advising physicians of appropriate coding eliminates the tendency to "under code" just to be safe. The EHR allows for more accurate coding, with the ability to automate complete supporting documentation, and provides built-in coding assistants based on E/M guidelines.

Best of Breed versus One Throat to Choke

The concept of a fully integrated PM system was mentioned earlier in this chapter. Information technology was first introduced to health care to provide for patient registration and scheduling and to support the medical practice's billing functions. As EHRs have gained popularity, practices need to decide whether to maintain their legacy PM system and interface it to a best-of-breed electronic medical record or to replace the system with a single system that meets functionality requirements for both the business and clinical sides of the organization.

The benefits of a fully integrated system include the following:

- Fully integrated practice management and EHRs are on a single trajectory for upgrade and maintenance. The vendor ensures the systems will continue to work together to support the business and clinical functions required.

- Although they are generally more costly, fully integrated systems are less expensive to own because the vendor incurs the cost of maintaining integration and developing the products on the same trajectory.
- Fully integrated systems offer improved functionality. They support direct charge capture, a single master patient index, and direct interaction of the PM components with the clinical application. Direct charge capture gets charges into the PM system to be billed more quickly. Adding ICD-9 codes as discrete data in the clinical application makes it possible to populate the charges in the PM system and then pass them on to the clearinghouse. This practice all but eliminates manual charge entry. A single master patient index decreases error by having one database that houses all patient demographic and insurance information. In a fully integrated system, orders for ancillaries are entered and then tasked to the referral and prior authorization department, decreasing incidents where patients present for tests and consults without referrals or prior authorizations or without proper preparation for a test. A prepared, engaged patient is less costly to care for, more compliant with treatment options, and increases opportunity for pay for performance.

The disadvantage of a fully integrated system over interfacing a PM system with an EHR product is primarily cost and complexity. Fully integrated systems tend to be more expensive up front and require more server hardware and expertise to manage.

Managing a Conversion Successfully

The decision to implement a new application is significant, both as a financial investment and as an investment of resources to manage the transition from paper to electronic. For many practices, implementation is a defining moment in the practice life cycle. Assimilation of a conversion requires commitment from everyone: physicians, management personnel, and staff. It is a costly venture, from the up-front costs of hardware, software, networking, and support, to the disruption of the practice and potential lost income as the practice slows down while bringing various features "live." Yet, the return on investment (ROI) and potential for improved patient safety and reduced errors makes the endeavor worthwhile. Once a practice selects a vendor that is aligned with the practice's requirements, the success rides on the implementation. The ability to properly plan the implementation, knowing the strengths and understanding weaknesses of the practice, can make all the difference. A course of action that leads to a successful conversion encompasses the following:

- assembling a team,
- establishing buy-in,
- crafting an individualized implementation plan, and
- executing the plan.

Assembling an Implementation Team

A successful transition requires leadership from a team of people who will gather the institutional knowledge needed to make key decisions. Managing a successful conversion requires attention and intention directed at five basic components: technology, system design, implementation planning (which includes project timelines, system file-build, workflow reengineering, training, evaluation, and communication), support, and ongoing system development. A practice must assemble an implementation team to carry out its mission. Without a strong team as a foundation, all efforts will fail.

The transition process must be managed because it is during this time that the practice will move from a comfortable place of "knowing" to the new normal. During implementation, it is important to think beyond the way processes are performed today using old systems. It is the program manager's job to ensure the practice makes the transition and does not layer new processes on top of old one.

Successful organizations include members on the implementation team who can contribute knowledge about current processes and preserve what is working while remaining open to using the new system to make improvements. A typical implementation team includes the following functional roles:

- Program manager/consultant
    - Provides guidance and leadership related to overall project plan, system administrative file-build, training methodology and organization, system deployment, end-user hardware, and change management.
    - Assists the implementation team in interpreting project evaluation data, adjusting the project plan as necessary.
    - Provides guidance as to best practices in terms of the implementation and the system.
    - Keeps the project on task, on time, and on budget.

- Acts as a liaison to the vendor implementation staff as necessary.
- Project manager
  - Works directly with the program manager to organize, coordinate, and communicate progress at the practice.
  - Creates lines of accountability for the program manager to continuously monitor progress.
  - Informs the program manager of specific needs and requirements to ensure success and a quality product.
  - Creates accountability among project team members to assist in keeping the project on time, on budget, and true to project objectives.
- Physician leadership
  - Acts as a liaison with physicians as the team works to make the implementation plan operational.
  - Works closely with team members to provide leadership and guidance on all aspects of the project that require direct physician input and cooperation.
  - Acts as a liaison to governing boards to give regular project progress reports.
- Management Information Systems (MIS) director
  - Manages technology infrastructure and deployment, interface development and maintenance, and other information technology (IT) resources.
  - Purchases, configures, and deploys end-user hardware.
  - Configures and deploys networks, including wireless as needed.
  - Analyzes implementation evaluation data and adjusts project plan accordingly.
- Application specialists
  - Directs the initial build of the administrative tables that drive the system.
  - Modifies and customizes the system to meet practice requirements.
  - Prepares the system for training and live environment.
  - Manages and maintains all administrative tables.
  - Participates in development of workflows.
- Power users
  - Tests all content and workflows, the training environment, and training materials.
  - Reviews workflows, training methodologies, and plans.

- Puts into operation phases of the project plan; assist in progress evaluation; provide feedback related to additional training needs, workflow revision, and content revision.
- Provides classroom and "at-the-elbow" training for end-users.

Clinical Support

One might think that once a new PM system is in place, the business managers can relax. However, as the practice moves to using the system's EHR features, it is important to consider the impact on the business. Used correctly, an EHR system provides for the greatest opportunity to realize cost savings and efficiency. The clinical staff needs to become comfortable with the use of computers in order to document patient information as close to the encounter as possible. The practice must guard against using the EHR as a digitized paper repository and instead use it to support the workflow and workload of the clinical environment. Documenting family and social history, medical and surgical history, current medications and problems, history of the present illness, chief complaint, and vital signs at the point of care improves accuracy, efficiency, and quality of care and, ultimately, positively impacts the practice's bottom line.

Because physicians are usually the only revenue generator for the practice, freeing them up to see patients improves revenue generation and reduces the cost per visit. Tasks and workflow processes are shifted so that everyone on the clinical team is working at their level of their expertise and maximizing success.

Technical Resources

A strong technical team is a must for success. There needs to be a commitment of money, time, staff, and infrastructure. The group should be knowledgeable, flexible, and tenacious. These technical resources will be required to manage the hardware, software, and interfaces.

Establishing Buy-In

A successful conversion requires acceptance of the move to new processes and workflows involved in EHR technology applications. The practice must select a strong leader from each operational and clinical area in the practice to advocate for the new system. These champions should be computer-savvy and able to share the vision.

The planning should start early. It should include promoting the system at staff meetings and making sure everyone is as involved with the planning as they want to be. This part of the process may uncover some champions that could otherwise have been overlooked.

To ensure that everyone is comfortable having a computer on his or her desk, get the hardware early and introduce it into everyone's work space. Train staff to use Microsoft Windows by allowing them to play solitaire, if that helps—whatever improves eye/hand/mouse coordination.

Train! Train! Train! At first glance, the training sessions may seem to be keeping staff away from the office for too long. Don't worry! The investment of time up front will save many headaches down the road. The practice cannot afford to skimp on training for the administrator, managers, clinicians, and staff. Everyone needs it and will benefit from it. Simulations are also valuable and enable staff to deal with situations that may not otherwise be thought of without the pressure of being "live."

It is essential to stop every now and then to see how everyone is doing with the process. Mechanically, this can be staged and organized. How are people reacting to the change? Does anyone need extra training or support? Is anyone going to torpedo the efforts due to a lack of information or desire? With the right champions, and by checking in with everyone regularly, big surprises will be averted.

The champions should continue to convene in order to review progress and share new ideas. By working together, they are a great resource for the entire staff. The champions should be encouraged to teach informally and ensure buy-in continues to be strong and to make the needed adjustments.

The Implementation Plan

It is necessary to follow a disciplined project management process when working through the implementation plan. The steps are as follows:

1. Create a plan.
2. Share the plan.
3. Follow the plan.
4. Evaluate the plan's effectiveness.
5. Revise the plan.

The next step in successful conversion is to define what needs to be accomplished, set a timeline to accomplish these goals, and establish a strategy for successful implementation of new technology. Listen to the vendor, successful users, and experts. Work with the vendor's implementation team and empower your project manager. Start with the vendor's statement of work (SOW) and progress to a detailed project plan.

There are various ways to implement a new PM and EHR software solution. Following is a recommended method that will minimize the number of interruptions to the practice and ease physicians into going electronic.

If implementing a fully integrated PM and EMR system, it is recommended that the PM system be installed first and that 60 to 90 days pass before rolling out the EMR system. The rationale is to train the front office staff so that they are available for the medical staff to begin navigating the new system. It also gives the practice two monthly cycles to work out any issues and ensure cash flow is maintained.

Make key decisions early. Some areas include:

- Import. Decide what information from the current system should be imported to the new system. This can include demographics, payer files, scheduling, and more. Begin to clean up old files before sending them over to be imported.

- Timing. Decide when is the best time to go live. Most practices set a date that is at the end of a quarter and at the first of the month. If possible (and highly recommended), have physicians take vacation and/or reduce the work load. Optimally, close the office for the first day and turn off phones, or see patients in the afternoon only. This can reduce tension and reduce distractions, allowing staff to focus and adjust to the new system. Tell the staff well in advance to not take vacations or make personal appointments for the week or two before and after "going live." Be realistic and have staff understand that a system installation is above their regular duties and will require longer hours and possibly time on weekends. Although this may not be received well, it is better to set the expectation up front. Encourage staff by reassuring them of the benefits of the new system.

- Training. Decide who should be trained on what. First, make sure the workflow is correct for the new system. Ask the question, are the proper personnel in the correct jobs? With a new system, an opportunity opens to evaluate the practice's workflow. Think of how a patient will be seen and map out what type of staff member should be handling that task. Accomplish this by making a list of employees and their current job functions. Then shuffle staff around as needed and list the training that will be needed. One option is to assign those who are more computer savvy to be the point persons (or trainers) for that area; then, "train the trainers." It would be helpful for these trainers to have an understanding of how the system is loaded, know from where the data for specific fields are being pulled, and gain an overall view of how it fits together. That way, if something is not performing properly, problems usually can be solved. Those who are not comfortable with computers should familiarize themselves with a mouse by playing games or generating e-mails ahead of time. These individuals will be better prepared to learn the system and not be learning how to navigate a more modern system at the same time.

While the PM system is being established, preparations for EHR system implementation can begin. Form a committee with one person designated to work with the vendor and physicians. This person should look at patient files and group sections where specific information will be placed the new system. Also, the group should decide what information in the current files should be scanned. Interfaces such as labs should also begin. As the process progresses, documentation and templates can be built.

Following are recommendations for implementing an EMR system.

EHR Implementation Strategy

Managing the transition is another key element in successful implementation; it is important to be realistic as to how much change the practice and staff can manage at one time. Often, groups allow the vendor to impose an implementation strategy that is not aligned with the group's capability. It is acceptable and advisable for the practice to push back on a vendor plan if it feels like it is too much too soon. The vendor knows the product but they do not know the practice and how to best phase in the application. A primary goal for the vendor is to get a client's practice live as efficiently as possible in order to move on to the next practice. In this way, the vendor limits their costs of implementation and maximizes their revenues. Their recommended method, therefore, may or may not be the best method for the practice. Consideration must be given to the amount of time that the group can spend on the project, the practice's tolerance of risk, the staff's ability to adapt to change, and the degree of disruption the practice can tolerate while continuing to meet the needs of patients.

To implement at a more gradual pace, follow the four phases in Figure 11-1.

Set Expectations

Many implementations are perceived as a failure when in reality the expectations were unrealistic. Before the practice undertakes the venture, list why the group is implementing electronic charting. Some examples are to stay ahead of government regulations, participate in a patient quality reporting initiative (PQRI), gain efficiencies in the practice, improve the patient experience, maintain a competitive edge with community members, and gain better access to patient information. Set a time frame to achieve applicable goals. Examine the goals to make sure they are realistic and get buy-in along the way. Keep staff aware of these goals and revisit them prior to going live. Give quarterly or monthly feedback as the goals are tracked. Further develop and communicate the evaluation metrics associated with each phase of the project. When staff knows what is expected of them, they can better hit their marks.

Phase 1: Chart Access/Messaging/e-prescribing

- Begin scanning parts of the existing paper chart and preloading abstract patient information, using the future schedule.
- Have providers and nursing staff who access patient information use the electronic chart.
- Start using the messaging for interoffice communication such as phone notes and patient questions.
- Begin using e-prescribing as soon as possible to realize its advantages and incentives from Medicare.

Phase 2: Order Interfacing

The next phase allows for needed functionality from the new product.
- Begin managing orders for lab and diagnostic testing. Instead of looking at scanned paper responses for labs and results, medical staff can begin managing orders for lab and diagnostic testing. This functionality also allows for orders and results reconciliation to ensure that orders are completed properly.
- Results can go right to the physician's desktop for sign-off and management of subsequent studies that may be indicated. The practice can receive information directly with the interface and reduce handling time and expense.

Phase 3: Point-of-Care Documentation

- Begin to document patient visits using predefined templates in order to eliminate dictation.
- The practice can further break down this phase by separating the type of patient visit. For example, only begin electronic charting for new patient appointments. The key to this roll-out is to make sure that once a patient is "electronic," all health care providers document electronically going forward for that patient.

Physicians will begin to see the benefit of having documentation completed at the time of a visit along with immediate access to previous patient notes.

Phase 4: Charge Capture

Use of the four-phase approach separates direct charge capture from the documentation phase. This technique allows for minimal disruption of cash flow and lessens the financial impact to the practice while the glitches are worked out in the templates. This time period should be limited to 45 days because it slows down the ability to be efficient and get to ROI. In addition, most practices experience more accurate coding by using the direct charge capture function. During this period, physician input is monitored to ensure all charges are being entered accurately and completely. Be sure to ask your vendor if charge capture is an "all or nothing proposition." It is best if it can be turned on by the provider so that it can be tested before it is implemented practice wide.

FIGURE 11-1 Four Phases of Implementation

EMR "Roll-Out" Timing

Timing of the implementation plan is another vital consideration. Some implementations fail or struggle because the product was rolled out at the wrong time. Timing could mean the time of year. For example, implementing an EHR at a pediatric practice during flu season would likely not be successful. If the practice is in Florida, the "off season" or summer might be a better fit. Also, if the phased-in approach is being used, consider conducting the first phase of scanning during the summer when college students are available to assist at a reduced labor cost.

EHR Specialist Role

Some practices state that one reason for their smooth implementation was that they appointed a medically trained employee as the EHR specialist. This person's role is to work with physicians and other staff members in developing the workflows and templates. During training, the EHR specialist will assist the vendor in training and work with any physicians or nurses who need additional help. After implementation, this position transitions to being an advocate for the product. The EHR specialist answers questions, alters templates, and makes sure that all functionality is being used to its full potential. This person is aware of the new enhancements and will train the staff after the vendor sends the latest version update. This avoids the natural reaction to stay where the group is comfortable and not fully utilize the system. This is a way to stay current and truly recognize the ROI.

Training

Training is a key element in successful implementation. Having staff with knowledge of the product, as well as software trainers to assist and be ready to implement, minimizes confusion when the product is first being used. What can the practice do?

- Contractually require the vendor to appoint a trainer with a minimum of two years of experience with the product.
- Ensure there are enough hours budgeted for training of nursing staff, providers, and other employees who will be accessing the EHR (eg, the billing department).
- Practice, practice, practice. Hold a dress rehearsal prior to the go-live day and simulate patient visits for various diagnoses to aid in training and memory recall. During the mock visit, include the usual "oh, by the way" comments from patients that will drive a change in documentation. This will give the staff confidence in their ability to add things "on the fly" in a real situation.

Transforming Workflow

When implementing new technology, the temptation is to layer the new electronic processes over the older, more manual processes. A critical success factor in implementing new systems is to reengineer the manual processes in the context of the new electronic system.

Reflect on how patients and information flow through the organization before going through the paper to electronic transformation. It is essential to optimizing workflow processes and managing the transition. A tool for documenting and recognizing areas for improvement is called process mapping. When properly used, management can find opportunities to make the practice more efficient, usually reducing full-time equivalents (FTEs) and improving patient satisfaction. This section focuses on why process mapping is important, when it should be used, how to map processes, and the processes that are typically reengineered as part of the transformation from paper to electronic health records.

Why, When, and How to Improve Workflow

Workflow improvement becomes even more important when moving from a paper to an electronic environment. Methods that work well on paper may not transfer to an electronic process. Additionally, a practice that automates a bad workflow is guaranteeing that it will repeat that same error more efficiently and consistently than ever before.

Workflow analysis is a discipline. Some workflows are badly planned and should be corrected. Other workflows are adequate in a nonautomated setting but are inefficient or value-limiting when maintained in an electronic environment. Some workflows are hidden "best practices" used in portions of a practice, unknown to the rest of the organization. In an electronic environment, workflow standardization is crucial to the success of the transformation. Most practices use personnel and additional paper forms to solve problems. Workflow analysis and redesign has the additional benefit of streamlining processes, improving efficiency, and lowering costs.

The desire to hold on to individualization in a medical practice is strong. Often, long-term employees are wedded to processes for job security or because they have never completed a particular process in any other way. Fear of the unknown is a big hindrance. Particularly in multisite, multispecialty practices, standardization improves quality, ensures a unified patient and provider experience, and allows for more efficient and effective use of staff.

Workflow analysis and reengineering is a part of any sensible, well-thought-out implementation plan. In a phased approach, workflows are addressed at each phase. Introducing change in small increments both to the organization and the infrastructure ensures resources are in place and adequate to support the new environment. This approach also enhances the assimilation of new workflows and clinical functionality of the electronic chart. Do not expect workflow reengineering to happen overnight or without some disruption. Balancing the amount of disruption is critical to successful transformation. With too little disruption, change will not happen and things will slide back into the old and comfortable processes. Too much disruption and the practice will be so stressed that change will be resisted and the temptation to remove the conflict and return to the comfortable processes will be too great for the initiative to succeed.

Setting expectations that all processes will be reviewed and reengineered during implementation planning is the best and most successful technique. Communicating expectations to staff, training staff in the context of the reengineered workflows, and evaluating success within that context is critical to implementation success. Workflow transformation begins with understanding the elements of health care delivery.

The health care delivery model consists of six elements: care acquisition; patient record; test, and examination; diagnosis; treatment; and monitor, evaluate, and revise (Table 11-1). Each element has tasks associated with it, and each task requires review and ultimate reengineering. Mapping current process flow, diagramming each area, and assessing its efficiency will provide the practice with a better understanding of each area and the opportunity to improve practice productivity. The process map shown in Figure 11-2 was created using Microsoft Visio. It is an easy-to-use and valuable program to have when implementing an EHR.

Approach each area of function, including patient and information flow. Begin with a patient entry point, such as a new patient appointment call or a referral to the practice. Create various scenarios, branching off each situation on the process map. Identify stakeholder interaction, bottlenecks, time analysis, triggers, error rates, and more.

What Needs to Change

The tasks that typically need refinement during an EHR implementation are listed as follows:

- Internal messaging
- Phone system procedures
- Centralized check-in
- Prescription refills
- Lab and test order management
- Documenting an encounter
- Centralized check-out

Each task is addressed by examining how most practices perform current procedures, recommended best practice, the benefits of changing, and the potential issues the practice may incur during the reengineering process.

Internal Messaging

Current Procedure. Most practices use various paper methods to communicate within the office, such as sticky notes, writing on patient fee tickets, and scrap paper. Papers can be misplaced and are not conducive to communicating instructions between provider and support staff. Also, the information may need to become part of the patient record. Legibility, spelling, and the appropriateness of the documentation are common issues in the paper environment.

TABLE 11-1 Six Elements of the Health Care Delivery Model

Patient process begins with the patient needing health care.

Element 1	Seeking care	Events that precipitate entry to or exit from the health care delivery system
Element 2	Patient record	Create and maintain documentation of patient–provider encounters
Element 3	Test and examination	Assess, examine, perform diagnostic tests (invasive or noninvasive)
Element 4	Diagnosis	Apply analysis and clinical judgment to the data collected through examination, assessment, and diagnostic testing
Element 5	Treatment	Treat diagnosed illness; provide preventive and health promotion measures to ensure health and/or prevent illness or complication; administer therapeutics
Element 6	Monitor, evaluate, revise	Provide ongoing supervision of an acute illness or chronic disease based on patient outcomes and standards of care

Adapted from J.S. Maehling, Process re-engineering: Strategies for analysis and redesign in reengineering nursing and health care. In *The Handbook for Organizational Transformation*, S. Smith Blancett and D.L. Flarey, eds. p. 64, 1995, Aspen Publishers, Inc.

Recommended Procedure. Begin to use electronic messaging. Most document management and electronic medical records systems have a mechanism for electronic communication. This allows messages to flow between needed parties with documentation. Most systems feature the ability to place priority on the issue and make the communication part of the patient record. Electronic messaging allows providers and staff to communicate without leaving their respective work areas, thus improving workflow and efficiency. Providers can also easily communicate with staff when they are off site, improving patient satisfaction and staff efficiency. Electronic documentation can follow a template, which improves legibility and spelling compared to paper records. Templates provide decision support that encourages the gathering of pertinent information during the initial patient contact. Again, efficiency is improved, the patient gets feedback much quicker, and the likelihood of each task getting touched once and resolved improves.

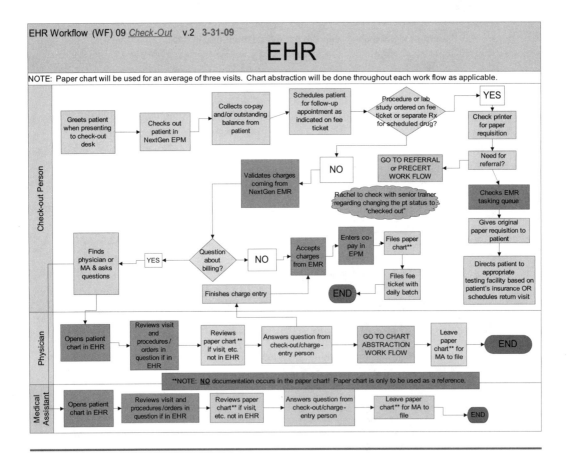

FIGURE 11-2 Process Map Workflow Example

It may take some time for staff to become comfortable with electronic messaging. Old habits can be hard to break, particularly if staff members are not comfortable with computers. Typically, staff does not trust the system and need several positive experiences to "believe" messages are getting to the intended recipient and are not being lost into the ether. The most effective technique is to require that all messages be communicated electronically from the time of go-live and afterward. Removal of the entire paper processes is the fastest route to electronic messaging.

Phone System Procedures

Current Procedure. In many practices, the front desk staff field all phone calls, greet patients, check patients in, register patients, and route patients to the clinical area. This constant interruption of workflow leads to errors, results in poor job satisfaction, and leaves patients with a bad impression.

Recommended Procedure. Isolate and centralize a phone center to allow personnel to perform tasks at the point of call. Use electronic messaging to distribute messages, which will foster more efficient patient care, a quieter work environment, and improved staff productivity. Although relocating the operator function and personnel may be a significant process, having a centralized phone center is worthwhile.

The two main areas of resistance to changing to centralized phone centers are the fact that only the specialized staff in a particular pod can assist a patient because of the nuances of the practice and cost. Standardization and electronic communication improve the success of centralized phone centers. Decreased errors, improved patient communication and satisfaction, and resolution of patient issues by a single staff member saves money and, in many cases, covers the costs of the call center.

Centralized Check-In

Current Procedure. Most offices have a check-in procedure at the front desk. Using process mapping, the practice can determine if the front desk staff is performing other miscellaneous tasks that distract from their primary focus, causing interruptions and errors in registration. A patient's first impression of the group is formed at this point of entry. Further, the first step in the revenue cycle is registration; if it is done incorrectly, the claim will be denied.

Recommended Procedure. When possible, centralize the check-in function and use a queuing procedure for patients to expedite the flow. Consider the cost and ROI of transitioning to kiosks as an adjunct for patient check-in. The patient is more likely to enter his or her information correctly. Plus, staff that are focused on the registration process at check-in will improve the patient experience and the revenue cycle.

Cost is the main cause for resistance to changes in front desk procedures. However, as mentioned earlier, costs are easily covered by improvements in the revenue cycle.

Prescription Refills

Current Procedure. Traditionally, prescriptions refill requests are communicated via a phone call and written down on paper. This paper trail is given to a nurse who attaches it to the patient file for physician review. The physician decision is written on the request and handed back to the nurse to call the pharmacy and notify the patient.

Recommended Procedure. With an electronic system, phone messages can be captured directly into the EHR to notify the physician. The physician receives the request electronically and prescribes the medication electronically, when possible. The pharmacy is notified though the electronic submission. If a patient is to be called back, the nurse is prompted through the EHR.

The practice should also consider patient portal access for refill requests to further streamline the workflow. Inherently, this electronic method has less steps and less room for error. Additionally, the requests and actions taken are noted in the patient file. The benefit of tracking prescription refills and refill requests easily outweighs the learning curve related to electronic prescribing and overcoming comfortable habits of verbal requests and verbal orders.

Lab and Test Order Management

Current Procedure. Labs and tests are ordered by a physician on paper or given verbally to a nurse by a physician. The patient is then asked to schedule the lab or test or the patient is assisted with scheduling by someone in the office. The requested orders are noted in the patient's chart. Some offices have a paper system to watch for orders to be returned. Other offices check for any outstanding orders prior to a patient visit.

Recommended Procedure. Lab and test orders are entered at the time of the patient visit through documentation in the EHR. The system is set up with specific time for each test or lab work to be returned and reminders are sent to a coordinator to track. Designated staff monitor outstanding test and lab work electronically and follow up with incomplete orders by running and analyzing a weekly orders reconciliation report. This workflow allows for better compliance through orders management and less paper, thus reducing errors. The challenge is in training and monitoring work queues as part of a new responsibility.

Charting

Current Procedure. A patient's chart is pulled one to two days prior to the appointment. The fee ticket and other paperwork are placed on top of the paper file. The chart is retrieved and placed with the patient in a room, usually in an outside holder. The physician reviews the chart prior to entering the room. As the patient is seen, notes are taken on paper, with dictation to follow.

Recommended Procedure. The patient is marked as having arrived in the EHR and roomed by a medical assistant or nurse. Vitals, past medical history, and reason for visit details are entered into the system. The physician reviews the information prior to entering the room. The physician documents the visit as the patient is seen, with test and lab work requested and prescriptions written in real time.

This workflow facilitates efficiency and reduced effort in getting patient information to the physician. As an added benefit, documentation is complete at the end of the patient visit. Some aspects of this recommended workflow need to be managed, including initial additional time to enter information, training on software navigation, comfort level difference between providers, and properly designed templates for usability.

Centralized Check-Out

Current Procedure. Traditionally, the fee ticket is collected at check-out and either entered or held for entry by the billing office. If charges are held for the billing office, these charges can take up to two days after the visit to be entered. Collection of a copayment occurs either at the front desk or at check-out and can be set up as unallocated money. Sometimes, past-due balances are collected. The next appointment is then made, if applicable.

Recommended Procedure. Charges are entered upon check-out by knowledgeable staff or at the time of physician documentation. The payer plan has been loaded into the PM system in order to collect the patient-responsible charges. Payment is posted immediately. Any patient material is distributed, such as patient education, orders, or prescriptions. The next appointment is made, if requested. Also, consider locating the check-out desk with business office/patient accounts in order to handle past-due balances and payment terms.

The benefits of this procedure are avoidance of double handling of fee tickets, quick turnaround of electronic charge submissions, and an increase in the amount of money collected at the time of service. However, it may require reassigning personnel and responsibilities, placing knowledgeable staff at check-out, and potentially increasing patient wait time.

Overall, by examining the practice's workflow and implementing well-thought-out changes, the benefits can include:

- better overall workflow;
- reduced errors and improved patient safety;
- improved patient experience;

- improved staff satisfaction due to clearly defined responsibilities and having just enough information at just the right time to assist a patient;
- improved physician experience as a result of efficient staff utilization;
- staff working up to the level of their license or defined role;
- cost reductions through elimination of redundant operations and duplicative staff;
- improved cash flow;
- improved medication management as well as improved management of drug-seeking behaviors;
- automated referral and diagnostic test tracking and management;
- improved disease management; and
- improved uniform delivery of gold standard care.

Implementing an EHR can be transformational for a practice but only if clinical and business processes are assessed, analyzed, and reengineered. Expect the possibility of personnel turnover and the need to manage behavioral change of staff and physicians. Allowing staff the opportunity to express opinions or concerns about the new methodologies, communicating expectations of commitment to the new methodologies, holding staff accountable, and focusing on results will improve the chances for success. Most patients will be very supportive and welcome the process improvements. Communication with patients is prudent in order to give them an opportunity to adjust to the new procedures.

Conclusion

EHR system implementation can be an intimidating endeavor. For the active practice leader faced with the ongoing challenges of daily practice operations, the thought of starting a new initiative can seem overwhelming. However, by gathering sufficient information to lay the foundation and by following a step-by-step plan of action, the busiest executive can be empowered to successfully manage a conversion.

Reference

1. Wang, S.J., Middleton, B., et al. A Cost-Benefit Analysis of Electronic Medical Records in Primary Care. *American Journal of Medicine*, April 1, 2003. Accessed 1/7/2010 at www.amjmed.com/article/PIIS0002934303000573/fulltext.

APPENDIX A

Online Resources

Abundant quantities of health care–specific resources are available via the Internet. This includes information from federal and state governments, regulatory agencies, professional societies, and other organizations. The following list of Web-based resources is useful for health care organizations and providers.

1. www.cms.hhs.gov

The Centers for Medicare and Medicaid Services' (CMS) Website contains a vast array of information regarding the agency, the Medicare www.cms.hhs.gov/home/medicare.asp) and Medicaid (www.cms.hhs.gov/home/medicaid.asp) programs, current research, and educational programming. One valuable tool on the CMS Website is the Physician Fee Schedule (www.cms.hhs.gov/PhysicianFeeSched/), which is updated and posted at least once per year. Another valuable tool on the CMS Website is the information regarding PQRI (www.cms.hhs.gov/pqri/), which includes annual updates on the program and reporting structure.

2. www.hhs.gov/oig

The role of the Office of the Inspector General (OIG), as posted on its Website, is "to protect the integrity of Department of Health and Human Services (HHS) programs, as well as the health and welfare of the beneficiaries of those programs." The Website provides details regarding the OIG's advisory opinions (http://oig.hhs.gov/fraud/advisoryopinions/opinions.asp). Although the opinions are not law, they generally set the market standard for the subject on which they are based. Recent opinion topics include compensated call coverage, ambulatory surgery centers, joint venturing, and other physician/hospital alignment arrangements.

3. www.medicare.gov/default.asp

The Medicare Website is designed to be a resource for people with Medicare coverage, including information regarding billing, appeals, reporting fraud, and other consumer-driven topics. One detailed resource on this Website is the contact database (www.medicare.gov/contacts/default.aspx), which can be queried to provide information specific to each of the 50 states.

4. www.irs.gov/index.html

The Internal Revenue Service Website provides information for individuals, businesses, and non-profit/charity organizations. Current and historical IRS regulations are archived on the site, and many of the forms that health care organizations (and other businesses) must complete are also available online.

5. www.naic.org

The National Association of Insurance Commissioners' Website provides contact information for the insurance regulatory agency in each state.

6. www.cms.hhs.gov/PhysicianSelfReferral/ and http://oig.hhs.gov/fraud.asp

Information regarding physician self-referral regulations (ie, Stark Law) and the Anti-Kickback Statute are available on the CMS and OIG Websites. (Note: Although these Websites provide detailed and valuable information, it is also often necessary for a health care organization to engage legal counsel to ensure compliance with all applicable regulatory and legal terms and conditions.)

7. Professional Society Websites

Most professional societies and medical organizations have Websites that provide information regarding eligibility and membership, and many of these Websites also provide insights regarding the current health care environment, upcoming seminars the organization is hosting, publications they offer, and other beneficial information. There are national specialty societies as well as state, regional, and local organizations. Some of these organizations are designed to be of greatest use to providers, others are centered on health care administrators and executives, and still others are applicable to anyone involved in health care. A selection of these organizations and their Websites is listed as follows.

- Aerospace Medical Association: www.asma.org
- American Academy of Allergy, Asthma & Immunology: www.aaaai.org
- The American Academy of Child and Adolescent Psychiatry: www.aacap.org
- American Academy of Cosmetic Surgery: www.cosmeticsurgery.org
- The American Academy of Dermatology: www.aad.org
- American Academy of Facial Plastic and Reconstructive Surgery: www.facial-plastic-surgery.org
- American Academy of Family Physicians: www.aafp.org

American Academy of Hospice and Palliative Care: www.aahpm.org

American Academy of Insurance Medicine: www.aaimedicine.org

American Academy of Neurology: www.aan.com

American Academy of Nurse Practitioners: www.aanp.org

American Academy of Ophthalmology: www.aao.org

American Academy of Orthopaedic Surgeons: www.aaos.org

American Academy of Otolaryngic Allergy: www.aaoaf.org

American Academy of Otolaryngology—Head and Neck Surgery: www.entnet.org

American Academy of Pain Medicine: www.painmed.org

American Academy of Pediatrics: www.aap.org

American Academy of Pharmaceutical Physicians: www.aapp.org

American Academy of Physical Medicine and Rehabilitation: www.aapmr.org

American Academy of Physician Assistants: www.aapa.org

American Academy of Psychiatry & the Law: www.aapl.org

American Academy of Sleep Medicine: www.aasmnet.org

American Association for Hand Surgery: www.handsurgery.org

American Association for Thoracic Surgery: www.aats.org

American Association of Clinical Endocrinologists: www.aace.com

American Association of Clinical Urologists: www.aacuweb.org

American Association of Gynecologic Laparoscopists: www.aagl.com

American Association of Hip and Knee Surgeons: www.aahks.org

American Association of Neurological Surgeons: www.neurosurgery.org/aans

American Association of Neuromuscular and Electrodiagnostic Medicine: www.aaem.net

American Association of Plastic Surgeons: www.aaps1921.org

American Association of Public Health Physicians: www.aaphp.org

American Clinical Neurophysiology Society: www.acns.org

American College of Cardiology: www.acc.org

American College of Chest Physicians: www.chestnet.org

American College of Emergency Physicians: www.acep.org

American College of Gastroenterology: www.acg.gi.org

American College of Healthcare Executives: www.ache.org

American College of Medical Genetics: www.acmg.net

American College of Medical Quality: www.acmq.org

American College of Nuclear Medicine: www.acnucmed.com

American College of Nuclear Physicians: www.acnponline.org

American College of Obstetricians and Gynecologists: www.acog.com

American College of Occupational and Environmental Medicine: www.acoem.org

American College of Physician Executives: www.acpe.org

American College of Physicians—American Society of Internal Medicine: www.acponline.org

American College of Preventative Medicine: www.acpm.org

American College of Radiation Oncology: www.acro.org

American College of Radiology: www.acr.org

American College of Rheumatology: www.rheumatology.org

American College of Surgeons: www.facs.org

American Gastroenterological Association: www.gastro.org

American Geriatrics Society: www.americangeriatrics.org

American Medical Association: www.ama-assn.org

American Medical Group Association: www.amga.org

American Orthopaedic Association: www.aoassn.org

American Orthopaedic Foot and Ankle Society: www.aofas.org

American Pediatric Surgical Association: www.eapsa.org

American Psychiatric Association: www.psych.org

American Roentgen Ray Society: www.arrs.org

American Society for Aesthetic Plastic Surgery: www.surgery.org

American Society for Clinical Pathology: www.ascp.org

American Society for Dermatologic Surgery: www.asds-net.org

American Society for Gastrointestinal Endoscopy: www.asge.org

American Society for Reproductive Medicine: www.asrm.org

American Society for Surgery of the Hand: www.hand-surg.org

American Society for Therapeutic Radiology and Oncology: www.atro.org

American Society of Abdominal Surgeons: www.gis.net/~absurg/

American Society of Addiction Medicine: www.asam.org

American Society of Anesthesiologists: www.asahq.org

The American Society of Bariatric Physicians: www.asbp.org

American Society of Cataract and Refractive Surgery: www.ascrs.org

American Society of Clinical Oncology: www.asco.org

American Society of Colon and Rectal Surgeons: www.fascrs.org

American Society of General Surgeons: www.theasgs.org

American Society of Hematology: www.hematology.org

American Society of Maxillofacial Surgeons: www.maxface.org

American Society of Neuroradiology: www.asnr.org

American Society of Plastic Surgeons: www.plasticsurgery.org

American Society of Retina Specialists: www.vitreoussociety.org

American Thoracic Society: www.thoracic.org

American Urological Association: www.auanet.org

Association of Military Surgeons of the United States: www.amsus.org

Association of University Radiologists: www.aur.org

College of American Pathologists: www.cap.org

Congress of Neurological Surgeons: www.cns.org

The Endocrine Society: www.endo-society.org

National Association of Medical Examiners: www.thename.org

National Medical Association: www.nmanet.org

North American Spine Society: www.spine.org

Radiological Society of North America: www.rsna.org

Renal Physicians Association: www.renalmd.org

Society of American Gastrointestinal Endoscopic Surgeons: www.sages.org

Society of Cardiovascular & Interventional Radiology: www.scvir.org

Society of Critical Care Medicine: www.sccm.org

Society of Interventional Radiology: www.sirweb.org

Society of Nuclear Medicine: www.snm.org
Society of Thoracic Surgeons: www.sts.org

8. www.ama-assn.org/go/pmc

The American Medical Association Practice Management Center Website provides updated information regarding issues that impact health care practices. (In addition to the Website, AMA members can e-mail practicemanagementcenter@ama-assn.org for assistance.)

APPENDIX B

Section I—Medicare Part A Intermediary and Part B Carrier by State

		REGIONAL OFFICE
Alabama		Atlanta
Part A	Blue Cross and Blue Shield of Alabama Mutual of Omaha Insurance Company	
Part B	Blue Cross and Blue Shield of Alabama	
RHHI	Palmetto GBA, LLC	
DMERC	Palmetto GBA, LLC	
Alaska		Seattle
Part A	Noridian Mutual Insurance Company Mutual of Omaha Insurance Company	
Part B	Noridian Mutual Insurance Company	
RHHI	United Government Services, LLC	
DME MAC	Noridian Mutual Insurance Company	
American Samoa		
Part A	United Government Services, LLC Mutual of Omaha Insurance Company	
Part B	Noridian Mutual Insurance Company	
RHHI	United Government Services, LLC	
DME MAC	Noridian Mutual Insurance Company	
Arizona		San Francisco
Part A	Noridian Administrative Services, LLC Mutual of Omaha Insurance Company	
Part B	Noridian Administrative Services, LLC Mutual of Omaha Insurance Company	
RHHI	United Government Services, LLC	
DME MAC	Noridian Mutual Insurance Company	

continued

		REGIONAL OFFICE
Arkansas		Dallas
Part A	Arkansas Blue Cross and Blue Shield, A Mutual Insurance Company Mutual of Omaha Insurance Company	
Part B	Arkansas Blue Cross and Blue Shield, A Mutual Insurance Company	
RHHI	Palmetto GBA, LLC	
DME MAC	Palmetto GBA, LLC	
California		San Francisco
Part A	United Government Services, LLC Mutual of Omaha Insurance Company	
Part B	National Heritage Insurance Company	
RHHI	United Government Services, LLC	
DME MAC	Noridian Mutual Insurance Company	
Colorado		Denver
Part A	TrailBlazer Health Enterprises, LLC Mutual of Omaha Insurance Company	
Part B	Noridian Mutual Insurance Company	
RHHI	Blue Cross and Blue Shield of Alabama	
DMERC	Palmetto GBA, LLC	
Connecticut		Boston
Part A	Empire HealthChoice Assurance, Inc. Mutual of Omaha Insurance Company	
Part B	First Coast Service Options, Inc.	
RHHI	Anthem Health Plans of Maine, Inc.	
DME MAC	National Heritage Insurance Company	
Delaware		Philadelphia
Part A	Empire HealthChoice Assurance, Inc. Mutual of Omaha Insurance Company	
Part B	TrailBlazer Health Enterprises, LLC	
RHHI	Blue Cross and Blue Shield of Alabama	
DME MAC	National Heritage Insurance Company	
District of Columbia		Philadelphia
Part A	Highmark Inc. Mutual of Omaha Insurance Company	
Part B	TrailBlazer Health Enterprises, LLC	
RHHI	Blue Cross and Blue Shield of Alabama	
DME MAC	National Heritage Insurance Company	

		REGIONAL OFFICE
Florida		Philadelphia
Part A	First Coast Service Options Mutual of Omaha Insurance Company	
Part B	First Coast Service Options	
RHHI	Palmetto GBA, LLC	
DMERC	Palmetto GBA, LLC	
Georgia		Atlanta
Part A	Blue Cross and Blue Shield of Georgia, Inc. Mutual of Omaha Insurance Company	
Part B	Blue Cross and Blue Shield of Alabama	
RHHI	Palmetto GBA, LLC	
DMERC	Palmetto GBA, LLC	
Guam		San Francisco
Part A	United Government Services, LLC Mutual of Omaha Insurance Company	
Part B	Noridian Mutual Insurance Company	
RHHI	United Government Services, LLC	
DME MAC	Noridian Mutual Insurance Company	
Hawaii		San Francisco
Part A	United Government Services, LLC Mutual of Omaha Insurance Company	
Part B	Noridian Mutual Insurance Company	
RHHI	United Government Services, LLC	
DME MAC	Noridian Mutual Insurance Company	
Idaho		Seattle
Part A	Noridian Mutual Insurance Company Mutual of Omaha Insurance Company	
Part B	Connecticut General Life Insurance Company	
RHHI	United Government Services, LLC	
DME MAC	Noridian Mutual Insurance Company	
Illinois		Chicago
Part A	Anthem Insurance Companies, Inc. Mutual of Omaha Insurance Company	
Part B	Wisconsin Physicians Service	
RHHI	Palmetto GBA, LLC	
DMERC	Palmetto GBA, LLC	

continued

		REGIONAL OFFICE
Indiana		**Chicago**
Part A	Anthem Insurance Companies, Inc. Mutual of Omaha Insurance Company	
Part B	AdminaStar Federal, Inc.	
RHHI	Palmetto GBA, LLC	
DME MAC	AdminaStar Federal, Inc.	
Iowa		**Kansas City**
Part A	Blue Cross and Blue Shield of Alabama Mutual of Omaha Insurance Company	
Part B	Noridian Mutual Insurance Company	
RHHI	Blue Cross and Blue Shield of Alabama	
DME MAC	Noridian Mutual Insurance Company	
Kansas		**Kansas City**
Part A	Blue Cross and Blue Shield of Kansas, Inc. Mutual of Omaha Insurance Company	
Part B	Blue Cross and Blue Shield of Kansas, Inc.	
RHHI	Blue Cross and Blue Shield of Alabama	
DME MAC	Noridian Mutual Insurance Company	
Kentucky		**Atlanta**
Part A	Anthem Insurance Companies, Inc. Mutual of Omaha Insurance Company	
Part B	AdminaStar Federal, Inc.	
RHHI	Palmetto GBA, LLC	
DME MAC	AdminaStar Federal, Inc.	
Louisiana		**Dallas**
Part A	Blue Cross and Blue Shield of Mississippi Mutual of Omaha Insurance Company	
Part B	Arkansas Blue Cross and Blue Shield, A Mutual Insurance Company	
RHHI	Palmetto GBA, LLC	
DMERC	Palmetto GBA, LLC	
Maine		**Boston**
Part A	Anthem Health Plans of Maine, Inc. Mutual of Omaha Insurance Company	
Part B	National Heritage Insurance Company	
RHHI	Anthem Health Plans of Maine, Inc.	
DME MAC	National Heritage Insurance Company	

		REGIONAL OFFICE
Maryland		Philadelphia
Part A	Highmark, Inc. Mutual of Omaha Insurance Company	
Part B	TrailBlazer Health Enterprises, LLC	
RHHI	Blue Cross and Blue Shield of Alabama	
DME MAC	National Heritage Insurance Company	
Massachusetts		Boston
Part A	Anthem Health Plans of Maine, Inc. Mutual of Omaha Insurance Company	
Part B	National Heritage Insurance Company	
RHHI	Anthem Health Plans of Maine, Inc.	
DME MAC	National Heritage Insurance Company	
Michigan		Chicago
Part A	United Government Services, LLC Mutual of Omaha Insurance Company	
Part B	Wisconsin Physicians Service	
RHHI	Palmetto GBA, LLC	
DME MAC	AdminaStar Federal, Inc.	
Minnesota		Chicago
Part A	Noridian Mutual Insurance Company Mutual of Omaha Insurance Company	
Part B	Wisconsin Physicians Service	
RHHI	United Government Services, LLC	
DME MAC	AdminaStar Federal, Inc.	
Mississippi		Atlanta
Part A	Blue Cross and Blue Shield of Mississippi Mutual of Omaha Insurance Company	
Part B	Blue Cross and Blue Shield of Alabama	
RHHI	Palmetto GBA, LLC	
DMERC	Palmetto GBA, LLC	
Missouri		Kansas City
Part A	Blue Cross and Blue Shield of Mississippi Mutual of Omaha Insurance Company	
Part B	Blue Cross and Blue Shield of Kansas, Inc. (Western Missouri) Arkansas Blue Cross and Blue Shield, A Mutual Insurance Company (Eastern Missouri)	

continued

		REGIONAL OFFICE
RHHI	Blue Cross and Blue Shield of Alabama	
MAC	Noridian Mutual Insurance Company	
Montana		**Denver**
Part A/B MAC	Noridian Administrative Services, LLC Mutual of Omaha Insurance Company	
Part B	Noridian Administrative Services, LLC Mutual of Omaha Insurance Company	
RHHI	Blue Cross and Blue Shield of Alabama	
DME MAC	Noridian Mutual Insurance Company	
Nebraska		**Kansas City**
Part A	Blue Cross and Blue Shield of Nebraska Mutual of Omaha Insurance Company	
Part B	Blue Cross and Blue Shield of Kansas, Inc.	
RHHI	Blue Cross and Blue Shield of Alabama	
DME MAC	Noridian Mutual Insurance Company	
Nevada		**San Francisco**
Part A	United Government Services, LLC Mutual of Omaha Insurance Company	
Part B	Noridian Mutual Insurance Company	
RHHI	United Government Services, LLC	
DME MAC	Noridian Mutual Insurance Company	
New Hampshire		**Boston/San Francisco**
Part A	Anthem Health Plans of New Hampshire, Inc. Mutual of Omaha Insurance Company	
Part B	National Heritage Insurance Company	
RHHI	Anthem Health Plans of New Hampshire, Inc.	
DME MAC	National Heritage Insurance Company	
New Jersey		**New York**
Part A	Blue Cross Blue Shield of Tennessee Mutual of Omaha Insurance Company	
Part B	Empire HealthChoice, Inc.	
RHHI	United Government Services, LLC	
DME MAC	National Heritage Insurance Company	

		REGIONAL OFFICE
New Mexico		Dallas
Part A	TrailBlazer Health Enterprises, LLC Mutual of Omaha Insurance Company	
Part B	Arkansas Blue Cross and Blue Shield, A Mutual Insurance Company	
RHHI	Palmetto GBA, LLC	
DMERC	Palmetto GBA, LLC	
New York		New York
Part A	Empire HealthChoice Assurance, Inc.	
Part B	HealthNow New York, Inc. Empire HealthChoice Assurance, Inc. Group Health Incorporated	
RHHI	United Government Services, LLC	
DME MAC	National Heritage Insurance Company	
North Carolina		Atlanta
Part A	Blue Cross and Blue Shield of South Carolina Mutual of Omaha Insurance Company	
Part B	Connecticut General Life Insurance Company	
RHHI	Palmetto GBA, LLC	
DMERC	Palmetto GBA, LLC	
North Dakota		Denver
Part A/B MAC	Noridian Administrative Services, LLC Mutual of Omaha Insurance Company	
Part B	Noridian Administrative Services, LLC Mutual of Omaha Insurance Company	
RHHI	Blue Cross and Blue Shield of Alabama	
DME MAC	Noridian Mutual Insurance Company	
Northern Marianna Islands		San Francisco
Part A	United Government Services, LLC Mutual of Omaha Insurance Company	
Part B	Noridian Mutual Insurance Company	
RHHI	United Government Services, LLC	
DME MAC	Noridian Mutual Insurance Company	

continued

		REGIONAL OFFICE
Ohio		Chicago
Part A	Anthem Insurance Companies, Inc. Mutual of Omaha Insurance Company	
Part B	Palmetto GBA, LLC	
RHHI	Palmetto GBA, LLC	
DME MAC	AdminaStar Federal, Inc.	
Oklahoma		Dallas
Part A	Group Health Service of Oklahoma, Inc. Mutual of Omaha Insurance Company	
Part B	Arkansas Blue Cross and Blue Shield, A Mutual Insurance Company	
RHHI	Palmetto GBA, LLC	
DMERC	Palmetto GBA, LLC	
Oregon		Seattle
Part A	Noridian Mutual Insurance Company Mutual of Omaha Insurance Company	
Part B	Noridian Mutual Insurance Company	
RHHI	United Government Services, LLC	
DME MAC	Noridian Mutual Insurance Company	
Pennsylvania		Philadelphia
Part A	Highmark, Inc. Mutual of Omaha Insurance Company	
Part B	Highmark, Inc.	
RHHI	Blue Cross and Blue Shield of Alabama	
DME MAC	National Heritage Insurance Company	
Puerto Rico		New York
Part A	Cooperative de Seguros de Vida de Puerto Rico Mutual of Omaha Insurance Company	
Part B	Triple-S, Inc.	
RHHI	United Government Services, LLC	
DMERC	Palmetto GBA, LLC	
Rhode Island		Boston
Part A	Arkansas Blue Cross and Blue Shield, A Mutual Insurance Company Mutual of Omaha Insurance Company	
Part B	Arkansas Blue Cross and Blue Shield, A Mutual Insurance Company	

		REGIONAL OFFICE
RHHI	Anthem Health Plans of Maine, Inc.	
DME MAC	National Heritage Insurance Company	
South Carolina		**Atlanta**
Part A	Palmetto GBA, LLC Mutual of Omaha Insurance Company	
Part B	Palmetto GBA, LLC	
RHHI	Palmetto GBA, LLC	
DMERC	Palmetto GBA, LLC	
South Dakota		**Denver**
Part A	Blue Cross and Blue Shield of Alabama Mutual of Omaha Insurance Company	
Part B	Noridian Administrative Services, LLC	
RHHI	Blue Cross and Blue Shield of Alabama	
DME MAC	Noridian Mutual Insurance Company	
Tennessee		**Atlanta**
Part A	Blue Cross and Blue Shield of Tennessee Mutual of Omaha Insurance Company	
Part B	Connecticut General Life Insurance Company	
RHHI	Palmetto GBA, LLC	
DMERC	Palmetto GBA, LLC	
Texas		**Dallas**
Part A	TrailBlazer Health Enterprises, LLC Mutual of Omaha Insurance Company	
Part B	TrailBlazer Health Enterprises, LLC	
RHHI	Palmetto GBA, LLC	
DMERC	Palmetto GBA, LLC	
U.S. Virgin Islands		**New York**
Part A	Cooperative de Seguros de Vida de Puerto Rico Mutual of Omaha Insurance Company	
Part B	Triple-S, Inc.	
RHHI	United Government Services, LLC	
DMERC	Palmetto GBA, LLC	
Utah		**Denver**
Part A/B MAC	Noridian Administrative Services, LLC Mutual of Omaha Insurance Company	
Part B	Noridian Mutual Insurance Company	

continued

		REGIONAL OFFICE
RHHI	Blue Cross and Blue Shield of Alabama	
DME MAC	Noridian Mutual Insurance Company	
Vermont		Boston/San Francisco
Part A	Anthem Health Plans of New Hampshire, Inc. Mutual of Omaha Insurance Company	
Part B	National Heritage Insurance Company	
RHHI	Anthem Health Plans of Maine, Inc.	
DME MAC	National Heritage Insurance Company	
Virginia		Philadelphia
Part A	United Government Services, LLC Mutual of Omaha Insurance Company	
Part B	TrailBlazer Health Enterprises, LLC	
RHHI	Blue Cross and Blue Shield of Alabama	
DMERC	Palmetto GBA, LLC	
Washington		Seattle
Part A	Noridian Mutual Insurance Company Mutual of Omaha Insurance Company	
Part B	Noridian Mutual Insurance Company	
RHHI	United Government Services, LLC	
DME MAC	Noridian Mutual Insurance Company	
West Virginia		Philadelphia
Part A	United Government Services, LLC Mutual of Omaha Insurance Company	
Part B	Blue Cross Blue Shield of South Carolina	
RHHI	Blue Cross and Blue Shield of Alabama	
DMERC	Palmetto GBA, LLC	
Wisconsin		Chicago
Part A	United Government Services, LLC Mutual of Omaha Insurance Company	
Part B	Wisconsin Physicians Service	
RHHI	United Government Services, LLC	
DME MAC	AdminaStar Federal, Inc.	

		REGIONAL OFFICE
Wyoming		Denver
Part A/B MAC	Noridian Administrative Services, LLC Mutual of Omaha Insurance Company	
Part B	Noridian Mutual Insurance Company	
RHHI	Blue Cross and Blue Shield of Alabama	
DME MAC	Noridian Mutual Insurance Company	

Source: Intermediary Carrier Directory. U.S. Department of Health and Human Services Centers for Medicare & Medicaid Services.

Any inquiries regarding the content of this directory or changes to the information contained herein should be referred to the Centers for Medicare & Medicaid Services, Office of Acquisition and Grants Management, Division of Medicare Contracts, 7500 Security Boulevard - C2-21-15, Baltimore, Maryland 21244.

COMMUNICATING WITH INTERMEDIARIES AND CARRIERS

Medicare contracts cover the rights and obligations of Intermediaries, Carriers, and the Secretary of Health and Human Services.

Requests for action or information not specifically authorized by such contracts should not be made.

APPENDIX C

Prompt Pay Statutes and Regulations by State

State	Status/Terms of Law	State Authority	How to Contact
Alabama	Payment within 45 days of receipt of clean written claim or 30 calendar days of clean electronic claim. Interest payment of 1.5% per month prorated daily, accruing from date payment overdue.	Alabama Department of Insurance	www.aldoi.gov PO Box 303351 Montgomery, AL 36130-3351 Phone: 334-269-3550 Fax: 334-241-4192 E-mail: Insdept@insurance.alabama.gov
Alaska	Clean claims must be paid within 30 days.	Alaska Division of Insurance	www.commerce.state.ak.us/ins/home.htm PO Box 110805 Juneau, AK 99811-0805 Phone: 907-465-2515 Fax: 907-465-3422
Arizona	Adjudication and payment of clean claims are two separate steps. Insurers must adjudicate clean claims with 30 days of receipt or within time frame designated by contract. Insurers must pay any approved portions of the clean claims within 30 days of adjudication, or within a time frame designated by contract.	Arizona Department of Insurance	www.id.state.az.us/ 2910 N. 44th St. #210 Phoenix, AZ 85018 Phone: 602-364-2394 Fax: 602-364-2175 E-mail: providerinfo@id.state.az.us

continued

State	Status/Terms of Law	State Authority	How to Contact
	Penalty for late payment is 10% per annum or another amount designated by contract, with interest accruing from date payment is due.		
Arkansas	Clean, electronic claims must be paid or denied in 30 calendar days, 45 if paper. Late penalty 12% per annum times the number of days in the delinquent payment period divided by 365.	Arkansas Insurance Department	http://insurance.arkansas.gov/Administration/contact.html 1200 West Third St. Little Rock, AR 72201 Phone: 501-371-2600 Toll Free: 800-282-9134 Fax: 501-371-2618
California	Claims must be paid within 45 working days for an HMO, 30 days for a health service plan. Interest accrues at 15% per annum.	California HMO Help Center	www.hmohelp.ca.gov California Department of Managed Health Care 980 9th Street, Suite 500 Sacramento, CA 95814-2725 Toll Free: 877-525-1295 Fax: 916-255-5241 E-mail: plans-providers@dmhc.ca.gov
Colorado	Claims must be paid in 30 days if submitted electronically, 45 if paper. Penalty is 10% annually, with an additional penalty of 10% of the total claim after 90 days.	Colorado Division of Insurance	www.dora.state.co.us/insurance 1560 Broadway, Suite 850 Denver, CO 80202 Phone: 303-894-7499 Toll Free: 800-930-3745 Fax: 303-894-7455 E-mail: helpdesk@dora.state.co.us.

State	Status/Terms of Law	State Authority	How to Contact
Connecticut	Claims must be paid within 45 working days. Interest accrues at 15% per annum.	Connecticut Insurance Department	www.ct.gov/cid/site/default.asp Consumer Affairs Unit PO Box 816 Hartford, CT 06142-0816 Phone: 860-297-3900 Toll Free: 800-203-3447 Fax: 860-97-3872 E-mail: cid.ca@ct.gov
Delaware	Clean claims must be paid in 45 days. Penalty for late payment is interest at the maximum rate allowable to lenders under Del.C. 2301 (a), computed from the date the claim or bill for services first became due.	Delaware Insurance Department	www.delawareinsurance.gov/ 841 Silver Lake Blvd Dover, DE 19904 Phone: 302 674-7300 Toll Free: 800-282-8611 E-mail: consumer@state.de.us
Distirct of Columbia	Clean claims must be paid in 30 days. Interest penalty for overdue claims: 1.5% from day 31–60; 2% from day 61–120; 2.5% from 121 and after.	District of Columbia Department of Insurance, Securities, and Banking	www.disr.dc.gov/disr/site/default.asp 810 First Street, NE, Suite 701 Washington, DC 20002 Phone: 202-727-8000
Florida	Electronic clean claims must be paid in 20 days, 40 days if paper. Interest penalty for late payments is 12% per year.	Florida Department of Financial Services	http://www.myfloridacfo.com/ 200 East Gaines St. Tallahassee, FL 32399-4228 Phone: 850-413-5923 E-mail: insurance consumer-advocate@myfloridacfo.com

continued

State	Status/Terms of Law	State Authority	How to Contact
Georgia	Claims must be paid within 15 working days. Interest accrues at 18% per annum.	Georgia Office of Insurance and Safety Fire Commissioner	www.gainsurance.org Georgia Insurance Commissioner Consumer Services Division 2 M.L.K. Jr. Drive West Tower, Suite 716 Atlanta, GA 30334 Phone: 404-656-2070 Toll Free: 800-656-2298 Fax: 404-657-8542
Hawaii	Clean, paper claims must be paid in 30 days, electronic claims within 15 days. Interest accrues at 15% per annum. Commissioner may impose fines.	State of Hawaii Insurance Division	http://hawaii.gov/dcca/ins P.O. Box 3614 Honolulu, HI 96811 Phone: 808-586-2790 or 808-586-2799 Fax: 808-586-2806 E-mail: ihealth@dcca.hawaii.gov
Idaho	Paper claims due in 45 days; electronic claims due 30 days from receipt. Penalties: Legal rate of interest in accordance with section 28-22-104, Idaho Code.	Idaho Department of Insurance	www.doi.idaho.gov/ 700 West State Street PO Box 83720 Boise, ID 83720-0043 Phone: 208-334-4250 Fax: 208-334-4398
Illinois	Clean claims must be paid in 30 days. Interest accrues at 9% per annum.	Illinois Department of Insurance	www.idfpr.com/DOI/default2.asp 320 West Washington Street Springfield, IL 62767-0001 Phone: 312-814-2427 Toll Free: 877-527-9431 Fax: 217-558-2083 E-mail: DOI.Director@illinois.gov

State	Status/Terms of Law	State Authority	How to Contact
Indiana	Paper claims must be paid in 45 days; 30 days for electronic claims. Interest payable at rate provided under IC 12-15-21-3(7)(A).	Indiana Department of Insurance	www.in.gov/idoi Consumer Services Division 311 W Washington Street, Suite 300 Indianapolis IN 46204-2787 Phone: 317-232-2385 Toll Free: 800-622-4461 Fax: 317-234-2103 E-mail: idoi@IN.gov
Iowa	Clean claims must be paid within 30 days. Penalty of 10% for late payment.	Iowa Insurance Division	www.iid.state.ia.us/ 330 Maple St. Des Moines, IA 50319-0065 Phone: 515-281-5705 Toll Free: 877-955-1212 Fax: 515-281-3059
Kansas	Claims will be paid in 30 days. Interest accrues at a rate of 1% per month.	Kansas Insurance Department	www.kslegislature.org/legsrv-statutes/getStatuteInfo.do 420 SW 9th Street Topeka, KS 66612 Phone: 785-296-3071 Toll Free: 800-432-2484 Fax: 785-296-7805 E-mail: commissioner@ksinsurance.org
Kentucky	Claims must be paid or denied within 30 working days. Interest accrues at 12% per annum when 31–60 days late; 18% when 61–90 days late; and 21% when 91+ days late.	Kentucky Department of Insurance	http://insurance.ky.gov/ Commissioner's Office PO Box 517 Frankfort, KY 40602-0517 Phone: 502-564-3630 Toll Free: 800-595-6053 Fax: 502-564-1453 E-mail: Debbie.Stamper@ky.gov

continued

State	Status/Terms of Law	State Authority	How to Contact
Louisiana	A health insurer must pay a clean claim filed electronically in 25 days, unless the insurer chose a 30-day across the board standard for both electronic and non-electronic claims. A non-electronic clean claim submitted by a non-contracted provider must be paid with 30 days of submission. A non-electronic clean claim submitted by a contracted provider within 45 days of date of service must be paid within 45 days. A non-electronic clean claim submitted by a contracted provider within 60 days of date of service must be paid within 60 days. Penalty is 1% of unpaid balance.	Louisiana Department of Insurance	www.ldi.state.la.us 1702 N. 3rd Street Baton Rouge, LA 70802 Phone: 225-342-5900 Toll Free: 800-259-5300 Fax: 225-342-3078 E-mail: public@ldi.state.la.us
Maine	Clean claims must be paid within 30 days. Interest accrues at 1.5% per month.	Maine Bureau of Insurance	www.maine.gov/pfr/insurance/ #34 State House Station Augusta, ME 04333-0034 Phone: 207-624-8475 Toll Free: 800-300-5000 Fax: 207-624-8599 E-mail: Insurance.PFR@maine.gov
Maryland	Clean claims must be paid within 30 days. Interest accrues at 1.5% (31–60 days late), 2% (61–120), and 2.5% (121+).	Maryland Insurance Administration	www.mdinsurance.state.md.us 200 St. Paul Place, Suite 2700 Baltimore, MD 21202

State	Status/Terms of Law	State Authority	How to Contact
			Phone: 410-468-2000 Toll Free: 800-492-6116 Fax: 410-468-2020
Massachusetts	Clean claims must be paid 45 days after receipt. Interest penalty of 1.5% per month.	Massachusetts Division of Insurance	www.mass.gov/doi 1000 Washington Street, Suite 810 Boston MA 02118-6200 Phone: 617-521-7794 Fax: 617-521-7575
Michigan	Claims must be paid in 45 days with an interest penalty of 12% per annum. (This law applies only to non-contracted providers)	Michigan Department of Energy, Labor, & Economic Growth, Office of Financial and Insurance Regulation	www.michigan.gov/dleg/0,1607,7-154-10555---,00.html PO Box 30165 Lansing, MI 48909-7665 Phone: 517-373-0220 Toll Free: 877-999-644 Fax: 517-335-4978 E-mail: ofir-ins-info@michigan.gov
Minnesota	Clean claims must be paid in 30 days. Interest accrues at 1.5% per month if not paid or denied.	Minnesota Department of Health	www.health.state.mn.us/ PO Box 64975 St. Paul, MN 55164-0975 Phone: 651-201-5000 Toll Free: 888-345-0823
Mississippi	Clean claims must be paid within 45 days. Interest accrues at 1.5% per month.	Mississippi Insurance Department	www.mid.state.ms.us/ PO Box 79 Jackson, MS 39205-0079 Phone: 601-359-3569 Toll Free: 800-562-2957 Fax: 601-359-1077

continued

State	Status/Terms of Law	State Authority	How to Contact
Missouri	Claims must be acknowledged within 10 days and paid within 45 days. Interest accrues at a monthly rate of 1%. After 40 processing days, entitled to an additional penalty of 50% of claim, not to exceed $20.	Missouri Department of Insurance	http://insurance.mo.gov/ PO Box 690 Jefferson City, MO 65102-0690 Phone: 573-751-4126
Montana	Clean claims must be paid within 30 days. Interest accrues at 10% per annum.	Office of the Commissioner of Securities and Insurance, Montana's State Auditor	www.sao.state.mt.us 840 Helena Ave. Helena, MT 59601 Phone: 406-444-2040 Toll Free: 800-332-6148 Fax: 406-444-3497 E-mail: stateauditor@mt.gov
Nebraska	Paper claims must be paid within 45 days and electronic claims must be paid within 30 days of receipt.	Nebraska Department of Insurance	www.doi.ne.gov Terminal Building 941 O Street, Suite 400 Lincoln, NE 68508-3690 Phone: 402-471-2201 Toll Free: 877-564-7323 E-mail: www.doi.ne.gov/forms/complaint.htm
Nevada	Claims must be paid in 30 days. Penalty interest accrues at rate set forth in Nevada Revised Statute 99.040.	Nevada Division of Insurance	http://doi.state.nv.us 788 Fairview Dr., Suite 300 Carson City, NV 89701 Phone: 775-687-4270 Toll Free: 800-992-0900 Fax: 775-687-3937 E-mail: cscc@doi.state.nv.us

State	Status/Terms of Law	State Authority	How to Contact
New Hampshire	Clean paper claims must be paid in 30 days, electronic in 15. 1.5% monthly interest penalty.	New Hampshire Insurance Department	www.state.nh.us/insurance 21 South Fruit Street, Suite 14 Concord, NH 03301 Phone: 603-271-2261 Toll Free: 800-852-3416 Fax: 603-271-1406 E-mail: consumerservices@ins.nh.gov
New Jersey	Clean, electronic claims must be paid within 30 days, paper claims within 40 days. Penalty of 10% simple interest.	New Jersey Department of Banking and Insurance, Division of Insurance	www.state.nj.us/dobi/insmnu.shtml Veronica Schmitt, RN, BSN, MSA Special Investigator Provider Prompt Pay Review State of New Jersey PO Box 329 Trenton, NJ 08625-0329 Phone: 609-292-7272 Toll Free: 800-446-7467
New Mexico	Clean claims must be paid within 30 days if electronic, 45 days if paper. Interest accrues at 1.5% per month.	New Mexico Public Regulation Commission, Insurance Division	www.nmprc.state.nm.us/id.htm PO Box 1269 Santa Fe, NM 87504-1269 Phone: 505-827-4601 Toll Free: 800-947-4722 Fax: 505-827-4734
New York	Claims must be paid with 45 days. Interest accrues at greater of 12% per year or corporate tax rate determined by Commissioner. Fines up to $500/day may also be imposed.	New York State Insurance Department	www.ins.state.ny.us One Commerce Plaza Albany, NY 12257 Phone: 518-474-6600 (Albany); 212-480-6400 (New York City) Toll Free: 800-342-3736

continued

State	Status/Terms of Law	State Authority	How to Contact
North Carolina	Paper and electronic claims must be paid or denied within 30 days. Annual interest penalty of 18%.	North Carolina Department of Insurance	www.ncdoi.com/ 1201 Mail Service Center Raleigh, NC 27699-1201 Phone: 919-807-6750 Toll Free: 800-546-5664
North Dakota	Claims must be paid within 15 days.	North Dakota Insurance Department	www.nd.gov/ndins State Capitol, 5th Floor 600 E. Boulevard Ave. Bismarck, ND 58505-0320 Phone: 701-328-2440 Toll Free: 800-247-0560 Fax: 701-328-4880 E-mail: insurance@nd.gov
Ohio	Clean claims must be paid within 30 days. Interest penalty of 18% per annum.	Ohio Department of Insurance	www.insurance.ohio.gov 50 W. Town Street Third Floor, Suite 300 Columbus, OH 43215 Phone: 614-644-2658 Toll Free: 800-686-1526
Oklahoma	Clean claims must be paid within 45 days. Penalty of 10% of claim as interest for late claims.	Oklahoma Insurance Department	www.oid.state.ok.us PO Box 53408 Oklahoma City, OK 73152-3408 Phone: 405-521-2828 Toll Free: 800-522-0071 Fax: 405-521-6635 E-mail: www.ok.gov/oid/contact.html
Oregon	Clean claims must be paid in 30 days. 12% interest penalty applies.	Oregon Insurance Division	www.cbs.state.or.us/external/ins PO Box 14480 Salem, OR 97309-0405 Phone: 503-947-7980 Toll Free: 888-877-4894 Fax: 503-378-4351 E-mail: dcbs.insmail@state.or.us

State	Status/Terms of Law	State Authority	How to Contact
Pennsylvania	Clean claims must be paid in 45 days. Interest accrues at 10% per annum.	Pennsylvania Insurance Department	www.insurance.pa.gov 1209 Strawberry Square Harrisburg, PA 17120 Phone: 717-787-2317 Fax: 717-787-8585
Rhode Island	Clean claims must be paid in 30 days, 40 days for paper claims. 12% interest per annum penalty applies.	State of Rhode Island Department of Business Regulation	www.dbr.ri.gov/divisions/insurance/ 1511 Pontiac Avenue Cranston, RI 02920 Phone: 401-462-9520 Fax: 401-462-9532 E-mail: InsuranceInquiry@dbr.state.ri.us
South Carolina	Health insurers must pay clean claims in 45 days for paper and 30 days from receipt of electronic claim. Interest penalty is 50% of the difference between the billed charges, as submitted on the claim and the contracted rate or $100 000, whichever is less.	South Carolina Department of Insurance	www.doi.sc.gov/ 1201 Main Street, Suite 1000 Columbia, SC 29201 Phone: 803-737-6200 Fax: 803-737-6205 E-mail: sdubois@doi.sc.gov
South Dakota	Electronic claims must be paid in 30 days; paper claims in 45.	South Dakota Department of Insurance	www.state.sd.us/drr2/reg/insurance 445 East Capitol Avenue Pierre, SD 57501 Phone: 605-773-3563 Fax: 605-773-5369 E-mail: insurance@state.sd.us

continued

State	Status/Terms of Law	State Authority	How to Contact
Tennessee	Clean electronic claims must be paid within 21 days, paper in 30 days. Interest accrues at 1% per month.	Tennessee Department of Commerce and Insurance	www.state.tn.us/commerce/insurance/index.html Insurance Division 500 James Robertson Parkway Nashville, TN 37243 Phone: 615-741-2176 Toll Free: 800-342-4029 E-mail: Insurance.Info@TN.Gov
Texas	Claims must be paid within 45 days (HMOs only). Interest accrues at 18% per annum.	Texas Department of Insurance	www.texashealthoptions.com/cp2/askus.html PO Box 149104 Austin, TX 78714-9104 Phone: 512-463-6169 Toll Free: 800-578-4677 Fax: 512-475-1771 E-mail: ConsumerProtection@tdi.state.tx.us
Utah	Claims must be paid or denied in 30 days. Penalty interest may be applied according to formula: first 90 days, late fee determined by multiplying together total amount of the claim, total number of days the payment is late, and .1%; 91+ days, late fee shall be determined by adding together the late fee for 90-day period and multiplying together the following: total amount of the claim and total number of days the payment was late beyond the initial 90-day period; interest penalty is 10% per annum.	Utah Insurance Department	www.insurance.utah.gov 3110 State Office Building Salt Lake City, UT 84114 Phone: 801-538-3800 Toll Free: 800-439-3805 Fax: 801-538-3829 E-mail: administration.uid@utah.gov

State	Status/Terms of Law	State Authority	How to Contact
Vermont	Claims must be paid or denied in 45 days. Interest penalty is 12% per annum.	Vermont Department of Banking, Insurance, Securities, & Health Care Administration (BISHCA)	www.bishca.state.vt.us 89 Main Street Montpelier, VT 05620-3101 Phone: 802-828-3301 E-mail: Bishca-PubInfo@state.vt.us
Virginia	Clean claims must be paid within 40 days. Penalty interest is legal rate of 6%.	Virginia State Corporation Commission Bureau of Insurance	www.scc.virginia.gov/division/boi/index.htm Tyler Building, PO Box 1157 Richmond, VA 23218 Phone: 804-371-9741 Toll Free: 800-552-7945 E-mail: bureauofinsurance@scc.virginia.gov
Washington	95% of the monthly volume of clean claims of each provider shall be paid in 30 days. 95% of the monthly volume of all claims of each provider shall be paid or denied within 60 days.	Washington State Office of the Insurance Commissioner	www.insurance.wa.gov PO Box 40256 Olympia, WA 98504-0256 Phone: 360-725-7000 Toll Free: 800-562-6900 Fax: 360-586-2018 E-mail: cap@oic.wa.gov
West Virginia	Claims must be paid in 30 days if electronic, 40 days if paper. Interest penalty of 10% per annum.	West Virginia Insurance Commission	www.wvinsurance.gov/ PO Box 50540 Charleston, WV 25305-0540 Phone: 304-558-3386 Toll Free: 888-879-9842 E-mail: Consumer.Service@wvinsurance.gov

continued

State	Status/Terms of Law	State Authority	How to Contact
Wisconsin	If clean claims are not paid within 30 days they are subject to a penalty interest rate of 12% per year.	Office of the Commissioner of Insurance	www.legis.state.wi.us/rsb/statutes.html http://oci.wi.gov/ PO Box 7873 Madison, WI 53707-7873 Phone: 608-266-3585 Toll Free: 800-236-8517 Fax: 608-266-5648 E-mail: ocicomplaints@wisconsin.gov
Wyoming	Claims must be paid within 45 days. Interest penalty is 10% per year.	Wyoming Insurance Department	http://insurance.state.wy.us/ 106 East 6th Avenue Cheyenne, WY 82002 Phone: 307 777-7401 Toll Free: 800-438-5768 Fax: 307-777-2446 E-mail: wyinsdep@state.wy.us

APPENDIX D

Refund Recoupment Statutes by State

State	Statute/URL	Explanation	Period
Alabama	Code of AL 27-1-17 (Section 7, Item 3e) www.legislature.state.al.us/codeofAlabama/1975/27-1-17.htm	An insurer, health service corporation, and health benefit plan shall not retroactively deny, adjust, or seek recoupment or refund of a paid claim for health care expenses submitted by a health care provider for any reason, other than fraud or coordination of benefits or for duplicate payments on claims received from the same insurer, health service corporation, or health benefit plan for the same service, after the expiration of one year from the date that the initial claim was paid, or after the expiration of the same period of time that the health care provider is required to submit claims pursuant to a contract between the health care provider and an insurer, health service corporation, or health benefit plan, whichever date occurs first. Retroactive denials, adjustments, recoupments, or refunds based on coordination of benefits shall be governed by subsection (f). Notwithstanding any other provision of law or contract to the contrary, if an insurer, health service corporation, or health benefit plan retroactively denies, adjusts, or seeks recoupment or refund of a paid claim, the health care provider shall have an additional period of six months from the date that the notice required by subsection (g) was	12 months

continued

State	Statute/URL	Explanation	Period
		received within which to file either a revised claim or a request for reconsideration with additional medical records or information, and the insurer, health service corporation, or health benefit plan shall process the revised claim or request for reconsideration in accordance with the requirements of subsections (a), (b), and (c), or in accordance with U.S. Department of Labor regulations governing the resolution of claims disputes and time for appeals, if applicable.	
Alaska	AS 21.54.020 http://touchngo.com/lglcntr/akstats/Statutes/Title21/Chapter54/Section020.htm	Regarding Direct Payment to Providers, this statute does not prohibit a health care insurer from recovering an amount mistakenly paid to a provider or a covered person.	None
Arizona	20-3102 www.azleg.gov/ars/20/03102.htm	Payment Adjustments – ARS § 20-3102(l) provides that an insurer or provider shall not adjust or request adjustment of a payment or denial of a claim more than one year after the insurer has paid or denied the claim.	12 months
Arkansas	Code Ann. §§ 23-61-108, 23-63-1806, 25-15-201, et seq www.insurance.arkansas.gov/Legal%20Dataservices/rulesandregs/rnr85_May_1_2006.doc	Section 3. Time a. Except in cases of fraud committed by the health care provider, a health care insurer may only exercise recoupment from a provider during the 18-month period after the date that the health care insurer paid the claim submitted by the health care provider. The exception for fraud means fraud that the insurer discovered after the 18-month period and could not have discovered prior to the end of the 18-month period by the	18 months

State	Statute/URL	Explanation	Period
		exercise of reasonable diligence; it does not permit a health care insurer to extend the 18-month period under the rationale that it is still investigating a claim for fraud or any similar reason.	
California	SB 634 10133.66.(b) http://info.sen.ca.gov/pub/05-06/bill/sen/sb_0601-0650/sb_634_bill_20050411_amended_sen.html	(b) Reimbursement requests for the overpayment of a claim shall not be made, including requests made pursuant to Section 10123.145, unless a written request for reimbursement is sent to the provider within 365 days of the date of payment on the overpaid claim. The written notice shall clearly identify the claim, the name of the patient, and the date of service, and shall include a clear explanation of the basis upon which it is believed the amount paid on the claim was in excess of the amount due, including interest and penalties on the claim. The 365-day time limit shall not apply if the overpayment was caused in whole or in part by fraud or misrepresentation on the part of the provider.	365 days
Colorado	Colo. Rev. Stat. § 10-16-106.5 (HB 99-1250, 1999) and (H.B. 02-1353, 2003) www.state.co.us/gov_dir/leg_dir/olls/digest2002a/INSURANCE.htm	Managed care plans—adjustments to health care claims. Requires that adjustments to health care claims be made within 12 months after the date of the original explanation of benefits except in the case of adjustments to claims paid under a risk assumption or risk sharing agreement, which must be made within six months after the last date of service. Requires adjustments to claims related to coordination of benefits with federally funded health plans to be made within 36 months after the date of service.	12 months

continued

State	Statute/URL	Explanation	Period
		Prohibits retroactive adjustment of claims based on eligibility for coverage if the health care provider (provider) received eligibility verification within two business days prior to delivery of service.	
Connecticut	www.cga.ct.gov/ 2005/fc/2005SB-00764-R000156-FC.htm	Effective October 1, 2005, this bill prohibits insurers and HMOs from seeking to recover an overpayment for a claim paid under a health insurance policy unless the insurer or HMO provides written notice to the person from whom recovery is sought within five years after receiving the initial claim. By law, a "person" is an individual, corporation, partnership, limited liability company, association, joint stock company, business trust, unincorporated organization, or other legal entity.	Within 5 years
Delaware	http://delcode.delaware.gov/ title18/c033/ index.shtml	Per Insurance Code, CHAPTER 33. HEALTH INSURANCE CONTRACTS, Delaware's insurance code does not list refund recoupment laws.	None
District of Columbia	D.C. Code Ann.§ 31-3133(a)(b) www.msdc.org/ pp_and_ summary.pdf	(a) A health insurer may only retroactively deny reimbursement to a provider (1) for services subject to coordination of benefits with another health insurer during the 18-month period after the date that the health insurer paid the health care provider; or (2) except as provided in paragraph (1) of this subsection, during the six-month period after the date that the health insurer paid the health care provider. (b)(1) A health insurer that retroactively denies reimbursement to a health care provider under subsection (a)(1) of this section shall	6 months

State	Statute/URL	Explanation	Period
		provide the health care provider with a written statement specifying the basis for the retroactive denial. If the retroactive denial of reimbursement results from coordination of benefits, the written statement shall provide the name and address of the entity acknowledging responsibility for payment of the denied claim.	
Florida	www.flsenate .gov/Statutes/ indes.cfm?App_ mode=Display_ Statute& Search_String =&URL=Ch0627 /Sec6131.htm	a) If an overpayment determination is the result of retroactive review or audit of coverage decisions or payment levels not related to fraud, a health insurer shall adhere to the following procedures: 1. All claims for overpayment must be submitted to a provider within 30 months after the health insurer's payment of the claim. A provider must pay, deny, or contest the health insurer's claim for overpayment within 40 days after the receipt of the claim. All contested claims for overpayment must be paid or denied within 120 days after receipt of the claim. Failure to pay or deny overpayment and claim within 140 days after receipt creates an uncontestable obligation to pay the claim.	30 months
Georgia	www.legis.state .ga.us/legis/ 2001_02/fulltext/ sb476.htm	(a) No carrier, plan, network, panel, or any agent thereof may conduct a post-payment audit or impose a retroactive denial of payment on any claim by any claimant relating to the provision of health care services that was submitted within 90 days of the last date of service or discharge covered by such claim unless: (1) The carrier, plan, network, panel, or agent thereof has provided to the claimant in writing	18 months

continued

State	Statute/URL	Explanation	Period
		notice of the intent to conduct such an audit or impose such a retroactive denial of payment of such claim or any part thereof and has provided in such notice the specific claim and the specific reason for the audit or retroactive denial of payment; (2) Not more than 12 months have elapsed since the last date of service or discharge covered by the claim prior to the delivery to the claimant of such written notice; and (3) Any such audit or retroactive denial of payment must be completed and notice provided to the claimant of any payment or refund due within 18 months of the last date of service or discharge covered by such claim.	
Hawaii		No refund recoupment law	
Idaho		No refund recoupment law	
Illinois		No refund recoupment law	
Indiana	C 27-8-5.7-10 www.in.gov/ legislative/ic/ code/title27/ar8/ ch5.7.html	C 27-8-5.7-10 Claim Payment Errors Sec. 10. (a) An insurer may not, more than two (2) years after the date on which an overpayment on a provider claim was made to the provider by the insurer: (1) request that the provider repay the overpayment; or (2) adjust a subsequent claim filed by the provider as a method of obtaining reimbursement of the overpayment from the provider. (b) An insurer may not be required to correct a payment error to a provider more than two (2) years after the date on which a payment on a provider claim was made to the provider by the insurer. (c) This section does not apply in cases of fraud by the provider, the insured, or the insurer with respect	2 years

State	Statute/URL	Explanation	Period
		to the claim on which the overpayment or underpayment was made. As added by P.L.55-2006, SEC.1.	
Iowa	Admin. Code 191-15.33(507B) www4.legis.state.ia.us/ IAChtml/191.htm#rule_191_15_32	191—15.33(507B) Audit Procedures for Medical Claims 15.33(1) Prohibitions. This rule applies to all claims paid on or after January 1, 2002: a. Absent a reasonable basis to suspect fraud, an insurer may not audit a claim more than two years after the submission of the claim to the insurer. Nothing in this rule prohibits an insurer from requesting all records associated with the claim. b. Absent a reasonable basis to suspect fraud, an insurer may not audit a claim with a billed charge of less than $25.	2 years
Kansas	40-2442 Chapter 40.—INSURANCE, Article 24.—REGULATION OF CERTAIN TRADE PRACTICES www.ksinsurance.org/consumers/pp_statutes.htm	No refund recoupment law	
Kentucky	KY Rev. Stat. Ann.§§ 304.17A et seq. www.lrc.state.ky.us/KRS/304-17A/708.pdf	An insurer shall not be required to correct a payment error to a provider if the provider's request for a payment correction is filed more than 24 months after the date that the provider received payment for the claim from the insurer (except in cases of fraud).	24 months
Louisiana	Regulation 74 and R.S. 22:250.34 B. and	According to Regulation 74 and R.S. 22:250.34 B., "Health insurance issuers that limit the period	Same deadline as for

continued

State	Statute/URL	Explanation	Period
	Louisiana (HB 2052, 1999) www.ldi.state.la.us/Health/Quality_Assurance/frequently_asked_questions.htm	of time that a preferred provider or entity under contract for delivery of covered benefits has to submit claims for payment under R.S. 22:250.32 or 250.33 shall have the same limited period of time following payment of such claims to perform any review or audit for purposes of reconsidering the validity of such claims".	submitting claims
Maine	Me. Rev. Stat. Ann. Tit. 24-A, § 4303 (10A & B) www.mainelegislature.org/legis/statutes/24-A/title24-Asec4303.html	10. Limits on Retrospective Denials. A carrier offering a health plan in this State may not impose on any provider any retrospective denial of a previously paid claim or any part of that previously paid claim unless: A. The carrier has provided the reason for the retrospective denial in writing to the provider [2003, c. 218, §9(NEW)]; and B. The time that has elapsed since the date of payment of the previously paid claim does not exceed 12 months. The retrospective denial of a previously paid claim may be permitted beyond 12 months from the date of payment only for the following reasons: (1) The claim was submitted fraudulently; (2) The claim payment was incorrect because the provider or the insured was already paid for the health care services identified in the claim; (3) The health care services identified in the claim were not delivered by the provider; (4) The claim payment was for services covered by Title XVIII, Title XIX, or Title XXI of the Social Security Act; (5) The claim payment is the subject of adjustment with another	12 months

State	Statute/URL	Explanation	Period
		insurer, administrator or payor; or (6) The claim payment is the subject of legal action. [2007, c. 106, §1 (AMD).]	
Maryland	MD Insurance Code Ann. § 15-1003 et seq. Md. Code Ann., Hlth § 15-102.3 Md. Regs. Code tit. 31, Subtitle 10, § 11 www.michie.com/maryland/lpext.dll?f=templates&fn=main-h.htm&2.0	MD Insurance Code Ann. § 15-1008. "(1) If a carrier retroactively denies reimbursement to a health care provider, the carrier: (i) may only retroactively deny reimbursement for services subject to coordination of benefits with another carrier, the Maryland Medical Assistance Program, or the Medicare Program during the 18-month period after the date that the carrier paid the claim submitted by the health care provider; and (ii) except as provided in item (i) of this paragraph, may only retroactively deny reimbursement during the six-month period after the date that the carrier paid the claim submitted by the health care provider."	6 months
Massachusetts	H.B. 3906 Amended: MGL 176G Section 6 (Managed Care) www.mass.gov/legis/bills/house/ht03pdf/ht03906.pdf	No insurer shall impose on any health care provider any retroactive denial of a previously paid claim or any part thereof unless: (a) The insurer has provided the reason for the retroactive denial in writing to the health care provider; and (b) The time which has elapsed since the date of payment of the challenged claim does not exceed 12 months. The retroactive denial of a previously paid claim may be permitted beyond 12 months from the date of payment only for the following reasons: (see Statute)	12 months
Michigan		No refund recoupment law	
Minnesota	www.revisor.leg.state.mn.us/bin/bldbill.php?bill=H2438.0&session=ls84	No refund recoupment law	

continued

State	Statute/URL	Explanation	Period
Mississippi		No refund recoupment law	
Missouri	Missouri (HB 328 & 88, 2001) Sect. 376.384 www.moga.state.mo.us/statutes/C300-399/3760000384	376.384. 1. All health carriers shall: (3) Not request a refund or offset against a claim more than 12 months after a health carrier has paid a claim except in cases of fraud or misrepresentation by the health care provider;	12 months
Montana	Montana Code Annotated 33-22-150 http://data.opi.state.mt.us/bills/mca/33/22/33-22-150.htm	33-22-150. Reciprocal limitations on claim filing and claim audits—time limit for reimbursements or offsets —exceptions. (1) Except as provided in subsection (3), (4), or (5), if a health insurance issuer limits the time in which a health care provider or other person is required to submit a claim for payment, the health insurance issuer has the same time limit following payment of the claim to perform any review or audit for reconsidering the validity of the claim and requesting reimbursement for payment of an invalid claim or overpayment of a claim. (2) Except as provided in subsection (3), (4), or (5), if a health insurance issuer does not limit the time in which a health care provider or other person is required to submit a claim for payment, a health insurance issuer may not request reimbursement or offset another claim payment for reimbursement of an invalid claim or overpayment of a claim more than 12 months after the payment of an invalid or overpaid claim.	12 months
Nebraska	Title 210 – NEB. DEPT of INS. Chapter 60 (011-011.01(B))	011.01(B)(3) The insurer has notified the claimant within six (6) months of the date of the error, except that in instances of error	6 months

State	Statute/URL	Explanation	Period
	www.sos.ne.gov/rules-and-regs/reg-search/Rules/Insurance_Dept_of/Title-210/Chapter-60.pdf	prompted by representations or nondisclosures of claimants, the insurer notifies the claimant within fifteen (15) days after the date that clear, documented evidence of discovery of such error is included in its file; and 011.01(B)(4) Such notice states clearly the nature of the error, the amount of the overpayment, and the 3-year limitation as provided in subsection 011.01(C).	
Nevada	www.leg.state.nv.us/NAC/NAC-686A.html#NAC686ASec304	No refund recoupment law	
New Hampshire	NH (Ins. Code 420-J:8-b) and eff. 4/9/2006 (HB 1652) www.gencourt.state.nh.us/rsa/html/XXXVII/420-J/420-J-8-b.htm	II. No health carrier shall impose on any health care provider any retroactive denial of a previously paid claim or any part thereof unless: (a) The carrier has provided the reason for the retroactive denial in writing to the health care provider; and (b) The time which has elapsed since the date of payment of the challenged claim does not exceed 18 months. The retroactive denial of a previously paid claim may be permitted beyond 18 months from the date of payment only for the following reasons: (1) The claim was submitted fraudulently; (2) The claim payment was incorrect because the provider or the insured was already paid for the health care services identified in the claim; (3) The health care services identified in the claim were not delivered by the physician/provider;	18 months

continued

State	Statute/URL	Explanation	Period
		(4) The claim payment was for services covered by Title XVIII, Title XIX, or Title XXI of the Social Security Act; (5) The claim payment is the subject of an adjustment with a different insurer, administrator, or payor and such adjustment is not affected by a contractual relationship, association, or affiliation involving claims payment, processing, or pricing; or (6) The claim payment is the subject of legal action.	
New Jersey	P.L. 2005 c.352 (52824 1R)10(a)-10(d), 11(a)(b) www.njleg.state.nj.us/2004/Bills/PL05/352_.HTM	(10) With the exception of claims that were submitted fraudulently or submitted by health care providers that have a pattern of inappropriate billing or claims that were subject to coordination of benefits, no payer shall seek reimbursement for overpayment of a claim previously paid pursuant to this section later than 18 months after the date the first payment on the claim was made. No payer shall seek more than one reimbursement for overpayment of a particular claim. At the time the reimbursement request is submitted to the health care provider, the payer shall provide written documentation that identifies the error made by the payer in the processing or payment of the claim that justifies the reimbursement request. No payer shall base a reimbursement request for a particular claim on extrapolation of other claims, except under the following circumstances: (a) in judicial or quasi-judicial proceedings, including arbitration; (b) in administrative proceedings; (c) in which relevant records required to be maintained by	18 months

State	Statute/URL	Explanation	Period
		the health care provider have been improperly altered or reconstructed, or a material number of the relevant records are otherwise unavailable; or (d) in which there is clear evidence of fraud by the health care provider and the payer has investigated the claim in accordance with its fraud prevention plan established pursuant to section 1 of P.L.1993, c.362 (C.17:33A-15), and referred the claim, together with supporting documentation, to the Office of the Insurance Fraud Prosecutor in the Department of Law and Public Safety established pursuant to section 32 of P.L.1998, c.21 (C.17:33A-16).	
New Mexico		No refund recoupment law	
New York	Managed Care Reform S.8417/A.11996 http://image.iarchives.nysed.gov/images/images/80838.pdf	This legislation sets rules for the recoupment of overpayments by health plans to physicians, including limiting overpayment recovery efforts to two years after the original payment of the claim (with exceptions for fraud, abusive billing, self funded programs, and government programs).	24 months
North Carolina	G.S. 58-3-225(h) www.ncdoi.com/LH/Documents/Checklists/NorthCarolina Department OfInsurance PrompPay Guidance.pdf	The prompt pay law does not specify a time limit within which insurers can recoup overpayments made to providers but states that the time period for recoveries can be established in the contract between the insurer and the provider. If this is not specifically addressed in the provider contract, then the appropriate statute of limitations would apply. [Refer to G.S. 58-3-225(h)]	Per contract
North Dakota		No refund recoupment law	

continued

State	Statute/URL	Explanation	Period
Ohio	Ohio Rev Code Ann. §§3901.38.1 et seq. http://codes.ohio.gov/orc/3901.388	A) A payment made by a third-party payer to a provider in accordance with sections 3901.381 to 3901.386 of the Revised Code shall be considered final two years after payment is made. After that date, the amount of the payment is not subject to adjustment, except in the case of fraud by the provider. (B) A third-party payer may recover the amount of any part of a payment that the third-party payer determines to be an overpayment if the recovery process is initiated not later than two years after the payment was made to the provider. The third-party payer shall inform the provider of its determination of overpayment by providing notice in accordance with division (C) of this section. The third-party payer shall give the provider an opportunity to appeal the determination. If the provider fails to respond to the notice sooner than thirty days after the notice is made, elects not to appeal the determination, or appeals the determination but the appeal is not upheld, the third-party payer may initiate recovery of the overpayment. When a provider has failed to make a timely response to the notice of the third-party payer's determination of overpayment, the third-party payer may recover the overpayment by deducting the amount of the overpayment from other payments the third-party payer owes the provider or by taking action pursuant to any other remedy available under the Revised Code. When a provider elects not to appeal a determination of overpayment or appeals the determination but the appeal is not upheld, the	24 months

State	Statute/URL	Explanation	Period
		third-party payer shall permit a provider to repay the amount by making one or more direct payments to the third-party payer or by having the amount deducted from other payments the third-party payer owes the provider.	
Oklahoma	Title 36, Chapter 1, Art. 12-A 1, Sect 1250.5 www.oscn.net/ applications/ oscn/Deliver Document.asp? citeid=445085	The following act by an insurer constitutes an unfair claim settlement practice: 14. Requesting a refund of all or a portion of a payment of a claim made to a claimant or health care provided more than twenty-four (24) months after the payment is made. This paragraph shall not apply: a. if the payment was made because of fraud committed by the claimant or health care provided, or b. if the claimant or health care provider has otherwise agreed to make a refund to the insurer for overpayment of a claim.	24 months
Oregon		No refund recoupment law	
Pennsylvania	HB 1850 – Session 2005, Subsect 603-B www2.legis.state.pa.us/WU01/LI/BI/BR/2005/O/HB1850P2486.pdf	§ 603-B. Retroactive Denial of Reimbursement (a) General rule—If an insurer retroactively denies reimbursement to a health care provider, the insurer may only: (1) retroactively deny reimbursement for services subject to coordination of benefits with another insurer, the medical assistance program, or the Medicare program during the 12-month period after the date that the insurer paid the health care provider; and (2) except as provided in paragraph (1), retroactively deny reimbursement during a 12-month period after the date that the insurer paid the health care provider.	12 months

continued

State	Statute/URL	Explanation	Period
		(Referred to Committee on Insurance, July 2, 2005)	
Rhode Island		No refund recoupment law	Bill pending
South Carolina	Section 38-94-20 www.scstatehouse.net/sess116_2005-2006/bills/53.htm	If the provider does not supply information reasonably requested by the insurer in connection with the audit, the insurer may: (1) notify the provider in writing that the provider shall provide the information not later than the 45th day after the date of the notice or forfeit the amount of the claim; and (2) if the provider does not provide the information required by this subsection, recover the amount of the claim. (G) The insurer shall complete the audit on or before the 180th day after the date the clean claim is received by the insurer, and any additional payment due a provider or any refund due the insurer must be made not later than the 30th day after the completion of the audit. If a provider disagrees with a refund request made by an insurer based on the audit, the insurer shall provide the provider with an opportunity to appeal, and the insurer may not attempt to recover the payment until all appeal rights are exhausted. (01/11/05 Senate Referred to Committee on Banking and Insurance SJ-105)	
South Dakota		No refund recoupment law	
Tennessee	Pub. Acts, 2003, (SB 460, Chapter #257) Tenn. Code Annotated, Title 56, Chapter 7	56-7-110. (f) Notwithstanding subsection (c), if a health insurance entity or an agent contracted to provide eligibility verification, verifies that an individual is a covered person and if the health	6 months

State	Statute/URL	Explanation	Period
	www.state.tn.us.sos/acts/103/pub/pc0257.pdf	care provider provides services to the individual in reliance on such verification, the health insurance entity may not thereafter retroactively deny a claim on the basis that the individual is not a covered person unless such retroactive denial occurs within six (6) months of the date that the health insurance entity paid the claim; otherwise, the health insurance entity is barred from making such recoupment unless there was fraud by the health care provider.	
Texas	Tex. Ins. Code Ann. § 3.70-3C and §§ 843.000 et seq.**§ 3.70-3C is entitled Preferred Provider Benefits Plans, while §§ 843.000 et seq. is entitled Health Maintenance Organizations www.statutes.legis.state.tx.us/Docs/IN/htm/IN.843.htm	Under § 3.70-3C, the insurer has no later than the 180th day after provider receives payment to recover an "overpayment" (must provide written notice re specific reasons for request of recovery of funds).	180 days
Utah	Utah Code § 31A-26-301.6 http://le.utah.gov/~code/TITLE31A/htm/31A26_030106.htm	(14) Nothing in this section may be construed as limiting the ability of an insurer to: (a) recover any amount improperly paid to a provider or an insured: (i) in accordance with Section 31A-31-103 or any other provision of state or federal law; (ii) within 24 months of the amount improperly paid for a coordination of benefits error;	12 months

continued

State	Statute/URL	Explanation	Period
		(iii) within 12 months of the amount improperly paid for any other reason not identified in Subsection (14)(a)(i) or (ii); or (iv) within 36 months of the amount improperly paid when the improper payment was due to a recovery by Medicaid, Medicare, the Children's Health Insurance Program, or any other state or federal health care program; (b) take any action against a provider that is permitted under the terms of the provider contract and not prohibited by this section; (c) report the provider to a state or federal agency with regulatory authority over the provider for unprofessional, unlawful, or fraudulent conduct; or (d) enter into a mutual agreement with a provider to resolve alleged violations of this section through mediation or binding arbitration. (15) A health care provider may only seek recovery from the insurer for an amount improperly paid by the insurer within the same time frames as Subsections (14)(a) and (b). Amended by Chapter 11, 2009 General Session	
Vermont	18 V. S. A. § 9418 www.leg.state.vt.us/ statutes/ fullsection.cfm? title=18& chapter =221& section=09418	(h) A health plan in this state shall not impose on any provider any retrospective denial of a previously paid claim or any part of that previously paid claim, unless: (1) The health plan has provided at least 30 days' notice of any retrospective denial or overpayment recovery or both in writing to the provider. The notice must include: (A) the patient's name; (B) the service date; (C) the payment amount; (D) the proposed adjustment; and	12 months

Appendix D 257

State	Statute/URL	Explanation	Period
		(E) a reasonably specific explanation of the proposed adjustment. (2) The time that has elapsed since the date of payment of the previously paid claim does not exceed 12 months. (i) The retrospective denial of a previously paid claim shall be permitted beyond 12 months from the date of payment for any of the following reasons: (1) The plan has a reasonable belief that fraud or other intentional misconduct has occurred; (2) The claim payment was incorrect because the health care provider was already paid for the health services identified in the claim; (3) The health care services identified in the claim were not delivered by the provider; (4) The claim payment is the subject of adjustment with another health plan; or (5) The claim is the subject of legal action. (j)(1) For purposes of subsections (h) and (i) of this section, for routine recoveries as described in subdivisions (A) through (J) of this subdivision (1), retrospective denial or overpayment recovery of any or all of a previously paid claim shall not require 30 days' notice before recovery may be made.	
Virginia	Va. Code Ann § 38.2-3407.15 http://law.justia.com/virginia/codes/toc3802000/38.2-3407.15.html	6. No carrier may impose any retroactive denial of a previously paid claim unless the carrier has provided the reason for the retroactive denial and (i) the original claim was submitted fraudulently, (ii) the original claim payment was incorrect because the provider was already paid for the health care	12 months

continued

State	Statute/URL	Explanation	Period
		services identified on the claim or the health care services identified on the claim were not delivered by the provider, or (iii) the time which has elapsed since the date of the payment of the original challenged claim does not exceed the lesser of (a) 12 months or (b) the number of days within which the carrier requires under its provider contract that a claim be submitted by the provider following the date on which a health care service is provided. Effective July 1, 2000, a carrier shall notify a provider at least 30 days in advance of any retroactive denial of a claim. 7. Notwithstanding subdivision 6 of this subsection, with respect to provider contracts entered into, amended, extended, or renewed on or after July 1, 2004, no carrier shall impose any retroactive denial of payment or in any other way seek recovery or refund of a previously paid claim unless the carrier specifies in writing the specific claim or claims for which the retroactive denial is to be imposed or the recovery or refund is sought. The written communication shall also contain an explanation of why the claim is being retroactively adjusted.	
Washington	Chapter 48.43.600 http://law.onecle.com/washington/insurance/48.43.600.html	§ 48.43.600. Overpayment Recovery—Carrier (1) Except in the case of fraud, or as provided in subsections (2) and (3) of this section, a carrier may not: (a) Request a refund from a health care provider of a payment previously made to satisfy a claim unless it does so in writing to the provider within 24 months after the date that the payment	24 months

State	Statute/URL	Explanation	Period
		was made; or (b) request that a contested refund be paid any sooner than six months after receipt of the request. Any such request must specify why the carrier believes the provider owes the refund. If a provider fails to contest the request in writing to the carrier within 30 days of its receipt, the request is deemed accepted and the refund must be paid. (2) A carrier may not, if doing so for reasons related to coordination of benefits with another carrier or entity responsible for payment of a claim: (a) Request a refund from a health care provider of a payment previously made to satisfy a claim unless it does so in writing to the provider within 30 months after the date that the payment was made; or (b) request that a contested refund be paid any sooner than six months after receipt of the request. Any such request must specify why the carrier believes the provider owes the refund, and include the name and mailing address of the entity that has primary responsibility for payment of the claim. If a provider fails to contest the request in writing to the carrier within thirty days of its receipt, the request is deemed accepted and the refund must be paid. (3) A carrier may at any time request a refund from a health care provider of a payment previously made to satisfy a claim if: (a) A third party, including a government entity, is found responsible for satisfaction of the claim as a consequence of liability imposed by law, such as tort liability; and (b) the	

continued

State	Statute/URL	Explanation	Period
		carrier is unable to recover directly from the third party because the third party has either already paid or will pay the provider for the health services covered by the claim. (4) If a contract between a carrier and a health care provider conflicts with this section, this section shall prevail. However, nothing in this section prohibits a health care provider from choosing at any time to refund to a carrier any payment previously made to satisfy a claim. (5) For purposes of this section, "refund" means the return, either directly or through an offset to a future claim, of some or all of a payment already received by a health care provider. (6) This section neither permits nor precludes a carrier from recovering from a subscriber, enrollee, or beneficiary any amounts paid to a health care provider for benefits to which the subscriber, enrollee, or beneficiary was not entitled under the terms and conditions of the health plan, insurance policy, or other benefit agreement. (7) This section does not apply to claims for health care services provided through dental-only health carriers, health care services provided under Title XVIII (Medicare) of the social security act, or Medicare supplemental plans regulated under chapter 48.66 RCW. [2005 c 278 § 1.] Notes: Application—2005 c 278: "This act applies to contracts issued or renewed on or after January 1, 2006." [2005 c 278 § 3.]	

State	Statute/URL	Explanation	Period
West Virginia	HB 2486, Article 43, WV Code §33-45-7A www.legis.state.wv.us/Bill_Text_HTML/2001_SESSIONS/RS/BILLS/hb2486%20sub.htm	(7) (A) Effective the first day of July, 2001, a insurer shall notify a provider at least 30 days in advance of any retroactive denial of a claim. A provider to whom a previously paid claim has been denied by a health benefit plan in accordance with subsection (a) of this section shall, upon receipt of notice of retroactive denial by the plan, reimburse the health benefit plan for such payment within 30 calendar days of receipt of the notice. No insurer may deny payment of a claim for services preauthorized but not yet paid, unless the reason for denial is provided in writing and either the claim is not a clean claim or the claim is fraudulent or has a material misrepresentation. No insurer may impose any retroactive denial of a previously paid claim for services which were preauthorized unless the insurer has provided the reason for the retroactive denial in writing and: (i) The original claim was submitted fraudulently; or (ii) The original claim payment was incorrect because the provider was already paid for the health care services identified on the claim or the health care services identified on the claim were not delivered by the provider. (B) No insurer may impose any retroactive denial of a previously paid claim for services which were not preauthorized unless the insurer has provided the reason for the retroactive denial and: (i) The original claim was submitted fraudulently;	12 months

continued

State	Statute/URL	Explanation	Period
		(ii) The original claim payment was incorrect because the provider was already paid for the health care services identified on the claim or the health care services identified on the claim were not delivered by the provider; or
(iii) The time which has elapsed since the date of the payment of the original challenged claim does not exceed the lesser of: (I) 12 months; or (II) the number of days within which the insurer requires under its provider contract that a claim be submitted by the provider following the date on which a health care service is provided.	
Wisconsin	www.legis.state.wi.us/statutes/Stat0628.pdf	No refund recoupment law	
Wyoming	HB 0167 Section 26-15-124 http://legisweb.state.wy.us/2004/introduced/hb0167.pdf	Section 1. W.S. 26-15-124 by creating a new paragraph (d) is amended to read:
26-15-124. Claims to be accepted or rejected; attorney's fee.
(d) An issuer of health insurance, as defined in W.S.26-1-1-2(a)(xxxiii) or its assignee, may seek reimbursement of benefits paid in error to a health care provider on behalf of an insured, subject to the following conditions:
(i) The insurer gives written or electronic notice to the provider and the insured specifying the date of the payment, any identifying number associated with the payment, the amount of the alleged overpayment and the basis for the insurer's determination that the payment was made in error;
(ii) The notice required by paragraph (i) of this subsection is sent	18 or 24 months

State	Statute/URL	Explanation	Period
		by the insurer within eighteen (18) months after the date of payment or twenty-four (24) months after the date of service, whichever is sooner; (iii) The insurer shall have the burden of proof in the administration of a policy or judicial proceedings to collect the overpayment; (iv) The insurer may collect the overpayment by offsetting future payments to the same provider only if: (a) The provider has authorized the insurer in writing to recover the overpayment by offsetting future payments; or (b) The insurer has clear documentation that the payment was erroneous under the provisions of the policy, the provider has not responded to the insurer within thirty (30) days of the notice required by paragraph (i) of this subsection, and the payment to be offset is make within twelve (12) months of the notice required by paragraph (i) of this subsection. Section 2. This act is effective July 1, 2004.	

APPENDIX E

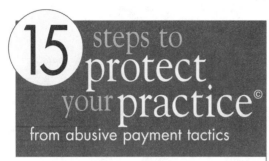

15 steps to protect your practice©
from abusive payment tactics

(1) Know the coverage terms of the patient's insurance policy.
- Maintain records of patient's employer including name, address and phone number.
- Maintain records of any secondary payor associated with patient, including Medicare, Medicaid and workers' compensation.

(2) Obtain and review your contract with the carrier for:
- The nature and scope of covered services;
- The fee-schedule;
- Claim submission requirements (including where and how to transmit);
- Standards for claim review (retrospective review, medical record requests, etc);
- Pre-certification requirement;
- Claim adjudication policies and procedures; and
- Coding guidelines or policies.

(3) Obtain all provider manuals, fee schedules, medical policy manuals and other documents referred to in the contract.

(4) Obtain a specific provider and customer service representative contact, and obtain the name and contact information of the health insurer's local medical director.

(5) Understand and comply with all documentation requirements.

(6) Stay informed of CPT®, ICD, and other code changes and requirements. Make sure you have the most current copies of all code books, standards, and guidelines.

(7) Prepare and submit timely, "clean" claims:
- Use appropriate CPT codes and modifiers;
- Identify and bill correct payor; and
- Comply with all payor requirements for claims submission (including method or mode of submission).

(8) Keep contemporaneous documents in patient files to support claims.

(9) Track submission of claims and receipt of EOB's. Keep records of:
- Date of service;
- Date of submission;
- Date of acknowledgement of receipt by billing entity, clearinghouse, and payor;
- Date of receipt of EOB or any other notice from payor;
- Date of payment (partial and/or final).

(10) Evaluate EOB's for accuracy to detect processing errors. Check for:
- Coding changes;
- Reimbursement rates and adjustments;
- Explanation and denial of benefits (including reason/explanation codes); and
- Interest payments (if applicable).

(11) Request written explanation for all claim delays, partial payments, and denials, and maintain follow-up log on all claims delayed beyond state law specifications.

(12) Submit timely formal appeal letter with supportive documentation as required by contract and request appeal to be reviewed by a practicing, board-certified specialist representing your practice area.

(13) File complaint with state insurance commissioner for claims that are delayed beyond state-required time frames.

(14) Inform county and state medical societies regarding the submission of any and all complaints against health insurers for contracting and payment related issues. Complete any complaint form offered by the medical society.

(15) Complete the AMA's online Health Plan Complaint Form. The data collected through the Health Plan Complaint Form will be used to identify trends and to facilitate discussions with national health insurers to resolve administrative hassles and physician complaints.

Information about the AMA's Private Sector Advocacy (PSA) Health Plan Complaint Form and all other PSA initiatives can be found at: www.ama-assn.org/go/psa.

American Medical Association
Physicians dedicated to the health of America

APPENDIX F

Disclosure of Security Breach by State

State	Statute	URL(s)
Alabama	No security breach law	
Alaska	Alaska Statute § 45.48.0101 et seq	www.legis.state.ak.us/basis/ folioproxy.asp?url=http://wwwjnu01 .legis.state.ak.us/cgi-bin/folioisa.dll/ stattx09/query=[JUMP:'AS4548010']/doc/ {@1}?firsthit
Arizona	Arizona Revised Statute § 44-7501	www.azleg.state.az.us/ FormatDocument.asp?inDoc=/ ars/44/07501.htm&Title=44
Arkansas	Arkansas Code § 4-110-101 et seq.	www.nacua.org/nacualert/docs/ SecurityBreach/arkcode.pdf
California	California Civil Code §§ 56.06, 1785.11.2, 1798.29, 1798.82	www.leginfo.ca.gov/cgi-bin/ displaycode?section=civ&group= 00001-01000&file=56-56.07 www.leginfo.ca.gov/cgi-bin/ displaycode?section=civ&group= 01001-02000&file=1785.10-1785.19.5 www.leginfo.ca.gov/cgi-bin/ displaycode?section=civ&group= 01001-02000&file=1798.25-1798.29 www.leginfo.ca.gov/cgi-bin/ displaycode?section=civ&group= 01001-02000&file=1798.80-1798.84
Colorado	Colorado Revised Statute § 6-1-716	www.state.co.us/gov_dir/leg_dir/olls/ sl2006a/sl_145.htm
Connecticut	Connecticut General Statute 361-701(b)	www.cga.ct.gov/2007/pub/Chap669 .htm#Sec36a-701b.htm
Delaware	Delaware Code tit. 6, § 12B-101 et seq.	http://delcode.delaware.gov/title6/c012b/ index.shtml

continued

State	Statute	URL(s)
District of Columbia	D.C. Code §28-3851 et seq.	http://weblinks.westlaw.com/result/ default.aspx?cite=UUID(N05E829E0EF-6811DBB3FFF-706A9038598)&db= 1000869&findtype=VQ&fn=_top&ifm= NotSet&pbc=4BF3FCBE&rlt=CLID_ FQRLT6034522412265&rp=/Search/ default.wl&rs=WEBL10.05&service=Find &spa=DCC-1000&sr=TC&vr=2.0
Florida	Florida Statute § 817.5681	www.flsenate.gov/Statutes/ index.cfm?App_mode=Display_ Statute&Search_String=&URL=Ch0817/ SEC5681.HTM&Title=->2007-> Ch0817->Section%205681
Georgia	Georgia Code §§ 10-1-910, -911	http://law.justia.com/georgia/codes/ 10/10-1-910.html
		http://law.justia.com/georgia/codes/ 10/10-1-911.html
Hawaii	Hawaii Revised Statute § 487N-2	www.capitol.hawaii.gov/ hrscurrent/Vol11_Ch0476-0490/ HRS0487N/HRS_0487N-0002.htm
Idaho	Idaho Code §§ 28-51-104 to 28-51-107, 2010 H.B. 566	www.legislature.idaho.gov/idstat/Title28/ T28CH51SECT28-51-104.htm
		www.legislature.idaho.gov/idstat/Title28/ T28CH51SECT28-51-105.htm
		www.legislature.idaho.gov/idstat/Title28/ T28CH51SECT28-51-106.htm
		www.legislature.idaho.gov/idstat/Title28/ T28CH51SECT28-51-107.htm
		www.legislature.idaho.gov/legislation/ 2010/H0566.pdf
Illinois	Illinois 815 ILCS 530/1 et seq.	www.ilga.gov/legislation/ilcs/ ilcs3.asp?ActID=2702&ChapAct=815 ILCS 530/&ChapterID=67&ChapterName =BUSINESS+TRANSACTIONS&Act Name=Personal+Information+Protection +Act.
Indiana	Indiana Code §§ 24-4.9 et seq., 4-1-11 et seq., 2009 H.B. 1121	www.in.gov/legislative/ic/code/title24/ ar4.9/ch1.pdf
		www.in.gov/legislative/ic/code/title4/ar1/ ch11.html
		www.in.gov/legislative/bills/2009/HE/ HE1121.1.html

State	Statute	URL(s)
Iowa	Iowa Code § 715C.1 (2008 S.F. 2308)	www.iowa.gov/tax/taxlaw/08legsum.html#SF2308
Kansas	Kansas Statute 50-7a01, 50-7a02	http://privacylaw.proskauer.com/Kansas_Complete.pdf www.kslegislature.org/legsrv-statutes/getStatuteFile.do?number=/50-7a02.html
Kentucky	No security breach law	
Louisiana	Louisiana Revised Statute § 51:3071 et seq.	www.legis.state.la.us/lss/lss.asp?doc=322027
Maine	Maine Revised Statute tit. 10 §§ 1347 et seq., 2009 Public Law 161	www.mainelegislature.org/legis/statutes/10/title10sec1346.html www.mainelegislature.org/legis/statutes/10/title10sec1347.html www.mainelegislature.org/legis/statutes/10/title10sec1348.html http://mainelegislature.org/legis/bills/bills_124th/chapters/PUBLIC161.asp
Maryland	Maryland Code Commercial Law § 14-3501 et seq.	www.michie.com/maryland/lpext.dll?f=templates&fn=main-h.htm&cp=mdcode
Massachusetts	Massachusetts General Laws § 93H-1 et seq.	www.mass.gov/legis/laws/mgl/93h-1.htm
Michigan	Michigan Comp. Laws §445.72	www.legislature.mi.gov/(S(bknenk55qp1tbs45dbhdmf55))/mileg.aspx?page=GetObject&objectname=mcl-445-72
Minnesota	Minnesota Statute §§ 325E.61, 325E.64	www.revisor.mn.gov/bin/getpub.php?type=s&num=325E.61&year=2007 www.revisor.mn.gov/bin/getpub.php?pubtype=STAT_CHAP&year=2007&section=325E#stat.325E.64.0
Mississippi	Mississippi 2010 H. B. 583 (effective July 1, 2011)	http://billstatus.ls.state.ms.us/documents/2010/pdf/HB/0500-0599/HB0583SG.pdf
Missouri	Missouri. Revised Statute § 407.1500	www.moga.mo.gov/statutes/c400-499/4070001500.htm

continued

State	Statute	URL(s)
Montana	Montana Code § 30-14-1701 et seq., 2009 H.B. 155, Chapter 163	http://law.justia.com/montana/codes/30/30-14-1705.html http://data.opi.mt.gov/bills/2009/billhtml/HB0155.htm
Nebraska	Nebraska Revised Statute §§ 87-801, -802, -803, -804, -805, -806, -807	http://uniweb.legislature.ne.gov/laws/statutes.php?statute=87-801&print=true http://uniweb.legislature.ne.gov/laws/statutes.php?statute=87-802&print=true http://uniweb.legislature.ne.gov/laws/statutes.php?statute=s8708003000 http://uniweb.legislature.ne.gov/laws/statutes.php?statute=87-804&print=true http://uniweb.legislature.ne.gov/laws/statutes.php?statute=87-805&print=true http://uniweb.legislature.ne.gov/laws/statutes.php?statute=87-806&print=true http://uniweb.legislature.ne.gov/laws/statutes.php?statute=87-807&print=true
Nevada	Nevada Revised Statute 603A.010 et seq.	www.leg.state.nv.us/nrs/NRS-603A.html
New Hampshire	New Hampshire Revised Statute §§ 359-C:19, -C:20, -C:21	www.gencourt.state.nh.us/rsa/html/XXXI/359-C/359-C-19.htm www.gencourt.state.nh.us/rsa/html/XXXI/359-C/359-C-20.htm www.gencourt.state.nh.us/rsa/html/XXXI/359-C/359-C-21.htm
New Jersey	New Jersey Statute 56:8-163	www.njleg.state.nj.us/2004/bills/pl05/226_.htm www.njleg.state.nj.us/2008/Bills/A2500/2270_I1.PDF
New Mexico	No security breach law	
New York	New York General Business Law § 899-aa	http://law.justia.com/newyork/codes/general-business/gbs0a39-f_article39-f.html http://law.justia.com/newyork/codes/general-business/gbs0899-aa_899-aa.html
North Carolina	North Carolina General Statute § 75-65	www.nacua.org/nacualert/docs/SecurityBreach/nccode.pdf

State	Statute	URL(s)
North Dakota	North Dakota Century Code § 51-30-01 et seq.	www.legis.nd.gov/cencode/t51c30.pdf
Ohio	Ohio Revised Code §§ 1347.12, 1349.19, 1349.191, 1349.192	http://codes.ohio.gov/orc/1347.12 http://codes.ohio.gov/orc/1349.19 http://codes.ohio.gov/orc/1349.191 http://codes.ohio.gov/orc/1349.192
Oklahoma	Oklahoma Statute § 74-3113.1 and 2008 H.B. 2245	www2.lsb.state.ok.us/os/os_74-3113.1.rtf. www.oml.org/npps/story.cfm?id=1254
Oregon	Oregon Revised Statute § 646A.600 et seq.	www.leg.state.or.us/ors/646a.html
Pennsylvania	Pennsylvania 73 Pa. Stat. § 2303	www.pacode.com/secure/data/001/chapter3/s3.13.html
Rhode Island	Rhode Island General Laws § 11-49.2-1 et seq.	www.rilin.state.ri.us/statutes/TITLE11/11-49.2/11-49.2-3.HTM
South Carolina	South Carolina Code § 39-1-90	www.scstatehouse.gov/code/t39c001.htm
South Dakota	No security breach law	
Tennessee	Tennessee Code § 47-18-2107, 2010 S.B. 2793	www.michie.com/tennessee/lpext.dll?f=templates&fn=main-h.htm&cp=tncode http://state.tn.us/sos/acts/106/pub/pc0650.pdf
Texas	Texas Business and Commerce Code § 521.03	www.statutes.legis.state.tx.us/Docs/BC/htm/BC.521.htm
Utah	Utah Code §§ 13-44-101, -102, -201, -202, -301	http://le.utah.gov/~code/TITLE13/htm/13_44_010100.htm http://le.utah.gov/~code/TITLE13/htm/13_44_010200.htm http://le.utah.gov/~code/TITLE13/htm/13_44_020100.htm http://le.utah.gov/~code/TITLE13/htm/13_44_020200.htm http://le.utah.gov/~code/TITLE13/htm/13_44_030100.htm
Vermont	Vermont Statute tit. 9 § 2430 et seq.	www.leg.state.vt.us/statutes/fullchapter.cfm?Title=09&Chapter=062

continued

State	Statute	URL(s)
Virginia	Virginia Code § 18.2-186.6, 2010 H.B. 1039 (effective January 1, 2011)	http://leg1.state.va.us/cgi-bin/legp504.exe?000+cod+18.2-186.6
Washington	Washington Revised Code § 19.255.010, 2010 H.B. 1149	http://apps.leg.wa.gov/rcw/default.aspx?cite=19.255.010 http://apps.leg.wa.gov/documents/WSLdocs/2009-10/Pdf/Bills/Session%20Law%202010/1149-S2.SL.pdf
West Virginia	West Virginia Code §§ 46A-2A-101 et seq.	www.legis.state.wv.us/WVCODE/Code.cfm?chap=46a&art=2A
Wisconsin	Wisconsin Statute § 134.98 et seq.	www.legis.state.wi.us/statutes/Stat0134.pdf
Wyoming	Wyoming Statute § 40-12-501 to -502	www.michie.com/wyoming/lpext.dll?f=templates&fn=main-h.htm

APPENDIX G

> These tools do not provide legal advice. Consultation with legal counsel may be appropriate to help identify and pursue claims that should be appealed. For additional information visit the Practice Management Center Website at www.ama-assn.org/go/pmc.

Sample letter for claims underpayment

[*Date*]
Attn: _____
Provider Appeals Department
[*Address*]
[*City, State, ZIP Code*]

Re: Claims underpayment
Insured/Plan Member: _____
Health Insurer Identification Number: _____
Group Number: _____
Patient Name: _____
Claim Number: _____
Claim Date: _____

Dear [*Health insurer*]:

I am writing on behalf of [*physician name*] to address claim adjudication errors involving the payment processed for [*patient name*]'s charges on [*date of service*].

[*Example bilateral denial text*]

Please be advised that the following services were provided and [*patient name*] received [*list of procedure(s) and/or service(s)*]. Each additional [*procedure*] was filed with the CPT modifier 50 to indicate a bilateral procedure was performed. Evidently, the additional procedures [*insert CPT codes*] were paid as unilateral in error, and CPT codes [*insert codes*] were erroneously denied as incidental, resulting in a total claim underpayment of [*$*].

[*Example partial payment text*]

According to our participating provider contract with [*health insurer*], all fees are subject to the negotiated fee schedule allowance. Since payment methodology is based on [*insert appropriate health insurer's payment methodology, eg, Medicare's RBRVS*], all fees are subject to [*insert appropriate health insurer's multiple payment guidelines and global periods, eg, CMS's multiple procedure payment guidelines and global periods*].

As such, the first procedure is to be paid at [%] of the fee allowance and the second through fifth procedures at [%] of the scheduled fee allowance. Therefore, as the contract provides, the following procedures should be paid as follows:

CPT Code	Our Fee	[*Health Insurer*] Rate	[*Health Insurer*] Paid	Amount Due
[*CPT code*] x2	$	$	$	$
[*CPT code*] x2	$	$	$	$
[*CPT code*] x2	$	$	$	$
			Total Due:	$

Other [*health insurer*] patient EOBs have been referenced that show past payment allowed for these exact procedures. Documentation is included revealing the correct [*health insurer*] rates as listed above were paid on other claims processed by [*health insurer*]. Apparently, claims are not being processed consistently for [*health insurer*].

[*The rationale for the appeal needs to be specific, similar to the following template for a separate procedure that also includes laboratory testing.*]

Concerning the denial of CPT [*code*]x2, this issue has been addressed numerous times by our office. The CPT modifier 59 was reported with CPT [*code*]x2 to alert that this procedure is separate from the other procedures and therefore, not inclusive to another procedure. As such, CPT [*codes*] are not subject to computer editing [*insert software package, if known*] and warrant manual review. Since CPT [*code*] was performed [*reason procedure or service was performed*], it cannot be denied as incidental. The operative report we provided clearly identifies [*reason procedure or service was performed*].

The ICD-9-CM codes reported, [*ICD-9-CM codes*], justify the medical necessity of this procedure. Therefore, the basis of [*health insurer*]'s denial of CPT [*code*] as incidental is not only invalid but also unsupported. Please refer this claim to a board-certified [*specialty*] physician for additional review.

We will expect payment in the amount of [*$*] to be released promptly in accordance with the [*state prompt payment act*].

Sincerely,

[*Practice Manager*]

The AMA Practice Management Center is a resource of the AMA Private Sector Advocacy unit.

© 2008 American Medical Association. Permission is granted to physicians to use this letter in connection with their practices. Any other use is prohibited.

> These tools do not provide legal advice. Consultation with legal counsel may be appropriate to help identify and pursue claims that should be appealed. For additional information visit the Private Sector Advocacy Website at www.ama-assn.org/go/psa.

Sample letter to patient's employer or health plan sponsor regarding late payment

[*Date*]
Attn: _____
Employer/Plan Sponsor
[*Address*]
[*City, State, ZIP Code*]

Re: Late payment of claims

Dear [*Employer*]:

I wanted to alert you to a situation occurring with [*health insurer*]. We treat a number of your employees under [*name of health insurer*]. Our practice is experiencing significant delays in payment of claims from [*name of health insurer*]. [*Add any details of your particular situation*]. As I am sure you can understand, this makes it very difficult to run a medical practice.

We are extremely concerned with our ability to continue to contract with health insurers that are seriously delinquent in payment of claims. This concerns us a great deal, for termination of our relationship with [*name of health insurer*] would interfere with established relationships with our patients, your employees. Why should premium-paying patients suffer because their payer fails to meet its obligations?

It would be very helpful to us if you could bring this issue to the attention of the representatives from [*health insurer*] with whom you contract. The problem is becoming increasingly chronic in our area.

Thank you for your consideration of this matter.

Sincerely,

[*Physician*]
    Or
[*Practice Manager*]

© 2008 American Medical Association. Permission is granted to physicians to use this letter in connection with their practices. Any other use is prohibited.

> These tools do not provide legal advice. Consultation with legal counsel may be appropriate to help identify and pursue claims that should be appealed. For additional information visit the Practice Management Center Website at www.ama-assn.org/go/pmc.

Sample letter to health insurer regarding late payment

[*Date*]
Attn: _____
[*Health Insurer*]
[*Address*]
[*City, State, ZIP Code*]

Re: Late payment of claims

Dear [*Health insurer*]:

I am writing in regards to the attached claims I have submitted to [*name of health insurer*]. These claims, which were submitted between [*date*] and [*date*], have not been paid, and I have not received any explanation for this delay in payment.

Please contact my office at your earliest convenience to explain the reason for this delay and to indicate when I will receive payment.

Optional sentence 1 (*For states with regulations/laws requiring payment within a specified timeframe*):

Under [*pertinent state law/regulation*], claims must be paid in [*x*] days or [*describe any penalty*]. Please include the appropriate interest amount in the payment.

[*Document any contact between your office and the health insurer about this matter*]

Note: The following sentences should be added only if the physician is comfortable with a more adversarial tone.

Optional sentence 2 (**Do not** *include this sentence if your contract prohibits you from billing patients directly for claims that are the payer's responsibility*):

I do not want to be put in the untenable position of billing my patients for the care they have contracted for through their insurance policy with [*state name of health insurer*].

Optional sentence 3:

Because I know the issue of delayed payment is of increasing concern to many physicians, I intend to report this delay and lack of explanatory information to the state insurance commissioner if the situation is not rectified within [*x*] days.

Thank you for your prompt attention to this matter.

Sincerely,

[*Physician*]
    Or
[*Practice Manager*]

(*optional cc: Patient/insured, patient's health insurer sponsor*)

The AMA Practice Management Center is a resource of the AMA Private Sector Advocacy unit.

© 2008 American Medical Association. Permission is granted to physicians to use this letter in connection with their practices. Any other use is prohibited.

> These tools do not provide legal advice. Consultation with legal counsel may be appropriate to help identify and pursue claims that should be appealed. For additional information visit the Practice Management Center Website at www.ama-assn.org/go/pmc.

Note: Many states have prompt payment requirements. Check your state law to determine whether it establishes a shorter period.

Sample letter to health insurer regarding late payment of claims in violation of contract

[*Date*]
Attn: _____
[*Health Insurer*]
[*Address*]
[*City, State, ZIP Code*]

Re: Late payment of claims

Dear [*Health insurer*]:

This letter is being sent to notify you of the prompt-payment provision agreed in our provider contract with [*health insurer*].

According to the contract, payment is to be issued within [*45*] days of receipt of a clean claim; otherwise, the provider discount is forfeited and full-billed charges are due. Attached is a copy of the [*claim form*] that has been reviewed for accuracy. Applicable medical record copies also are attached to prevent this claim from being delayed for additional information.

Please be advised that provider discounts applied on claims paid after the [*45*]-day requirement will not be honored. In such cases, the patient will be notified regarding the breach of contract.

We are willing to make every effort to ensure that you receive adequate claim information to facilitate the adjudication process. Likewise, we request your cooperation in paying our claims accurately and in a timely manner as the contract permits.

Thank you for your prompt attention to this matter.

Sincerely,

[*Physician*]
    Or
[*Practice Manager*]

The AMA Practice Management Center is a resource of the AMA Private Sector Advocacy unit.

© 2008 American Medical Association. Permission is granted to physicians to use this letter in connection with their practices. Any other use is prohibited.

> These tools do not provide legal advice. Consultation with legal counsel may be appropriate to help identify and pursue claims that should be appealed. For additional information visit the Private Sector Advocacy Website at www.ama-assn.org/go/psa.

Sample appeal letter for inappropriate E/M downcoding

[*Date*]
Attn: _____
Provider Appeals Department
[*Address*]
[*City, State, ZIP Code*]

Re: Inappropriate downcoding of CPT evaluation and management (E/M) code

Insured/Plan Member: _____
Health Plan Identification Number: _____
Group Number: _____
Patient Name: _____
Claim Number: _____
Claim Date: _____

Dear [*Health insurer*]:

[For E/M downcoding]

On the date of service listed above, the CPT E/M code for [*a/an*] [*name of service*] was reported with [*CPT code*]. [*Health insurer*] has inappropriately downcoded the CPT E/M code submitted and changed the code to [*new code*], resulting in the inappropriate reduction of payment for delivered medical care.

Under [*health insurer*] medical review guidelines, [*health insurer*] follows the CMS E/M coding guidelines [*1995 or 1997*] version. [*Physician name*] has billed according to the [*1995 or 1997*] CMS E/M guidelines accurately.

Downcoding of CPT E/M codes is not appropriate without review of medical record documentation. The American Medical Association (AMA) strongly opposes automatic downcoding and states:

> "The AMA vigorously opposes the practice of unilateral, arbitrary recoding and/or bundling by all payers."

The appropriateness on the reported level of the CPT E/M [*CPT code*] is clearly documented within the patient's chart (attached) and should be recognized by [*health insurer*]. Based on the circumstances of this case, we are requesting that CPT E/M code *[code]* be paid and not be inappropriately downcoded.

Thank you for your reconsideration. Please contact [contact name] at [telephone number] in our office should you have any questions regarding this claim.

Sincerely,

[Physician]
   Or
[Practice Manager]

[For procedure downcoding]

On the date of service listed above, the CPT code for [a/an] [name of procedure] was reported with [CPT code]. [Health insurer] has inappropriately downcoded the CPT code submitted and changed the code to [new code and name of procedure], resulting in the inappropriate reduction of payment for delivered medical care.

Downcoding of CPT codes is not appropriate without review of medical record documentation. The American Medical Association (AMA) strongly opposes automatic downcoding and states:

> "The AMA vigorously opposes the practice of unilateral, arbitrary recoding and/or bundling by all payers."

The level of complexity for the procedure performed CPT [code] was reported appropriately and is clearly documented within the patient's chart (attached) and should be recognized by [health insurer]. Based on the circumstances of this case, we are requesting that CPT code [code] be paid and not be inappropriately downcoded.

Thank you for your reconsideration. Please contact [contact name] at [telephone number] in our office should you have any questions regarding this claim.

Sincerely,

[Physician]
   Or
[Practice Manager]

© 2008 American Medical Association. Permission is granted to physicians to use this letter in connection with their practices. Any other use is prohibited.

Appendix G

> These tools do not provide legal advice. Consultation with legal counsel may be appropriate to help identify and pursue claims that should be appealed. For additional information visit the Private Sector Advocacy Website at www.ama-assn.org/go/psa.

Note: Physicians should check with their personal attorney before cashing a check that includes a restrictive endorsement such as "payment in full," as such language may be binding and prohibit the physician from seeking any further payment from the health insurer or the patient.

Sample appeal letter PPO discount taken when a contract does not exist

[*Date*]
Attn: _____
Provider Appeals Department
[*Address*]
[*City, State, ZIP Code*]

Re: PPO discount taken when a contract does not exist

Insured/Plan Member: _____
Health Plan Identification Number: _____
Group Number: _____
Patient Name: _____
Claim Number: _____
Claim Date: _____

Dear [*Health insurer*]:

For the date of service listed above, [*health insurer*] incorrectly applied a PPO discount to the claim when there is no contract between [*physician or group name*] and [*health insurer*]. Because [*physician or group name*] does not have a contract with [*health insurer*], we are under no obligation to accept a reduced payment and will not honor the PPO discount.

[When EOB states that the patient is not responsible for the balance]

The patient is legally responsible for payment of our services. We are accepting your payment as a partial payment on behalf of the patient. We intend to bill the patient for the balance. We request that you send a corrected EOB/RA to us and to the patient correctly stating that the patient is responsible for this remainder.

[For rental network]

[*Physician or group name*] has no record of a contract with the health insurer or network listed on the patient's identification card. If your records indicate otherwise, please provide a copy of the contract agreement which is being referenced.

Since [*physician or group name*] is an "out-of-network" provider, [*he/she*] is entitled to payment at our fee-for-service billed rate. We request that you send a corrected EOB/RA to the practice and to the patient.

Thank you for your consideration. Please contact [*staff name*] at [*telephone number*] in our office should you have any questions regarding this claim.

Sincerely,

[*Physician*]
    Or
[*Practice Manager*]

© 2008 American Medical Association. Permission is granted to physicians to use this letter in connection with their practices. Any other use is prohibited.

> These tools do not provide legal advice. Consultation with legal counsel may be appropriate to help identify and pursue claims that should be appealed. For additional information visit the Private Sector Advocacy Website at www.ama-assn.org/go/psa.

Note: If your state's Department of Insurance has a formal process for filing complaints, you should use that process rather than sending a letter.

Sample letter to state insurance commissioner or other entity that regulates various health insurers regarding late payment

[*Date*]
Attn: _____
[*Commissioner/Appropriate Contact State Regulatory Agency*]
[*Address*]
[*City, State, ZIP Code*]

Re: Late payment of claims

Dear [*Commissioner/Mr./Ms.*] _____:

Attached is correspondence I have sent to [*health insurer*] on [*date*] regarding the late payment of my claims. I have received no response from [*health insurer*].

As you may know, the physician community is increasingly concerned about the chronic late payment of claims. This is a troubling practice that makes it extremely difficult to run a practice. We are extremely concerned with our ability to continue to contract with payers that are seriously delinquent in claims payment. This concerns us a great deal, as a termination of our relationship with such payers would interfere with established relationships with patients. Why should premium-paying patients in this state suffer because their payer fails to meet its obligations?

Optional sentence *(for states with laws/regulations regarding late payment):*

Under [*cite law/regulation*], payment is required within [*x*] days. I am requesting that your agency enforce this provision as to [*health insurer*].

I hope your agency will act quickly to ensure an end is put to this practice. Thank you for your consideration of this matter.

Sincerely,

[*Physician*]
    Or
[*Practice Manager*]

Enclosure

(optional cc: Patient/insured, patient's health insurer sponsor)

© 2008 American Medical Association. Permission is granted to physicians to use this letter in connection with their practices. Any other use is prohibited.

GLOSSARY

This glossary serves as a reference relative to the terms and language associated with operations, reimbursement, and economic decision-making within a medical practice. These terms help to standardize and clarify the business aspect of clinical medicine.

A

account payable A *debt* owed to a creditor, often as a result of the purchase of merchandise, materials, supplies, or services. An account payable is normally a current *liability,* resulting from day-to-day operations of the practice.

account receivable A charge against a debtor, often from sales or services rendered. This receivable is not necessarily due or past due. An account receivable is the opposite of an *account payable*, and is normally a *current asset* arising from standard business operations.

accounting A service activity that provides quantitative information, most often financial in nature, regarding economic entities. The information from this service is intended to be used in economic decision-making.

accounting equation *Assets = Liabilities + Owners' Equity.*

accounting period The time period for which a *financial statement,* including an *income statement* or statement of *cash flows,* is prepared. The financial statements must clearly define the appropriate time period for which they are relevant. Normally, the time period is no less than one month and no more than one year.

accounting system The process, policies, and procedures used for collecting and summarizing financial data within a particular organization.

accounts receivable turnover The quotient of net *sales* and average *accounts receivable.*

accrual basis of accounting The method of recognizing *revenue* when goods are delivered or services are provided, regardless of when cash is received. *Expenses* are recognized in the same period the related revenue is recognized.

acquisition cost Cost of equipment or property plus all expenditures necessary to place and ready that asset for its intended use. Possible expenditures include legal fees, transportation charges, and installation costs.

adjusted bank balance of cash The balance shown on a bank statement. This value, when adjusted for the unrecorded deposits or outstanding checks, can be used to reconcile the bank's balance with the correct cash balance.

adjusted book balance of cash The balance shown in a practice's account for cash in the bank. When adjusted for any notes collected by the bank or bank service charges, this amount can be used to reconcile the account balance with the correct cash balance.

adjusting entry An entry made to correct an accounting event that has been improperly recorded or has not been recorded during the accounting period. This entry serves to update and correct the account.

administrative expense An *expense* related to the business as a whole, such as salaries of executives, office rental fee, or consulting fees.

admission of partner When a new partner joins a *partnership*, the old partnership is legally dissolved and a new one is formed. However, in actuality, many times the old accounting practices are sustained and adjusted only to reflect the newly joined partner. Should a new partner purchase the interest of a different partner, all that is changed is the name on one capital account. If *assets* and *liabilities* are contributed by the new partner, they must be recognized.

aging accounts receivable Management tool used to classify *accounts receivable* according to the time elapsed since the claim existed. This is used to determine an entity's uncollectible accounts receivable as of a specific date.

allocate To divide *revenues* or *expenses* from one account into several accounts, across several periods or among several cost centers.

Americans with Disability Act (ADA) The federal law that protects the rights of individuals with disabilities.

amortization The process of allocating a *debt* to different time periods, as often occurs with a loan, such as a mortgage. The term has also come to mean *writing off* (ie, liquidating) the cost of an asset. The amortization can be detailed through an "amortization schedule," which is a table detailing the allocation between *interest* and *principal*.

annuity Payments of equal amounts often made at equally spaced time intervals.

appraisal A valuation of an *asset* or *liability* that involves expert opinion.

appreciation An increase in the value of an asset. The opposite of *depreciation*.

arm's length Transaction conducted between two parties as though they were independent, even if they are related or otherwise affiliated. An arm's length transaction ensures an arrangement's compliance with legal guidelines. The basis for a *fair market value* determination.

articles of incorporation Document filed with a state or other regulatory authority by persons forming a corporation outlining the management of said corporation. When the document is returned with a certificate of incorporation, it becomes the corporation's charter.

assess To make an official valuation of an *asset*.

asset Everything of value owned by a person, company, or corporation. Assets are generally classified as either tangible assets (including current and fixed assets) or *intangible assets* (such as goodwill and accounts receivable).

assignment of accounts receivable Transfer of the legal ownership using *accounts receivable* as collateral. The assignment can be classified as general or specific, depending on the structure of the process.

audit Systematic inspection of a firm's accounting system and financial records. Also, assessment of a firm's compliance with generally accepted standards set forth by regulatory and governing bodies. See *internal audit*.

B

bad debt Portion of receivables that are uncollectible, usually from *accounts receivable* or loans. Bad debt is considered an expense for accounting purposes.

bad debt recovery Collection of an *account receivable* that was previously written off as uncollectible.

balance As a noun, the sum of *debit* entries minus the sum of *credit* entries in an account.

balance sheet Financial statement that lists a firm's assets, liabilities, and owners' equity at a specific point in time.

balloon Most *mortgage* and *installment loans* require relatively equal periodic payments. However, some loans do not fully amortize over the term of the note, thus requiring relatively equal periodic payments but a large final payment due at maturity. This large final payment is called a *balloon* payment. Such loans are called *balloon loans*.

bank balance The balance amount in a checking account, as shown on the *bank statement*.

bank reconciliation Process of comparing the book balance of the cash in a bank account and the bank's statement. Less items such as checks issued that have not cleared, deposits that have not cleared, deposits that have not been recorded by the bank, and free of errors made by the bank or the firm, the balance in a firm's accounting records should match the balance of the *bank statement*.

bank statement A summary statement sent by the bank to a customer that shows all financial transactions (including deposits, checks cleared, and service charges) for a given period of time, usually one month.

bankrupt Said of a company whose *liabilities* exceed the fair market value of its assets. A bankrupt firm is usually insolvent.

bill An itemized statement of the charges and terms of sale for goods shipped and services rendered. A bill is also a piece of paper currency.

bonus Premium over normal *wage* or *salary*; usually paid for meritorious performance or increased output.

book As a verb, to recognize a transaction in formal accounting records. As a noun, usually plural, the *journals* and *ledgers*. As an adjective, see *book value*.

book value The value of an *asset* as carried on the *balance sheet*. Book value is calculated as the cost of an asset less accumulated *depreciation*. Generally used to refer to the *net* amount of an *asset* or group of assets shown in the account.

branch A division of an organization; often refers to one that is physically separated from the home office of the enterprise, but not organized as a legally separate subsidiary.

breakeven point The point at which total *revenues* and total *expenses* are equal, where there is no net loss or gain.

budget Financial projection used to estimate and control the results of future operations.

burn rate Amount of *overhead costs* and other costs in excess of revenue that a firm will incur, usually at the onset of operations. It is ordinarily stated in terms of months.

bylaws Written rules adopted by the shareholders of a corporation that govern its internal management and specify the procedures for carrying out the functions of the organization.

C

capital Owners' investment into a business, either in the form of *equity* investment or long-term *debt*.

capital asset Generally, any item that is not bought or sold in standard business operations. This can include land, building, furniture, and equipment.

capital budget Plan of proposed outlays for acquiring long-term *assets* and the means by which these assets will be financed.

capital gain Profit that results when the selling price of a capital *asset* exceeds the purchase price. If the capital *asset* has been held for a sufficiently long period of time before sale, then the tax on the gain is computed at a rate lower than is used for other gains and ordinary income.

capital lease Generally used to finance an *asset* for the majority of its useful life. Both the *liability* and the *asset* are recognized on the lessee's *balance sheet*. Also called a finance lease.

capital loss Loss incurred when the selling price of a *capital asset* is less than the purchase price. Opposite of *capital gain*.

capitalization of earnings The process of valuing a business by computing the net present value of its predicted future *net income*.

cash Money in the form of currency such as coins, negotiable checks, balances in bank accounts, and marketable securities, such as government bonds.

cash basis of accounting In contrast to the *accrual basis of accounting*, a system of accounting in which *revenues* are recorded when cash is received and *expenses* are recognized as payments are made. No attempt is made to match *revenues* and *expenses* in determining *income* in a fixed *accounting period*.

cash budget Estimation of cash *receipts* and *disbursements* for a business for a specific period of time. This budget is used to determine whether a firm has enough cash to maintain standard operations and whether cash is being used in unproductive capacities.

cash flow Change in a cash account over a period of time, usually as the result of financing, operating, or investing. Measuring cash flow can be used for future planning and assessment of the financial health of an organization.

cash receipts journal A specialized *journal* used to record all *receipts* of cash.

certified check Type of check issued from a bank which guarantees there are sufficient reserves to fund the amount noted on the check. After it is issued, the check then becomes an obligation of the bank.

chart of accounts A systematic list of all accounts in a general ledger, each accompanied by a reference number.

check The Federal Reserve Board defines a check as "a draft or order upon a bank or banking house purporting to be drawn upon a deposit of funds for the payment at all events of a certain sum of money to a certain person therein named or to him or his order or to bearer and payable instantly on demand." It must contain the phrase "pay to the order of." The amount shown on the check's face must be clearly readable and it must have the signature of the drawer. Checks need not be dated, although they usually are. The *balance* in the *cash* account is usually reduced when a check is issued, not later when it clears the bank and reduces cash in bank.

check register A *journal* to record *checks* that are issued.

close As a verb, to transfer the balance of a temporary or contra or adjunct account to the main account to which it relates (eg, to transfer *revenue* and *expense* accounts directly, or through the income summary, to an owners' *equity* account, or to transfer purchase discounts to purchases). To *close* the books entails the above, usually done only once each year, at the end of the fiscal year.

closing entries At the end of the accounting period, the entries that accomplish the transfer of balances in temporary accounts to the related income summary account and *retained earnings* account.

coinsurance Insurance policy that protects against hazards, such as fire or water damage. In property insurance, coinsurance can take the form of a penalty by the insurance carrier wherein the insured may not collect the full amount of insurance for a loss unless the insurance policy covers at least some specified coinsurance percentage, usually about 80% of the replacement cost of the property. Coinsurance clauses induce the owner to carry full, or nearly full, coverage.

COLA Cost-of-Living Adjustment.

collateral Security or guarantee (often an *asset*) pledged by a borrower that will be given up if the *loan* is not repaid.

collectible Capable of being converted into *cash* now or at a later date.

commercial paper An unsecured, short-term note issued by corporate borrowers with a fixed maturity of one to 270 days. Corporations often use these notes for meeting short-term *liabilities* and financing *accounts receivable*.

commission Remuneration to employees based upon an activity rate, such as services rendered or products sold; usually expressed as a percentage.

comparative (financial) statements *Financial statements* in a consistent format showing information for the same company for different periods of time, usually two successive years. Nearly all published financial statements are in this form.

compound interest Accumulated interest calculated on *principal* plus previously undistributed interest.

consolidated financial statements Statements issued by legally separate companies who share common ownership. These statements show an aggregated financial position and income as it would appear if the companies were one economic entity.

contributed capital Amount paid to a company in exchange for ownership interest. Also called paid-in capital.

contribution margin *Revenue* less variable *expenses*. Gross operating margin per unit sold.

control system A device or set of devices for ensuring that actions are carried out according to plan or for safeguarding *assets*.

controller Person who manages accounting, financial reporting, and internal controls within an organization. This title is often given to the chief accountant of an organization. Also known as comptroller.

corporation Business organization authorized by a state (in a process called incorporation) to operate under the rules of the entity's charter.

correcting entry An *adjusting entry* where an improperly recorded transaction is properly recorded. The entry always involves an *income statement* account (*revenue* or *expense*) as well as a *balance sheet* account (*asset* or *liability*).

cost The value, measured by the price paid or required to be paid, needed to acquire goods or services.

cost center Part of an organization that does not directly increase profits but adds to the expense of running that organization.

Cost of goods sold (COGS) Figure on the income statement that reflects the cost of products sold to consumers in the primary business activity of an organization.

credit As a noun, an entry on the right-hand side of an account. As a verb, to make an entry on the right-hand side of an account. Records increases in *liabilities*, owner's equity, *revenues,* and *gains*; records decreases in *assets* and *expenses*. Also the ability or right to buy or borrow in return for a promise to pay later.

credit memorandum A commercial document used by a seller to inform a buyer that the buyer's *account receivable* is being credited (reduced) because of damages, errors, returns, or allowances. Also, the form provided to a depositor by a bank to indicate that the depositor's balance is being increased because of some event other than a deposit.

current asset *Balance sheet* item equaling cash and other *assets* that are expected to be converted into cash, usually within one year. Current *assets* include *cash*, cash equivalents, marketable securities, *accounts receivable, inventory,* and prepaid expenses.

current funds *Cash* and other *liquid assets* readily convertible into cash.

current liability An organization's debts or other obligations that must be discharged within a short time, usually the earnings cycle or one year. Current liabilities appear on the *balance sheet*.

current replacement cost The price paid to replace an existing *asset* with an identical asset (in the same condition and with the same service potential).

customers' ledger The *ledger* that shows *accounts receivable* of individual customers. It is the subsidiary ledger for the controlling account, *Accounts Receivable*.

D

debit As a noun, an entry on the left-hand side of an account. As a verb, to make an entry on the left-hand side of an account. Records increases in *assets* and decreases in *liabilities* and *net* worth. A debit is the opposite of a *credit*.

debit memorandum A document used by a seller to inform a buyer that the seller is debiting (increasing) the amount of the buyer's *account receivable*. Also, the document provided by a bank to a depositor to indicate that the depositor's *balance* is being decreased because of some event other than payment for a *check*, such as monthly service charges or the printing of checks. Also called a debit note.

debt An amount owed. The general name for *loans, notes*, bonds, and *mortgages* that are evidence of amounts owed and have definite payment dates.

deferral An accrual accounting process wherein past cash receipts and payments are not recognized on the *income statement* until some later period. Deferred revenues are recognized as *liabilities* and deferred expenses are recognized as *assets*.

defined contribution plan A *pension* or retirement plan, such as a 401(k) or 403(b) plan, where an employer makes cash contributions (either a set amount or a percentage) to eligible individual employee accounts under the terms of a formalized plan.

depreciation The process of allocating the cost of an *asset* across the time period it provides benefit (known as the asset's depreciable or useful life). Depreciation is a non-cash *expense*.

disbursement Payment of a *debt* or *expense* by *cash* or by *check*.

double entry The system of financial accounting wherein each transaction is recorded in at least two accounts to maintain the equality of the accounting equation; each entry results in recording equal amounts of *debits* and *credits*.

E

equity A claim to *assets*. Ownership interest in a corporation that takes the form of common or preferred stock.

ERISA Employment Retirement Income Security Act of 1974. The federal statute that sets minimum standards and other requirements for *pension plans*, as well as the rules on federal income tax effects related to these pension plans.

expense Outflow of cash or other *assets* in producing *revenue* or carrying out other activities that are part of an entity's operations. Expenses result in a decrease in owners' equity.

F

fair market value *Value* (price) negotiated at *arm's length* between a willing buyer and a willing seller, each acting rationally in his or her own self-interest with knowledge of all relevant facts.

FICA Federal Insurance Contributions Act. Social Security and Medicare payroll taxes and benefits are collected under this act.

financial projection Planning process that creates estimates regarding *sales* and *revenue, expenses, cost of goods sold,* and short and long-term *debt*. This process aids in budgeting and outlining future financing needs.

financial statements Documentation regarding an organization's financial activities. These statements include the *balance sheet, income statement,* statement of *retained earnings,* and statement of *cash flow,* as well as any notes thereto.

fiscal year A period of 12 consecutive months chosen by a business as the *accounting period* for annual reports. May or may not be aligned with the calendar year.

fixed cost (expense) An expenditure or *expense* that does not vary with production, sales, or volume of activity. Fixed costs include rent, insurance, property tax, and interest expense.

float *Checks* whose amounts have been added to depositor's bank account, but not yet subtracted from the drawer's bank account. "Free float" also refers to the number of shares of a publically owned company available for trading.

foreclosure The legal proceedings that can occur when a borrower fails to make a required payment on a *mortgage*. During these proceedings, the lender obtains a court ordered termination of the borrower's equitable right of redemption, and takes possession of the property for his or her use or sale.

fully vested Said of a *pension plan* when an employee (or his or her estate) has rights to all the benefits purchased with the employer's contributions to the plan, even if the employee is not employed by this employer at the time of death or retirement.

FUTA Federal Unemployment Tax Act. Payroll or employment tax paid only by an employer. While the tax is not deducted from the employee's *wage*, the amount paid by the employer is based on each employee's wages.

G

general journal The formal record where *double entry* bookkeeping entries are recognized through matching *debits* and *credits* (thus ensuring the maintenance of the *accounting equation*).

general ledger The formal *accounting* record containing all of an organization's financial statement accounts. Also called the nominal *ledger*.

goodwill *Intangible asset* listed on an organization's *balance sheet*. It represents the value of an organization's reputable brand name, positive customer relations, patents, and other non-physical assets. Goodwill can reflect the amount paid for an organization beyond its *book value* during an acquisition.

grandfather clause An exemption in new *accounting* pronouncements that renders transactions that occurred before a given date free from the new accounting requirements.

gross Not adjusted or reduced by deductions or subtractions. Contrast with *net*.

gross margin Total sales less the *cost of goods sold*. Also called gross profit.

H

holding company A company that confines its activities to owning other companies' outstanding stock. A holding company can supervise and manage other companies through ownership of a controlling interest in the companies whose stock it holds.

I

income Defined by the International Accounting Standards Board as "increases in economic benefits during the accounting period in the form of inflows or enhancements of assets or decreases in liabilities that result in increases in equity, other than those relating to contributions from equity participants." Income is synonymous with *revenue*, but is often used to as a shorthand reference for *net income*.

income accounts *Revenue* and *expense* accounts.

income statement The summary statement of *revenues* and *expenses* for a period of time, ending with *net income*. Also called the *profit and loss statement (P & L)*.

income tax An annual tax levied by the federal and other governments on the income of people, corporations, and other legal entities.

indexation Technique used to mitigate the effects of *inflation*. Income payments fixed in law or contracts are adjusted using a price index when they change as a given measure of price changes. This serves to transfer risk from the payee to the payer.

inflation Increase in the general price of products and services over a period of time.

information system A system, either formal or informal, for collecting, processing, storing, and communicating data. The people, records, and processes that comprise this system can be used to drive managerial decision making.

installment Portion of a *debt* often settled in successive payments at pre-determined intervals.

insurance A risk-reward relationship that awards reimbursement for specific, covered losses in exchange for the payment of premiums.

intangible asset A nonphysical *asset* that provides an organization exclusive or preferred position in the marketplace. Examples of intangible assets include copyrights, patents, trademarks, *goodwill*, organization costs, business methodologies, brand recognition, intellectual property, computer programs, government licenses, leases, franchises, mailing lists, exploration permits, import and export permits, construction permits, and marketing quotas.

interest The charge or cost for using borrowed *assets*. The interest rate (generally expressed as a percentage) is the fee paid per period, usually one year, for the use of the borrowed funds.

internal audit An analysis conducted by employees to evaluate an organization's compliance with business processes and procedures and to determine whether or not internal controls are effective. An external audit is conducted by a Certified Public Accountant.

Internal Revenue Service (IRS) Agency of the United States Department of the Treasury responsible for collecting *income* and certain other taxes and administering the Internal Revenue Code enacted by Congress.

in the black Operating at a profit.

in the red Operating at a *loss*.

inventory As a noun, the raw materials, supplies, work in process, and completely finished goods that serve as part of an organization's total *assets*. As a verb, to calculate the cost of goods on hand at a given time or to create a detailed list of all items on hand.

investment An expenditure to acquire property or other *assets* in order to produce *revenue*; a redirection of current resources made in anticipation of creating future benefits.

J

journal The place where business transactions are originally recorded as they occur. The book of entry prior to transfer to the *ledger*.

journal entry The initial recording of a business transaction in an organization's *accounting system*. Entries are made in a *journal*, and list equal *debits* and *credits*, with an explanation of the transaction, if necessary.

K

kiting Wrongful and illegal practice of taking advantage of the *float*, the time that elapses between the deposit of a *check* in one financial institution and its collection at another, for the purpose of increasing financial leverage.

L

lapping scheme Fraudulent accounting method wherein the *accounts receivable* section of an organization's *balance sheet* is altered to mask theft. For example, an employee could steal cash sent in by a customer. The theft from the first customer is concealed by using cash received from a second customer. The theft from the second customer is concealed by using the cash received from a third customer, and so on. The process could be continued until the thief returns the funds, makes the theft permanent by creating a fictitious *expense* or receivable write-off, or until the fraud is discovered.

lease A legal document or oral arrangement calling for the lessee (user) to pay the lessor (owner) for the possession and use of an *asset*.

leasehold improvement An improvement to a leased *asset* often resulting in an increase in that asset's value. It should be *depreciated* over the life of the *lease* or the improvement.

ledger The principal book for recording accounts and business transactions.

liability An obligation that requires an individual or company to pay a definite (or reasonably definite) amount at a definite (or reasonably definite) time in order to settle a *debt*. Liabilities are recorded on an organization's *balance sheet* and include *accounts payable,* notes payable, accrued expenses, deferred revenues, unearned revenue, bonds payable and payable for *wages,* taxes, and *interest*.

limited partner Member of a *partnership* who does not take part in the management of the organization and has limited personal *liability* for the *debts* of the partnership; every partnership must have at least one general partner who is fully liable. The limited partner is also called the nominal partner.

liquid assets *Cash,* current marketable securities, and sometimes current receivables; an *asset* that can be converted into *cash* quickly and easily.

loan *Debt* instrument wherein the owner of an *asset* (lender) allows another party (borrower) use of the asset for a period of time under an agreement that the borrower will return the asset and often make payments for the use of the asset. Generally the asset being lent is *cash* and the payment for its use is *interest*.

loss A condition where *expenses* exceed *revenues*. Negative *income* for a period or single transaction. An expenditure that produced no *revenue*.

M

margin *Revenue,* less specified *expenses*. Also known as profit margin.

merger The combining of two or more businesses into a single economic entity.

mortgage A legal contract between a borrower and lender wherein the lender provides a *loan* that is secured by the borrower's real estate.

N

negotiable Legally capable of being sold or transferred by endorsement and delivery. Usually said in reference to *checks* and *notes*.

net Remaining after all relevant deductions.

net income Gross profit less operating *expenses*, *costs*, and taxes. Also referred to as "the bottom line."

net loss A condition in which *expenses* and *losses* incurred in a given period exceed the *revenues* and gains of that same period.

nonprofit corporation An incorporated entity, such as a hospital, with shareholders who do not share in the earnings. This type of organization usually emphasizes providing programs and services (often for public benefit) rather than maximizing income.

note An unconditional written promise by the payee (borrower) to pay a specific sum on demand or at a certain future time. Also called a promissory note.

O

OASDHI Old Age, Survivors, Disability, and Health Insurance. Federal program created by the Social Security Act of 1935 to provide benefits to qualified retirees, their spouses and dependents, and some disabled workers.

operating An adjective used to refer to *revenue* and *expense* items relating to an organization's principal line of business.

OSHA Occupational Safety and Healthcare Administration. An agency of the United States Department of Labor created by Congress under the Occupational Safety and Health Act. This agency issues and enforces standards for safe and healthy working conditions in commerce and industry.

out-of-pocket Refers to an expenditure or outlay (usually in *cash*) that may or may not be reimbursed at a later time.

outstanding Amount left unpaid or uncollected. Value owed as a *debt*.

overdraft A withdrawal in excess of the available balance. Often refers to a *check* written on a checking account that contains insufficient funds to cover the amount of the check.

overhead costs Expenditures and *expenses* associated with the ongoing operations of a business. These costs are necessary to maintain the existence of a business, and are not directly associated with the production or *sale* of goods and services.

P

P & L Profit and loss statement. Another term for an *income statement*.

partnership Relationship between two or more people who share resources and operations in a jointly run organization. Partners (also called owners) share the profits and losses incurred for the business in which they have invested.

payable A *liability* that a company owes for goods or services purchased on *credit*.

payroll taxes A portion of the employee's *wages* or salary withheld by the employer for the purpose of paying local, state and federal taxing authorities to fund programs such Social Security, Medicare, and unemployment compensation.

pension fund A fund containing assets that are to be paid to retired, ex-employees as an *annuity* and that is typically held by an independent trustee and not to be considered as an *asset* of the employer.

pension plan Details or provisions of an employment contract for setting aside *annuities* or other benefits to be accessed by the employee after they retire to sustain their standard of living.

petty cash fund A small fund of *cash* maintained for incidental expenditures (eg, office supplies).

prime rate The *interest* rate charged by banks for *loans* to their stable and creditworthy customers.

principal The original amount of a *debt* on which *interest* is calculated. Also commonly used to describe the person that hires the agent when the owner is absent in a principal-agent relationship.

prior-period adjustment A *debit* or *credit* made directly to *retained earnings* prior to the start of the current period so that it has no direct impact on income for the current period.

pro forma statements Hypothetical statements. Financial statements as they would appear if some event, such as a *merger* or increased production and sales, had occurred or were to occur.

profit center A business unit or set of activities that generates *revenue*; contrast with *cost center*.

profit sharing plan An incentive plan, which can occur in various forms, where the employer contributes an amount for the benefit of the employee based on the *net income* of the company.

promissory note A written agreement in which a party agrees to pay a predetermined sum of money on demand or at a specified future date. See *note*.

prorate To *allocate* or assess in proportion to a baseline.

purchase order A document used to request that a *vendor* provide a good or a service in return for payment.

R

ratio The result of dividing one number by another. Ratios are generally used to assess aspects of profitability, solvency, and liquidity of a business entity. The three most commonly used financial ratios are to summarize some aspect of operations for a period, to summarize some aspect of financial position at a given point in time, and to relate some aspect of operations to a financial position.

receipt The act of obtaining *cash*.

rent A charge or payment, usually in a fixed amount and for a set period of time, for the occupancy or use of land or building belonging to another person or corporation.

retained earnings *Revenue* that is kept by a company for reinvestment in the company or to pay off *debt*. This money is not paid out to shareholders as dividends.

revenue The amount of money generated by the company from the sale of goods or property (tangible or intangible) or from services provided.

risk A measure of uncertainty and its impact on *return on investment*. Most people prefer less risk to more risk; therefore, in financial markets, investments with increased levels of risk are expected to return a higher yield or rate of return as compared to investments with lower levels of risk.

risk premium Extra compensation paid to an employee or additional *interest* paid to a lender, above the normal amounts, in return for their engaging in activities with greater than normal risk.

ROI Return on investment, a measure of profitability used to refer to a single project and expressed as a ratio; *revenue* generated divided by the average *cost* of *assets* consumed as part of the project.

S

salary Fixed compensation for services that is earned and paid on a regular basis but not based on an hourly rate. Contrast with *wage*.

sale A transaction where goods, services, or property (tangible or intangible) are delivered to a customer in return for *cash* or an obligation to pay; *revenue*.

simple interest *Interest* calculated only on *principal*, not compounded or added to the principal nor paid to the lender. *Interest = Principal × Interest rate × Time*. Contrast with *compound interest*.

Social Security taxes Taxes levied by the federal government on employers and employees to provide funds to pay retired persons, or their beneficiaries, who are entitled to receive such payments, either because they paid Social Security taxes themselves or they are eligible vis-à-vis determination by the federal government.

sole proprietorship A business structure in which owners' equity belongs to a single person.

spreadsheet A worksheet organized with columns and rows to enable two-way classification of financial data.

T

T-account Account formed by two perpendicular lines forming the letter "T" with the title above the horizontal line. *Debits* are captured to the left of the center line, and *credits* to the right.

take-home pay The amount of *wages* or *salary,* minus the deductions for *income taxes, Social Security taxes,* contributions to benefits plans, and dues.

tax credit A reduction in *liability* that is otherwise payable.

tax deduction A reduction from *revenues* and gains to determine *taxable income*. Tax deductions are technically different from tax exemptions, but both are used to reduce gross income in determining *taxable income.*

taxable income *Income* that is computed according to applicable local, state, or federal laws or regulations that is subject to taxation. Use the term pretax income to refer to income before taxes on the *income statement* in financial reports.

tickler file A collection of vouchers or other time sensitive document arranged chronologically in order remind the person in charge of certain duties to make payments (or to do other tasks) in their order of future occurrence.

trial balance A listing of all accounts with *debit* and *credit* balances in *double-entry* bookkeeping, that when totaled separately are equal.

U

underwriter An intermediary between the issuer of a security and the purchasing public. The intermediary agrees to purchase an entire security issue for a specified price to resale to others.

V

value Monetary worth; an amount of goods, services, or money, considered to be a reasonable equivalent for something else. See *fair market value.*

variance The discrepancy between actual and budgeted or planned *costs,* expenditures, or *expenses.*

vendor A party that provides a good or a service in return for money.

vested Said of an employee's *pension plan* benefits that are not contingent on the employee's continued employment for the employer because the employee has worked a minimum period for vesting set by the employer.

W

wage Compensation based on time worked or output of product by manual labor. See *take-home pay*.

warranty An obligation or guarantee that is factually stated or legally implied by the seller, and that often provides for a specific remedy such as repair or replacement in the event the article or service fails to meet a given standard.

weighted average An average computed by applying a weight to each value so that each value is not treated as an equal.

withholding A portion of an employee's *salary* or *wages*, usually for local, state, or federal *income taxes*, to be remitted by the employer, in the employee's name, to the taxing authority.

write down Downward revision of the value of an asset to reflect its market value, which has dropped below the *book value*. The amount by which the *book value* is reduced is charged against the earnings as an *expense* or *loss*.

write off To charge an asset to *expense* or *loss* in order to reduce the value of one's *assets* and earnings.

INDEX

A

Accounting terms (glossary), 285
Accounts receivable, 110
    days in, 130, *132*
    payer mix, 130
    turnover (glossary term), 285
Accreditation, National Committee for Quality Assurance, 34, 35
Accrual basis of accounting (glossary term), 285
Acquisition cost (glossary term), 285
Addiction medicine, American Society of Addiction Medicine, Website, 211
Adjusted bank balance of cash (glossary term), 285
Adjusted book balance of cash (glossary term), 285
Adjusting entry (glossary term), 286
Administrative expense (glossary term), 286
Administrative Simplification Provisions, *See* HIPAA regulations
Administrators
    American College of Healthcare Executives, Website, 210
    American College of Physician Executives, Website, 210
Admission of partner (glossary term), 286
Adolescent medicine, The American Academy of Child and Adolescent Psychiatry, Website, 208
Aerospace Medical Association, Website, 208
AF4Q, *See* Aligning Forces for Quality
Agency for Healthcare Research and Quality, 34–35
Aging accounts receivable (glossary term), 286
Aging reports, *See* Revenue
AHRQ, *See* Agency for Healthcare Research and Quality

Aligning Forces for Quality, 33–34
Allergy, American Academy of Allergy, Asthma & Immunology, Website, 208
Allied health professionals, Medicare PQRI eligible providers, 46
Allocate (glossary term), 286
The American Academy of Child and Adolescent Psychiatry, Website, 208
The American Academy of Dermatology, Website, 208
American Academy of Allergy, Asthma & Immunology, Website, 208
American Academy of Cosmetic Surgery, Website, 208
American Academy of Facial Plastic and Reconstructive Surgery, Website, 208
American Academy of Family Physicians
    policy on pay for performance, 38–39
    Website, 208
American Academy of Hospice and Palliative Care, Website, 209
American Academy of Insurance Medicine, Website, 209
American Academy of Neurology, Website, 209
American Academy of Nurse Practitioners, Website, 209
American Academy of Ophthalmology, Website, 209
American Academy of Orthopaedic Surgeons, Website, 209
American Academy of Otolaryngic Allergy, Website, 209
American Academy of Otolaryngology— Head and Neck Surgery, Website, 209
American Academy of Pain Medicine, Website, 209
American Academy of Pediatrics, Website, 209

American Academy of Pharmaceutical Physicians, Website, 209
American Academy of Physical Medicine and Rehabilitation, Website, 209
American Academy of Physician Assistants, Website, 209
American Academy of Psychiatry & the Law, Website, 209
American Academy of Sleep Medicine, Website, 209
American Association for Hand Surgery, Website, 209
American Association for Thoracic Surgery, Website, 209
American Association of Clinical Endocrinologists, Website, 209
American Association of Clinical Urologists, Website, 209
American Association of Gynecologic Laparoscopists, Website, 209
American Association of Hip and Knee Surgeons, Website, 209
American Association of Neurological Surgeons, Website, 209
American Association of Neuromuscular and Electrodiagnostic Medicine, Website, 209
American Association of Plastic Surgeons, Website, 209
American Association of Public Health Physicians, Website, 209
American Clinical Neurophysiology Society, Website, 209
American College of Cardiology
    Medicare PQRI successful reporting, 51
    Website, 209
American College of Chest Physicians, Website, 210
American College of Emergency Physicians, Website, 210
American College of Gastroenterology, Website, 210
American College of Healthcare Executives, Website, 210
American College of Medical Genetics, Website, 210
American College of Medical Quality, Website, 210
American College of Nuclear Medicine, Website, 210
American College of Nuclear Physicians, Website, 210
American College of Obstetricians and Gynecologists, Website, 210
American College of Occupational and Environmental Medicine, Website, 210
American College of Physician Executives, Website, 210
American College of Physicians—American Society of Internal Medicine, Website, 210
American College of Preventive Medicine, Website, 210
American College of Radiation Oncology, Website, 210
American College of Radiology, Website, 210
American College of Rheumatology, Website, 210
American College of Surgeons, Website, 210
American Gastroenterological Association, Website, 210
American Geriatrics Society, Website, 210
American Medical Association
    "Fifteen steps to protect your practice from abusive payment tactics," 265
    Health Plan Complaint Form, 265
    new CPT editions, 61
    policy and principles on pay for performance, 36, 39–40
    Practice Management Center Website, 212
    Private Sector Advocacy Website, 275
    Website, 210
American Medical Group Association, Website, 210
American Orthopaedic Association, Website, 210
American Orthopaedic Foot and Ankle Society, Website, 210
American Pediatric Surgical Association, Website, 210
American Psychiatric Association, Website, 210
American Roentgen Ray Society, Website, 210

American Society for Aesthetic Plastic
    Surgery, Website, 210
American Society for Clinical Pathology,
    Website, 210
American Society for Dermatologic Surgery,
    Website, 210
American Society for Gastrointestinal
    Endoscopy, Website, 210
American Society for Reproductive
    Medicine, Website, 210
American Society for Surgery of the Hand,
    Website, 210
American Society for Therapeutic Radiology
    and Oncology, Website, 211
American Society of Abdominal Surgeons,
    Website, 211
American Society of Addiction Medicine,
    Website, 211
American Society of Anesthesiologists,
    Website, 211
American Society of Bariatric Physicians,
    Website, 211
American Society of Cataract and Refractive
    Surgery, Website, 211
American Society of Clinical Oncology,
    Website, 211
American Society of Colon and Rectal
    Surgeons, Website, 211
American Society of General Surgeons,
    Website, 211
American Society of Hematology,
    Website, 211
American Society of Internal Medicine, *See*
    American College of Physicians—
    American Society of Internal Medicine
American Society of Maxillofacial Surgeons,
    Website, 211
American Society of Neuroradiology,
    Website, 211
American Society of Plastic Surgeons,
    Website, 211
American Society of Retina Specialists,
    Website, 211
American Thoracic Society, Website, 211
American Urological Association,
    Website, 211
Americans With Disability Act
    (glossary term), 286
Amortization (glossary term), 286
Ancillary charges, *See* Billing; Claims
Ancillary services, 135–144
    billing, 138–139
    "carve-outs," 141–142
    description and listing of, 136
    financial monitoring, 142–143
    implementing decision to provide,
        137–139
    quality delivered by private
        companies, 138
    Stark regulations, 139–141
Anesthesia, CPT codes, 62
Anesthesiology, American Society of
    Anesthesiologists, Website, 211
Annuity (glossary term), 286
Anti-Kickback Statute, 147, 148–150
    examples of violations, 149
    OIG Website, 208
Appeals, 110–116
    coding expert's role, 108–109, 110–112
    components of effective programs,
        111–113
    state processes, 114–115
    steps in, 113–115
Application specialists
    (IT conversions), 192
Appointments, *See* Patient appointments
Appraisal (glossary term), 286
Appreciation (glossary term), 286
Arm's length (glossary term), 286
Articles of incorporation
    (glossary term), 286
Assess (glossary term), 286
Asset (glossary term), 286
Assignment of accounts receivable
    (glossary term), 286
Association of Military Surgeons of the
    United States, Website, 211
Association of University Radiologists,
    Website, 211
Asthma, American Academy of Allergy,
    Asthma & Immunology,
    Website, 208
Audits, *See* Billing
    charts, 178, 180
    glossary term, 286
    internal, self-audits, 155, 174–181, 292

Audits *(continued)*
    Medicare recovery audit contractors, 156–157
Automobile insurance, 10

B

Bad debts, *See* Collections agencies
Balance (glossary term), 287
Balance billing, False Claims Act violations, 148
Balance sheet (glossary term), 287
Balanced Budget Act of 1997, 149, 150
Balloon (glossary term), 287
Bank balance (glossary term), 287
Bank reconciliation (glossary term), 287
Bank statement (glossary term), 287
Bankrupt (glossary term), 287
Bankruptcy, 95
Bariatric surgery, American Society of Bariatric Physicians, Website, 211
Benchmarks, 117–118, 119–123
    continuous monitoring and trending, 128–133
    data validity, 122
    E/M code utilization comparisons, 174, *175*
    essential components, 122–123
    external sources, 120, 122
    key ratios listed, 121
    usefulness of with continuous monitoring, 134
Bill (glossary term), 287
Billing
    ancillary charges, services, 88, 138–139, 143
    charge capture and entry, 88–89
    claims denials, appeals and reviews, 99–116
    coding, 57–74
    computerized, 15
    CPT modifier problems, 180
    cycle billing, 93
    EHR charge capture, 186–187
    EOBs (explanations of benefits), 109, 110, 111
    errors and refunding overpayments, 171, *172*
    evaluation of coding, *176*
    examples of False Claims Act violations, 147, 148
    explanations of benefits rejections, denials, etc., 180
    inaccuracies, 155
    "incident to" services, 179–180
    insurer fraud and abuse programs, 154–155
    internal audits, 155
    monitoring staff, 180
    payment posting, 15–16
    physician services in hospital setting, 89
    posting and balancing receipts and verifying charges, 85
    self-audits, 174–181
    software updates with new codes, 59
    support staff services, 179
    systems, 109–110
    written policies for compliance programs, 161, 163
Blackberry communication devices, 187
Blue Cross Blue Shield, Blue Distinction program, 35–36
Bonus (glossary term), 287
Book (glossary term), 287
Book value (glossary term), 287
Branch (glossary term), 287
Breakeven point (glossary term), 287
Budget (glossary term), 287
Budgeting, 123–128
    continuous monitoring and trending, 128–133
    expense-to-earnings percentages, 127–128
    physician buy-in, 127
    process, 124
    reality checks, 128
    sample dashboard report, *133*
    usefulness of with continuous monitoring, 134
Burn rate (glossary term), 287
Business relationships, 178–179
Bylaws (glossary term), 287

C

CAHPS, *See* Consumer Assessment of Healthcare Providers and Systems
Cancer, *See* Oncology Websites
Capital (glossary term), 287
Capital asset (glossary term), 287
Capital budget (glossary term), 288
Capital gain (glossary term), 288
Capital lease (glossary term), 288
Capital loss (glossary term), 288
Capitalization of earnings (glossary term), 288
Capitation, 14
    contract negotiations, 26–28
    HMOs, 4
Cardiovascular medicine Websites
    American College of Cardiology, 209
    Society of Cardiovascular & Interventional Radiology, 211
Carriers (term), 14
"Carve-outs," *See* Ancillary services
Cash (glossary term), 288
Cash basis of accounting (glossary term), 288
Cash budget (glossary term), 288
Cash flow (glossary term), 288
Cash receipts journal (glossary term), 288
Casualty insurance, 10
Cataract surgery, *See* Ophthalmology Websites
CCIP, *See* Chronic Care Improvement Program
Centers for Medicare and Medicaid Services, *See* US Centers for Medicare and Medicaid Services
Centers for Specialty Care, 36
CERT (comprehensive error rate testing), *See* Medicare
Certified check (glossary term), 288
Certified clinical nurse specialists, 179
Certified nurse midwives, 179
CHAMPUS, *See* TRICARE
Change management
    benefits of workflow analysis, 205–206
    successful IT implementation and conversions, 190–206

Charges, *See* Billing; Claims
Chart audits, 178, 180
Chart of accounts (glossary term), 288
Check (glossary term), 288
Check-out, *See* Patient appointments
Check register (glossary term), 288
Chest physicians, ACCP Website, 210
Children's Health Insurance Program, 8–9
CHIP, *See* Children's Health Insurance Program
Chronic Care Improvement Program, 43
CIGNA, 35
Civil Rights Office, *See* US Health and Human Services Department
Civilian Health and Medical Program for the Uniformed Services (CHAMPUS), *See* TRICARE
Claims
    allowable services in payer contracts, 100–105
    altering, falsifying, 148
    appeal of inappropriate E/M downcoding, sample letter for, 279–280
    appeals and reviews, 99, 110–116
    appeals of denials, 110–116
    charge capture and entry, 88–89
    clean, 106–108
    clean-claim laws, 90–91
    coding, 57–74
    coordination of benefits, 108
    denial and rejection tracking, 110
    denials, 110–116
    denials, acceptance of, 99
    denials as part of self-audit, 178
    denied, 92
    electronic, 15
    electronic clearinghouses, 15, 90
    error lists, 90
    evaluation of coding, *176*
    False Claims Act violations, 147–148
    "Fifteen steps to protect your practice from abusive payment tactics," 265
    follow-up, 93–95
    late-payment penalties, 108
    late payment, sample letters regarding, 275, 276–278
    monitoring, 176–178

Claims *(continued)*
   payment posting, 15–16
   processing, 105–110
   prompt-pay laws, 90–91, 107–108
   random sampling in self-audits, 174
   refunds, recoupments, 108
   rejected, 90
   remittances, 91–93
   sample appeal letter for PPO discount without contract, 281–282
   sample letter to state insurance commissioner regarding late payment, 283
   scrubber rejections, 178
   scrubbing, editing, 89–90
   secondary insurance, 92–93
   submission, 89–91
   terminology, 14–16
   underpayment, sample letter for, 273–274
   unpaid, 93–95
   zero payments, 92
Claims review, 99, 110–116
   insurer fraud and abuse programs, 154–155
   Medicaid Integrity Program, 158
   Medicare programs, 156–160
Clean-claim laws, 90–91
Clearinghouses, electronic, 15, 90
Clinical laboratory services, prohibitions on physician self-referrals, 150
Close (glossary term), 288
Closing entries (glossary term), 288–289
CMS, *See* US Centers for Medicare and Medicaid Services
Co-insurance, 12, 102, 104–105, 289
Coding, 57–74
   accuracy (choosing lower or higher codes), 59–60
   accuracy improvement with EHRs, 189
   CPT, 57–71
   current, up-to-date books and resources, 181
   evaluation, *176*
   Evaluation and Management (E/M) codes, 58, 61–62, 65–71
   "Fifteen steps to protect your practice from abusive payment tactics," 265
   folklore (information handed down by individuals), 59
   ICD-9-CM diagnosis codes, 71–72
   inappropriate E/M downcoding, sample appeal letter for, 279–280
   nonphysician providers using E/M codes, 179–180
   outdated codes, coding books, 59
   physician notes in medical records, 60–61
   physicians' knowledge of and training, 58–59
   role of experts in appeals process, 108–109, 110–112
   undercoding elimination, 189
   updating forms and billing software, 59
COGS (glossary term), 289
Coinsurance, 12, 102, 104–105, 289
COLA (glossary term), 289
Collateral (glossary term), 289
Collectible (glossary term), 289
Collections, *See also* Claims
   accounts receivable, 110, 130, *132*, 285
   agencies, 95–97
   bad debt (glossary term), 286
   bad debt recovery (glossary term), 287
   gross collection rate, 118–119, 130
   legal action, 96–97
   net, and actual revenue, 125
   net collection rate, 119, 130
   percentages, 130
   procedures, 94–95, 96–97
College of American Pathologists, Website, 211
Commercial paper (glossary term), 289
Commission (glossary term), 289
Communication, employee, compliance program incident reporting, 167–170
Community programs, Aligning Forces for Quality, 33–34
Comparative (financial) statements (glossary term), 289
Complaints
   "Fifteen steps to protect your practice from abusive payment tactics," 265
   Health Plan Complaint Form, 265
Compliance, meaning of the term, 146
Compliance officers, 160–161, *162*
   checklist of questions about, *162*

investigations of compliance violations, 171, *172*
ongoing training, 167
responsibilities, 161
Compliance programs, 145–183
  audit schedules, 174
  benefits of implementation, 160
  billing, claims coding and rejections, 174–178
  billing errors and refunding overpayments, 171, *172*
  business relationships, 178–179
  communication checklist, *170*
  compliance officer selection, 160–161, *162*
  disciplinary guidelines, 168, 170
  duty to report, 166
  effective plans, according to OIG, 160
  effective, successful plans, 181
  examples of False Claims Act violations, 147–148
  fraud alerts (OIG), 159
  functions to be monitored and audited, 174
  implementation responsibilities of compliance officers, 161
  incident reporting, anonymity, hot lines, 167
  incident reporting, non-retaliation, 166, 167–169
  "incident to" services, 179–180
  investigations of violations, 168, 170
  investigations of violations and corrective actions, 170–173
  legal counsel regarding self-disclosure of compliance violations, 173
  nonphysician providers using E/M codes, 179–180
  non-retaliation policy in reporting violations, 166
  OIG guidance, Web site, 159, 160
  ongoing training, 167
  periodic review of written policies and procedures, 164
  quiz on, 166
  repetitive training, 181
  sample report of suspected violation, *169*
  self-audits, 174–181
  self-disclosure of misconduct, violations, 171, 173
  staff training, education, 164–167, 180, 181
  standards of conduct, 161, 163
  steps, requirements for effective plans, 160
  training program evaluation tool, *166*
  typical training agenda, *165*
  violations, cost, 146
  written policies and procedures, 161, 163–164
Compound interest (glossary term), 289
Comprehensive error rate testing (CERT), *See* Medicare
Conduct standards, *See* Compliance programs
Congress of Neurological Surgeons, Website, 211
Consent for treatment, 82
Consolidated financial statements (glossary term), 289
Consultation codes, 70
Consumer Assessment of Healthcare Providers and Systems, 35
Consumers, Aligning Forces for Quality, 33–34
Contract Health Service, *See* Indian Health Services
Contract negotiations, 19–29
  ancillary services, 141–142
  basics, principles, 20–22
  capitation, 26–28
  checklists, do's and don'ts, 26–28
  claims appeals and, 100
  deal-breakers, 25–26
  due-diligence steps, 27–28
  evaluation of managed care plans, 22–25
  incremental and replacement pricing, 26–28
  negotiating team knowledge about MCOs, 20–21
  negotiating team leadership, 22
  take-it-or-leave-it positions, 22
  tie-breakers, 26
Contractual adjustments, 12
Contributed capital (glossary term), 289
Contribution margin (glossary term), 289

Control system (glossary term), 289
Controller (glossary term), 289
Coordination of benefits, 108
Copayments, 12, 83, 102, 104–105
    collection at time of patient registration, 83, 102
Corporation (glossary term), 289
Correcting entry (glossary term), 289
Cost (glossary term), 289
Cost center (glossary term), 289
Cost of goods sold (glossary term), 289
Cost-of-living adjustments, 125
"Covered entities" (HIPAA), 153
CPT (Current Procedural Terminology), 10, 58, 59
    add-on codes (Appendix D), 62
    changes (additions, deletions, revisions, Appendix B), 62
    chief complaint (CC) documentation, 66
    claims coding, 61–71
    clinical examples (Appendix C), 62
    codebook organization and sections described, 61–63
    codebook use and description, 63–64
    codes exempt from modifier 51 (Appendix E), 62
    codes exempt from modifier 63 (Appendix F), 62
    coding, 57–71
    crosswalked deleted codes (Appendix M), 63
    current, up-to-date manuals, 181
    descriptions of codes, 61
    E/M code components, 66–67
    E/M code guidelines, 65–66
    effective dates for new codes, 59
    electrodiagnostic medicine listing of sensory, motor and mixed nerves (Appendix J), 63
    examination levels, 68, *69*
    genetic testing code modifiers (Appendix I), 63
    history of present illness (HPI), 67
    index entries, 63, 64
    medical decision making (diagnosis, etc.), 68–69
    Medicare allowed amount, payment schedule, 11
    Medicare carrier updates, 70
    Medicare claims-based PQRI reporting, 49–50
    Medicare consultation codes, 70
    moderate/conscious sedation (Appendix G), 62–63
    modifier problems, 180
    modifiers (Appendix A), 62
    modifiers described, 64–65
    performance measures (Appendix H), 63
    PFSH (past family and social history), 68
    preventive services, 70–71
    product pending FDA approval (Appendix K), 63
    RBRVS and, 10–11
    resequenced codes (Appendix N), 63
    review of systems (ROS), 67–68
    time-based documentation, 69–70
    vascular families (Appendix L), 63
Credentialing, 16
Credit (glossary term), 289–290
Credit memorandum (glossary term), 290
Critical care medicine, Society of Critical Care Medicine, Website, 211
"Crossing the Quality Chasm: A New Health Care System for the 21st Century," 36–37
Current asset (glossary term), 290
Current funds (glossary term), 290
Current liability (glossary term), 290
Current Procedural Terminology, *See* CPT
Current replacement cost (glossary term), 290
Customers' ledger (glossary term), 290
Cycle billing, *See* Billing

D

Dashboard reports
    continuous monitoring and trending, 128–133
    description of, 130–131
    examples of, *131–133*
Data analysis
    continuous monitoring and trending, 128–133
    IT advantages in report generation, 188

DEA, *See* Drug Enforcement
    Administration
Debit (glossary term), 290
Debit memorandum (glossary term), 290
Debt (glossary term), 290
Debts, bad, *See* Collections agencies
Decision making, 68–69
Decision support, 186, 202
Deductibles, 12, 83
    waiver of, 155
Deferral (glossary term), 290
Defined contribution plan (glossary term),
    290
Depreciation (glossary term), 290
Dermatology Websites
    The American Academy of
        Dermatology, 208
    American Society for Dermatologic
        Surgery, 210
Diabetes educators, 179
Diagnosis and diagnostic services
    CPT codes, medical decision making,
        68–69
    examples of False Claims Act violations,
        147–148
    periodic monitoring of rejected claims, 178
    physician lab and test orders, *197*, 204
Dialysis Facility Compare, 43
Disbursement (glossary term), 290
Disease Management for Severely
    Chronically Ill, 43–44
Documentation, written policies for, 164
Double entry (glossary term), 290
Drug Enforcement Administration, 16
Drug benefit, *See* Prescription drug benefit
Drugs, *See* Pharmaceutical industry;
    Prescriptions
Dual eligibility, *See* Medicaid; Medicare
Due diligence, 178–181
Durable medical equipment and supplies,
    self-referrals, 150
Duty to report, *See* Compliance programs

E

E-mail, 188–189, *197*
    internal messaging, 201–203
    reminder systems, 188–189

Education, *See* Compliance programs
Electrodiagnosis, American Association of
    Neuromuscular and Electrodiagnostic
    Medicine, Website, 209
Electronic claims, *See* Claims
Electronic clearinghouse, *See*
    Clearinghouses
Electronic health records
    benefits of workflow analysis, 205–206
    charge capture, 186–187, *197*
    chart conversion from paper, *197*
    charting in real time, 204–205
    government assistance in purchasing
        information systems, 84
    implementation strategy, 196–198
    improved coding accuracy, 189
    Medicare PQRI reporting, 47–48, 51
    physician lab and test orders, *197*, 204
    point-of-care documentation, *197*
    prescription refills, 204
    proper uses, 193
    role of EHR specialist, 198
    staff training, 198
    timing of roll-out, 195, 196, 198
    workflow analysis, components (health
        care delivery model), 200, *201, 202*
Electronic mail, 188–189, *197*
    internal messaging, *197*
    reminder systems, 188–189
Electronic medical records, *See* Electronic
    health records
Electronic prescribing, *See* Prescriptions
Electronic protected health information, *See*
    Protected health information
Electronic remittances, 91–93
E-mail, 188–189, *197*
    internal messaging, 201–203
Emergency Medical Treatment and Labor
    Act, 147
Emergency medicine Websites, ACEP, 210
Employee benefits
    financial instruments (HRAs, HSAs), 5
    group health insurance coverage, 6
    Medicare supplemental coverage, 8
Employees, medical office, *See* Office staff
Employer health insurance plans, *See*
    Employee benefits
Employer-sponsored health plans, 105

EMTALA, *See* Emergency Medical Treatment and Labor Act
End Stage Renal Disease Quality Initiative, 43
Endocrinology Websites
   American Association of Clinical Endocrinologists, 209
   The Endocrine Society, 211
Endoscopy Websites
   American Society for Gastrointestinal Endoscopy, 210
   Society of American Gastrointestinal Endoscopic Surgeons, 211
Enteral nutrition, prohibitions on physician self-referrals, 150
Environmental medicine, American College of Occupational and Environmental Medicine, Website, 210
EOBs, *See* Explanations of benefits
Equipment, medical, *See* Durable medical equipment and supplies
Equity (glossary term), 290
ERISA (glossary term), 290–291
ESRD Disease Management Demonstration, 43
ESRDQI, *See* End Stage Renal Disease Quality Initiative
Evaluation and Management (E/M) codes, 58, 61–62, 65–71
   comparisons between physicians, 174, *175*
   nonphysician providers, 179–180
   periodic monitoring, 178
   sample letter for appeal of inappropriate downcoding, 279–280
Expense-to-earnings percentages, 127–128
Expenses
   budgeting process, 126–127
   glossary term, 291
   types of (fixed, variable, period), 126–127
Explanations of benefits, 109, 110, 111
   "Fifteen steps to protect your practice from abusive payment tactics," 265
   rejections, denials, etc., 180
   review, *177*, 178

F

Fair Debt Collection Practices Act, 94–95, 96
Fair market value (glossary term), 291
False Claims Act, 146, 147–148
Family medicine, American Academy of Family Physicians, Website, 208
Federal Employees Health Benefits Program, 6
Federal Trade Commission, *See* US Federal Trade Commission
Fee schedules and payment schedules
   CMS Website, 207
   contractual adjustments, 12
   cost-of-living adjustment, 125
   health plan reimbursement rates, 102–105
   increases in budgeting process (revenue), 124–125
   in-network, 14
   Medicare allowed amount, 11
   out-of-network, 14
   standard charge, 12
   usual and customary payment schedules, 11–12
   managed care, 11–12
Fee-for-service insurance plans, 3
FEHBP, *See* Federal Employees Health Benefits Program
FERA, *See* Fraud Enforcement and Recovery Act of 2009
FICA (glossary term), 291
Financial forecasting, *See* Budgeting
Financial management, *See* Benchmarks; Budgeting; Revenue cycle management
Financial performance, *See* Benchmarks
Financial projection (glossary term), 291
Financial statements (glossary term), 291
Fiscal year (glossary term), 291
Fistula First Breakthrough Initiative, 43
Fixed cost (expense) (glossary term), 291
Float (glossary term), 291
Forecasting, financial, *See* Budgeting
Foreclosure (glossary term), 291

Fraud, *See also* Compliance programs
  alerts (OIG), 159
  duty to report, 166
  examples of False Claims Act violations, 147–148
Fraud Enforcement and Recovery Act of 2009, 146
Fraud prevention, *See* Compliance programs
Free services, 155
Fully vested (glossary term), 291
FUTA (glossary term), 291

G

Gastroenterology Websites
  American College of Gastroenterology, 210
  American Gastroenterological Association, 210
  American Society for Gastrointestinal Endoscopy, 210
  American Society of Colon and Rectal Surgeons, 211
  Society of American Gastrointestinal Endoscopic Surgeons, 211
Gatekeepers, 4
General journal (glossary term), 291
General ledger (glossary term), 291
Geneticists, 179
Genetics, American College of Medical Genetics, Website, 210
Geriatric medicine, American Geriatrics Society, Website, 210
Glossary of terms, 285–297
Goodwill (glossary term), 291
GPRO, *See* Group Practice Reporting Option (PQRI)
Grandfather clause (glossary term), 291–292
Gross (glossary term), 292
Gross collection
  rate, 118–119, 130
  sample dashboard report, *131*
Gross margin (glossary term), 292
Group Practice Reporting Option (PQRI), 52–53

Group practices
  American Medical Group Association, Website, 210
  pay for performance (Physician Group Practice Demonstration), 41
  Stark regulations and ancillary services, 140
Gynecology Websites
  American Association of Gynecologic Laparoscopists, 209
  American College of Obstetricians and Gynecologists, 210

H

Hand surgery
  American Association for Hand Surgery, Website, 209
  American Society for Surgery of the Hand, Website, 210
HCFA 1500 form, 106
HCPCS, 58
  current, up-to-date manuals, 181
Head and neck surgery, *See* Otolaryngology Websites
Health administration
  American College of Healthcare Executives, Website, 210
  American College of Physician Executives, Website, 210
Healthcare Common Procedure Coding System, *See* HCPCS
Health care delivery model, 200, *201*
Health care fraud prevention, *See* Compliance programs
Health Effectiveness Data and Information Set, 34
Health insurance, *See* Insurance
Health Insurance Portability and Accountability Act, *See* HIPAA regulations
Health maintenance organizations, description of, 4
Health reimbursement accounts, 5
Health savings accounts, 5
Healthcare Common Procedure Coding System, *See* HCPCS

HEDIS, *See* Health Effectiveness Data and Information Set
Hematology, American Society of Hematology, Website, 211
High-deductible health insurance plans, 5
HIPAA regulations, 82, 152–153
   covered entities, 153
   penalties, 153
   Privacy Rule, 152
   Security Rule, 152, 153
History taking, 68
HMOs, *See* Health maintenance organizations
Holding company (glossary term), 292
Home health services, prohibitions on physician self-referrals, 150
Hospice, American Academy of Hospice and Palliative Care, Website, 209
Hospital Compare, Web address, 41–42
Hospitals
   ancillary services, 138
   charges, 89
   Premier Hospital Quality Initiative, 41–42
   services, Medicare Part A, 7
HRAs, *See* Health reimbursement accounts
HSAs, *See* Health savings accounts

I

ICD-9-CM, 10, 58, 59, 72–73
   current, up-to-date manuals, 181
   diagnosis coding, 71–72
   "E" codes, 72
   effective dates for new codes, 59
   "V" codes, 72
ICD-10-CM, preparing for, 73
Identity regulations, 80, 82
Identity theft, 80, 153–154
IHS, *See* Indian Health Services
Immunology, American Academy of Allergy, Asthma & Immunology, Website, 208
Improper Payments Information Act of 2002, 157
In-office charges, *See* Billing; Claims
In the black (glossary term), 293
In the red (glossary term), 293

Incident reporting, *See* Compliance programs
Income (glossary term), 292
Income accounts (glossary term), 292
Income statement (glossary term), 292
Income tax (glossary term), 292
Indemnity insurance plans, 3
Indexation (glossary term), 292
Indian Health Services, 9
Inflation (glossary term), 292
Information system (glossary term), 292
Information technology, 185–206, *See also* Electronic claims; Electronic health records; Electronic mail
   advantages of asynchronous communication, 188
   automated advanced beneficiary notice checks, 189
   conversion acceptance, buy-in, champions, 193–194
   conversion to electronic messaging, *197*
   e-prescribing, *197*
   EHR charge capture, *197*
   fully integrated systems, 187, 189–190
   going live with new systems, 195, 196
   health care delivery model, 200, *201*
   implementation plan, 194–196
   implementation team members, 191–193
   insurance verification in real time, 188
   internal messaging, 201–203
   management information systems director, 192
   mobile (portable) devices, 187
   patient portals and kiosks, 187–188, 203–204
   physician lab and test orders, *197*, 204
   point-of-service charge entry, 187
   project management in system conversions, 194–196
   replacing legacy systems, 186, 189–190
   reporting tools, 188
   return on investment, 186
   revenue-enhancing features, 186–189
   staff fears, responses, 199
   successful implementation and conversions, 190–206
   system testing by power users, 192–193

timing, disruptions, in EHR
  implementation, 196
timing of EHR roll-out, 195, 196, 198
training and simulations in preparation
  for conversions, 194
vendor selection and relationships,
  189–191, 196
workflow transformation, 199–206
Installment (glossary term), 292
Institute of Medicine, pay for performance
  and, 36–37
Insurance, 1–17; *See also* Billing; Claims;
  Explanations of benefits; Fee
  schedules and payment schedules;
  Medicare
  American Academy of Insurance
    Medicine, Website, 209
  authorizations, 78
  automated advanced beneficiary notice
    checks, 189
  automobile, 10
  casualty, 10
  co-insurance, 12, 102, 104–105
  coordination of benefits, 13
  copayment, 12, 83, 102, 104–105
  coverage, 3
  coverage determinations, 89–90
  coverage verification for patients,
    13, 16–17
  coverage verification in real time, 188
  covered services, 13
  customer service numbers, 77
  deductible, 12
  eligibility and verification, 104
  exclusions, 13
  fee-for-service plans, 3
  "Fifteen steps to protect your practice
    from abusive payment tactics," 265
  fraud and abuse prevention, 154–155
  indemnity plans, 3
  individually purchased policies, 6
  information when scheduling
    patients, 77
  liability, 10
  limitations, 13
  National Association of Insurance
    Commissioners, Website, 208
  out-of-pocket maximum, 13
  payment schedules, 12
  plan types and categories, 3–5
  pre-certifications, 78
  primary, 13
  secondary, 13, 92–93
  types of providers and programs, 5–10
  verification, 13
Intangible asset (glossary term), 292
Interest (glossary term), 292
Intermediaries (term), 14
Internal audit (glossary term), 292
Internal medicine, American College of
  Physicians—American Society of
  Internal Medicine, Website, 210
Internal Revenue Service, *See* US Internal
  Revenue Service
*International Classification of Diseases, 9th
  Revision, Clinical Modification, See*
  ICD-9-CM
Inventory (glossary term), 293
Investment (glossary term), 293
iPhones, 187
IRS, *See* US Internal Revenue Service

J

Journal (glossary term), 293
Journal entry (glossary term), 293

K

Kickbacks, 147, 148–150
  examples of violations, 149
  OIG advisory opinions, 159
  penalties, fines, 150
Kidney diseases, Renal Physicians
  Association, Website, 211
Kiosks, electronic, *See* Information
  technology
Kiting (glossary term), 293

L

Labor unions, Medicare supplemental
  coverage, 8
Laboratory services
  CPT codes, 62
  physician test orders, *197*, 204

Laboratory services *(continued)*
  prohibitions on physician self-referrals, 150
Laparoscopy, American Association of Gynecologic Laparoscopists, Website, 209
Lapping scheme (glossary term), 293
Laws, *See also* Anti-Kickback Statute; Compliance programs; HIPAA regulations; Stark Regulations
  American Academy of Psychiatry & the Law, Website, 209
  clean-claim laws, 90–91
  disclosure of security breach by state, 267–272
  health care fraud and abuse, 154–155
  legal representation in self-disclosure of compliance violations, 173
  primary health care-related statutes, 145–153
  prompt-pay laws, 90–91, 107–108
  prompt-pay statutes and regulations by state, 225–238
  refund recoupment statutes by state, 239–263
Lease (glossary term), 293
Leasehold improvement (glossary term), 293
Ledger (glossary term), 293
Legal representation, self-disclosure of compliance violations, 173
Level II codes, *See* HCPCS
Liability (glossary term), 293
Liability insurance, 10
Limited partner (glossary term), 293
Liquid assets (glossary term), 293
Loan (glossary term), 293–294
Lockbox payments, 16, 91
Loss (glossary term), 294

M

Managed care plans, 3–5
  administrative manuals, 101–102
  capitation contracts, 26–28
  cash posting and contract monitoring, 91
  claims denials, appeals and reviews, 99–116
  contract negotiations, 19–29
  contract renewals, 20
  credentialing, 16
  deal-breakers, 25–26
  evaluation by negotiating team, 22–25
  in-network and out-of-network, 14
  management of practice volumes and capacity, 28–29
  Medicare Advantage, 7, 8
  "national" rates, 21
  negotiated reimbursement rates, 102–105
  negotiating team knowledge about, 20–21
  negotiations regarding ancillary services, 141–142
  practice information sharing with patients, 28–29
  practice's leverage with, 29
  primary physician referral, 14
  reimbursement analysis, procedure frequency report, *23*, 24–25
  tie-breakers, 26
  usual and customary payment schedules, 11–12
  utilization review and quality assurance, 24
  weighted average reimbursement, 24–25, *25*
Management information systems director, *See* Information technology
Margin (glossary term), 294
Maxillofacial surgery, American Society of Maxillofacial Surgeons, Website, 211
MCMP, *See* Medicare Care Management Performance
Medicaid, 6, 8
  CMS Website, 207
  Disease Management for Chronically Ill Dual Eligible Beneficiaries, 44
  dual eligibility with Medicare, 8, 44
  MIP (integrity program), 158
Medicaid Integrity Program, 158
Medical equipment, *See* Durable medical equipment and supplies
Medical examiners, National Association of Medical Examiners, Website, 211

Medical Group Management Association,
  pay for performance standards, 37–38
Medical necessity, 58
Medical office staff, See Office staff
Medical records, See also Electronic
  health records
  notes, documentation, *60*, 60–61
Medical records, electronic, See Electronic
  health records
Medical specialty societies, online resources
  (Website addresses), 208–211
Medical supplies, See Durable medical
  equipment and supplies
Medically unlikely edits, *157*
Medicare, 6–8; See also Physician Quality
  Reporting Initiative
  Advantage plans (Part C), 7, 8
  allowed amount, 11
  audit receivables, recoveries,
    inappropriate reimbursements, 146
  balance billing violations, 148
  billing errors and refunding
    overpayments, 171, *172*
  Care Management Performance, 42
  carrier CPT updates, 70
  carriers, claims review programs, *157*
  claims review programs, 156–160
  claims scrubbing, editing, 89–90
  clean claims, 106
  CMS Website, 207
  comprehensive error rate testing (CERT),
    157–158
  consultation codes, 70
  contact database, 207
  coverage determination documents,
    Web site listing, 89–90
  dual eligibility with Medicaid, 8, 44
  electronic claims, 15
  electronic claims clearinghouses, 90
  Evaluation and Management (E/M)
    codes, 58, 61–62, 65–71
  excluded providers, 159
  excluding practitioners, 149
  fee schedule and health plan
    reimbursement rates, 102–105
  fee-for-service error rate, 157
  fee-for-service paid claims error rate, 158
  Health Care Quality Program, 42–43
  Health Support Program, 43
  ICD-9-CM and ICD-10-CM, 72–73
  limiting charge, 11
  MCMP (Medicare Care Management
    Performance), 42
  MHSP (Medicare Health Support
    Program), 43
  National Correct Coding Initiative,
    89, *157*
  *National Correct Coding Initiative
    Coding Policy Manual for Medicare
    Services*, 181
  newsletters, directives, 181
  open enrollment period, 8
  overpayments, violations of False Claims
    Act, 148
  Part A and Part B, 6–7
  Part A intermediary and Part B carriers
    by state, 213–223
  Part B and PQRI, 48
  participation, nonparticipation, 11
  pay for performance, 38
  pay for performance programs, 40–44
  payment schedule, 11
  Physician Quality Reporting Initiative,
    32, 43, 45–53
  prescription drug benefit (Part D), 7, 8
  Prescription Drug, Improvement and
    Modernization Act, 156
  preventive services covered by, 71
  RBRVS, 10–11
  recovery audit contractors, 156–157
  reimbursement standards and
    arrangements, 11–12
  supplemental plans (Medigap), 7, 8
Medicare and Medicaid Patient Protection
  Act of 1987, 146, 148–150
Medicare Care Management Performance, 42
Medicare Health Care Quality Program,
  42–43
Medicare Health Support Program, 43
Medicare Prescription Drug, Improvement
  and Modernization Act, 156
Medigap, 7
Merger (glossary term), 294
Messaging, See Electronic mail
MHSP, See Medicare Health Support
  Program

MIP, *See* Medicaid Integrity Program
Mobile communication devices, 187
Mortgage (glossary term), 294
MUEs, *See* Medically unlikely edits

N

National Association of Insurance Commissioners, Website, 208
National Association of Medical Examiners, Website, 211
National CAHPS Benchmarking Database, Web address, 35
National Committee for Quality Assurance, 34, 35
National Correct Coding Initiative, 89, *157*
National Correct Coding Initiative Coding Policy Manual for Medicare Services, 181
National Medical Association, Website, 211
NCQA, *See* National Committee for Quality Assurance
Negotiable (glossary term), 294
Negotiations, *See* Contract negotiations
Net (glossary term), 294
Net collection rate, 119, 125, 129, 130
Net income (glossary term), 294
Net loss (glossary term), 294
Neurology Websites
    American Academy of Neurology, 209
    American Association of Neuromuscular and Electrodiagnostic Medicine, 209
    American Society of Neuroradiology, 211
Neurophysiology, American Clinical Neurophysiology Society, Website, 209
Neurosurgery Websites
    American Association of Neurological Surgeons, 209
    Congress of Neurological Surgeons, 211
New patients, 76
Nonprofit corporation (glossary term), 294
North American Spine Society, Website, 211
Note (glossary term), 294
Notice of Privacy Practices, 82
Nuclear medicine Websites
    American College of Nuclear Physicians, 210
    American College of Nuclear Medicine, 210
    Society of Nuclear Medicine, 212
Nurse practitioners, 179
    American Academy of Nurse Practitioners, Website, 209
Nurses, Medicare PQRI eligible providers, 46
Nutritionists, 179

O

OASDHI (glossary term), 294
OBRA 1989, *See* Omnibus Budget Reconciliation Act of 1989
Obstetrics Websites, American College of Obstetricians and Gynecologists, Website, 210
Occupational medicine, American College of Occupational and Environmental Medicine, Website, 210
Occupational therapy services, prohibitions on physician self-referrals, 150
Office for Civil Rights, *See* US Health and Human Services Department
Office of Inspector General (OIG), 158–160
    advisory opinions, 207
    annual work plan (fraud and abuse concerns), 159
    audit receivables, recoveries, inappropriate reimbursements, 146
    compliance plan guidance, Web site, 159, 160
    excluding practitioners from Medicare, 149
    fraud alerts, 159
    kickback advisory opinions, 159
    Medicare excluded providers, 159
    Provider Self-Disclosure Protocol, 171, 173
    Website, 207
Office staff, *See also* Workflow
    annual compliance program refresher, 166
    billing department, 180
    cash gifts, 180
    checklist for effective communication of compliance program, *170*

comfort levels in computer use, 195
compliance needs assessment for specific positions, 167
compliance program training, education for, 164–167, 180, 181
compliance program training evaluation tool, *166*
disciplinary guidelines, 168, 170
duty to report, 166
education and training, 180
effectiveness of in-person and interactive training, 164, 166
EHR specialist, 198
EHR training, 198
fears, individual responses, in IT conversions, 199
front-desk protocols, 180
internal electronic messaging, 203
IT training, simulations in system conversions, 194, 195
non-retaliation policy in reporting violations, 166
quiz regarding practice's compliance program, 166
repetitive training in compliance program, 181
standards of conduct, 161, 163
training in IT conversions, 194, 195
turnover, 180
typical compliance program training agenda, *165*
workflow changes, adaptation, 205–206
OIG, *See* Office of Inspector General (OIG)
Omnibus Budget Reconciliation Act of 1989, 147, 150–152
Oncology Websites
American College of Radiation Oncology, 210
American Society for Therapeutic Radiology and Oncology, 211
American Society of Clinical Oncology, 211
Online resources, *See also* Information technology
professional society Web addresses listed, 208–211
Operating (glossary term), 294

Ophthalmology Websites
American Academy of Ophthalmology, 209
American Society of Cataract and Refractive Surgery, 211
American Society of Retina Specialists, 211
Orthopedic surgery Websites
American Academy of Orthopaedic Surgeons, 209
American Association of Hip and Knee Surgeons, 209
American Orthopaedic Association, 210
American Orthopaedic Foot and Ankle Society, 210
American Society for Surgery of the Hand, 210
Orthotics, prohibitions on physician self-referrals, 150
OSHA (glossary term), 294
Otolaryngology Websites
American Academy of Otolaryngic Allergy, 209
American Academy of Otolaryngology— Head and Neck Surgery, 209
Out-of-pocket (glossary term), 294
Out-of-pocket maximum, 13
Outstanding (glossary term), 294
Overdraft (glossary term), 294
Overhead costs (glossary term), 294

P

P & L (glossary term), 294
P4P, *See* Pay for performance
Pain medicine, American Academy of Pain Medicine, Website, 209
Pediatrics Websites, American Academy of Pediatrics, Website, 209
Palliative care, American Academy of Hospice and Palliative Care, Website, 209
Parenteral, enteral nutrition, prohibitions on physician self-referrals, 150
Partnership (glossary term), 294
Pathology
American Society for Clinical Pathology, Website, 210

Pathology *(continued)*
   College of American Pathologists, Website, 211
   CPT codes, 62
Patient appointments, 76–79
   check-out procedures, 83–84
   collecting copayments, 83
   confirmations, reminders, 78
   front-desk first impressions, 84
   missed appointments, no-shows, 79, 85
   new patients, 76
   registration process, checklist, 79–80, 81
   reminder systems, 188–189
Patient compliance, pay for performance and, 39
Patient volume
   forecasting, 126
   revenue component, 124
Patients
   bankruptcy, 95
   check-out procedures, 205
   communication of medical office policies, 79
   consent for treatment, 82
   demographic information, 76–78, 104
   driver's license copies, 155
   follow-up on unpaid claims, 93–95
   identity and privacy regulations, 80, 82
   insurance card copies, 155
   picture IDs, 80
   practice information sharing with, 28–29
   satisfaction surveys, 83–84
   self-check-in, 203–204
Pay for performance, 32, 36–44
   IOM principles, 37
   MGMA standards, 37–38
Payable (glossary term), 295
Payment posting, *See* Posting
Payment schedules, *See* Fee schedules and payment schedules
Payroll taxes (glossary term), 295
PCPI, *See* Physician Consortium for Performance Improvement
PCPs, *See* Primary care physicians
Pediatrics Websites
   The American Academy of Child and Adolescent Psychiatry, 208
   American Pediatric Surgical Association, 210
Pension fund (glossary term), 295
Pension plan (glossary term), 295
Per-click compensation, 151
Performance, financial, *See* Benchmarks
Performance measurement, *See also* Pay for performance
   Aligning Forces for Quality, 33–34
   data set (HEDIS), 34
   MGMA standards, 37
   non-adherent patients, 39
   Physician Consortium for Performance Improvement, 39–40
Petty cash fund (glossary term), 295
PGP, *See* Physician Group Practice Demonstration
Pharmaceutical industry, American Academy of Pharmaceutical Physicians, Website, 209
PHQI, *See* Premier Hospital Quality Initiative
Physical medicine Websites, American Academy of Physical Medicine and Rehabilitation, Website, 209
Physical therapy services, prohibitions on physician self-referrals, 150
Physician assistants, 179
   American Academy of Physician Assistants, Website, 209
Physician Consortium for Performance Improvement, 39–40
   successful Medicare PQRI reporting, 51
Physician Fee Lookup Tool, CMS Web site, 179
Physician Group Practice Demonstration, 41
Physician Quality Reporting Initiative, 32, 43, 45–53
   accurate coding, documentation, 52
   claims-based reporting, 49–50
   data collection, 51
   eligible providers, 46
   Group Practice Reporting Option, 52–53
   incentive payment, 47
   measures, 48–49
   Medicare Part B and, 48
   reporting periods and methods for 2010, 47–48

reporting via electronic health records, 47–48, 51
resources, participation tool kit, 52
satisfaction/dissatisfaction rates, *46*
successful reporting, 50–52
validation process, 48
Website, 207
Physician services, *See also* Billing; Claims; Evaluation and Management Codes
CPT codes, medicine section, 62
Medicare Part B, 7
Physician Voluntary Reporting Program, 45
Physicians
buy-in to budgeting process, 127
coding knowledge, training, 58–59
IT conversion leadership, 192
lab and test orders, *197*, 204
Medicare PQRI eligible providers, 46
oversight of compliance violation investigations, 171
provider numbers for satellite offices, 180
self-referral (Stark) regulations, 150–152
Plastic surgery Websites
American Academy of Cosmetic Surgery, 208
American Academy of Facial Plastic and Reconstructive Surgery, 208
American Association of Plastic Surgeons, 209
American Society for Aesthetic Plastic Surgery, 210
American Society of Maxillofacial Surgeons, 211
American Society of Plastic Surgeons, 211
Point-of-service plans, 5
Portable communication devices, 187
POSs, *See* Point-of-service plans
Post office boxes, lockbox payments, 16, 91
Posting, 15–16
Power users (IT conversions), 192–193
PPOs, *See* Preferred provider organizations
PQRI, *See* Physician Quality Reporting Initiative
Practice expenses, *See* Expenses
Practice management systems, *See* Information technology
Pre-certification, 13

Preferred provider organizations
description of, 4
sample appeal letter for PPO discount without contract, 281–282
silent, 103, 113
Premier Hospital Quality Initiative, 41–42
Prescription drug benefit, Medicare Part D, 7, 8
Prescriptions
American Academy of Pharmaceutical Physicians, Website, 209
e-prescribing, *197*
electronic refills, 204
refill requests, 79
Preventive medicine, American College of Preventative Medicine, Website, 210
Preventive services, CPT codes, 70–71
Primary care, American College of Physicians—American Society of Internal Medicine, Website, 210
Primary care physicians, 4
Prime rate (glossary term), 295
Principal (glossary term), 295
Prior-period adjustment (glossary term), 295
Privacy regulations, 80, 82, 152
Privacy Rule, *See* HIPAA regulations
Pro forma statements (glossary term), 295
Productivity, benchmark definition for, 121–122
Professional societies, online resources (Website addresses), 208–211
Profit center (glossary term), 295
Profit sharing plan (glossary term), 295
Program manager (IT conversions), 191–192
Project manager (IT conversions), 192
Promissory note (glossary term), 295
Prompt-pay laws, 90–91, 107–108
state-by-state descriptions, 225–238
Prorate (glossary term), 295
Prosthetics, prohibitions on physician self-referrals, 150
Protected health information, 82, 152, 153
safeguards against identity theft, 154
Provider identification numbers
misuse, 148
protection, confidentiality, 155
theft of, 180

Provider Self-Disclosure Protocol, 171, 173
Psychiatry Websites
    The American Academy of Child and Adolescent Psychiatry, 208
    American Academy of Psychiatry & the Law, 209
    American Psychiatric Association, 210
Public health Websites, American Association of Public Health Physicians, Website, 209
Public reporting, Aligning Forces for Quality, 33–34
Pulmonary diseases, American College of Chest Physicians, Website, 210
Purchase order (glossary term), 295

Q

Quality initiatives, 32–36
    accreditation, (NCQA), 34, 35
Quality of health care, American College of Medical Quality, Website, 210
Quality Plus standards, 35
Qui tam provision (False Claims Act), 147

R

Radiation medicine Websites
    American College of Radiation Oncology, 210
    American Society for Therapeutic Radiology and Oncology, 211
    Society of Cardiovascular & Interventional Radiology, 211
    Society of Interventional Radiology, 211
Radiation therapy services, prohibitions on physician self-referrals, 150
Radiological Society of North America, Website, 211
Radiology services
    CPT codes, 62
    prohibitions on physician self-referrals, 150
Radiology Websites
    American College of Radiology, 210
    American Roentgen Ray Society, 210
    American Society of Neuroradiology, 211
    Association of University Radiologists, 211
    Radiological Society of North America, 211
    Society of Interventional Radiology, 211
Railroad retirement health insurance, 8
Ratio (glossary term), 295
RBRVS, 10–11
Receipt (glossary term), 295
Reconstructive surgery, *See* Plastic surgery Websites
Recovery audit contractors, 156–157
    limits on requests for records, 156–157
Red Flags Rule, 80, 153–154
Reengineering, *See* Workflow
Referrals
    ancillary services and Stark regulations, 139–141
    gifts for, 180
    managed care plans, 14
    monitoring patterns, 178
    per-click compensation (self-referrals), 151
    physician self-referral violations, 150–152
    services for which physician self-referrals are prohibited, 150
Refractive surgery, *See* Ophthalmology Websites
Refund recoupment statutes by state, 239–263
Rehabilitation, American Academy of Physical Medicine and Rehabilitation, Website, 209
Reimbursement, *See also* Billing; Claims; Collections; Revenue cycle management
    terminology, 10–14
Relative value units, 120–121
    sample dashboard report, *132*
Reminder systems, 188–189
Remittances, *See* Revenue cycle management
Renal Physicians Association, Website, 211
Rent (glossary term), 295
Reproductive medicine, American Society for Reproductive Medicine, Website, 210
Resource-Based Relative Value Scale, *See* RBRVS
Retained earnings (glossary term), 295

Return on investment, information technology, 186
Revenue
  aging report, 129
  component in budgeting, 124–126
  enhancement, information technology contribution to, 186–189
  glossary term, 295
  gross, 124–125
  net collections, 125, 129
  per patient, 124
Revenue cycle management
  acceptable forms of payment, 93
  allowable services in payer contracts, 100–105
  appeals and reviews, 99, 110–116
  back-office processes, 87–97
  cash posting and contract monitoring, 91
  charge capture and entry, 88–89
  end-of-day balancing, processes, 84–85, 92
  front-end processes, 75–86
  payer internal claims processing and timelines, 105–110
  remittances, 91–93
  zero payments, 92
Rheumatology, American College of Rheumatology, Website, 210
Right to cure, 96
Risk (glossary term), 295–296
Risk premium (glossary term), 296
Robert Wood Johnson Foundation, Aligning Forces for Quality, 33–34
ROI (glossary term), 296

S

Safe harbors, 151
Salary (glossary term), 296
Sale (glossary term), 296
Scheduling, *See* Patient appointments
Security breaches, laws on disclosure of, by state, 267–272
Security Rule (HIPAA), 152, 153
  penalties on covered entities, 153
Self-audits, *See* Compliance programs
Self-disclosure, *See* Compliance programs
Self-insured employers, 6

Self-referral (Stark) regulations, 139–141, 150–152, 208
Simple interest (glossary term), 296
Sleep medicine, American Academy of Sleep Medicine, Website, 209
Social Security Act, 6
  violations by inducing referrals, 149
Social Security taxes (glossary term), 296
Society of American Gastrointestinal Endoscopic Surgeons, Website, 211
Society of Cardiovascular & Interventional Radiology, Website, 211
Society of Critical Care Medicine, Website, 211
Society of Interventional Radiology, Website, 211
Society of Nuclear Medicine, Website, 212
Society of Thoracic Surgeons, Website, 212
Sole proprietorship (glossary term), 296
Specialty societies, online resources (Website addresses), 208–211
Spine, North American Spine Society, Website, 211
Spreadsheet (glossary term), 296
Staff, *See* Office staff
Standard charge fee schedule, *See* Fee schedule
Standards of conduct, *See* Compliance programs
Stark regulations
  ancillary services, referrals, 139–141
  CMS Website, 208
  exceptions to, 151–152
  physician self-referral violations, 150–152
State-by-state listings
  disclosure of security breach, 267–272
  Medicare Part A intermediary and Part B carriers by state, 213–223
  prompt-pay laws, 225–238
  refund recoupment statutes by state, 239–263
State insurance commissioner, sample letter to, regarding late payment, 283
State insurance programs, *See* Medicaid; Workers' compensation insurance

States
- appeals processes, 114–115
- clean-claim laws, 90–91
- prompt-pay laws, 90–91, 107–108

Supplies, medical, *See* Durable medical equipment and supplies

Surgery, CPT codes, 62

Surgery Websites, *See also* Neurosurgery Websites; Ophthalmology Websites; Orthopedic surgery Websites; Otolaryngology Websites; Plastic surgery Websites; Thoracic surgery Websites
- American Association for Hand Surgery, 209
- American College of Surgeons, 210
- American Pediatric Surgical Association, 210
- American Society for Dermatologic Surgery, 210
- American Society for Surgery of the Hand, 210
- American Society of Abdominal Surgeons, 211
- American Society of Bariatric Physicians, 211
- American Society of Colon and Rectal Surgeons, 211
- American Society of General Surgeons, 211
- Association of Military Surgeons of the United States, 211
- Society of American Gastrointestinal Endoscopic Surgeons, 211

T

T-account (glossary term), 296
Take-home pay (glossary term), 296
Tax credit (glossary term), 296
Tax deduction (glossary term), 296
Taxable income (glossary term), 296
Telecommunication
- asynchronous, 188
- mobile (portable) devices, 187
- patient portals and kiosks, 187–188, 203–204
- telephone and e-mail reminder systems, 188–189

Telephones
- centralized phone center, 203
- reminder systems, 188–189

Terminology
- claims submission, 14–16
- reimbursement, 10–14

Test orders, *197*, 204
Third-party administrators, 15
Thoracic surgery Websites
- American Association for Thoracic Surgery, 209
- American Thoracic Society, 211
- Society of Thoracic Surgeons, 212

Tickler file (glossary term), 296
Time-based documentation, 69–70
Title XIX, *See* Social Security Act
Title XVIII, *See* Social Security Act
TPAs, *See* Third-party administrators
Training, *See* Compliance programs
Trial balance (glossary term), 296
TRICARE, 9

U

Underwriter (glossary term), 296
Unions, *See* Labor unions
Urology Websites
- American Association of Clinical Urologists, 209
- American Urological Association, 211

US Agency for Healthcare Research and Quality, 34–35
US Centers for Medicare and Medicaid Services, coverage determination documents, Web site listing, 89–90
US Centers for Medicare and Medicaid Services
- pay for performance programs, 40–44
- Physician Quality Reporting Initiative, 45–53
- Website, 207

US Federal Trade Commission, Red Flags Rule, 80, 153–154
US Health and Human Services Department, *See also* Office of Inspector General (OIG)
- Agency for Healthcare Research and Quality, 34–35
- Office for Civil Rights, 152, 153

US Internal Revenue Service
    glossary term, 292
    Website, 208
US Office of Inspector General, *See* Office of Inspector General (OIG)
Usual and customary payment schedules, *See* Payment schedules
Utilization review, 178

V

VA, *See* Veterans Administration
Value (glossary term), 296
Variance (glossary term), 296
Vendors, *See also* Information technology
    glossary term, 297
    kickback violations, 150
    selection and relationships with, 189–191, 196
Vested (glossary term), 297
Veterans Administration, 9

W

Wage (glossary term), 297
Warranty (glossary term), 297
Weighted average (glossary term), 297
Whistleblowers, qui tam provision (False Claims Act), 147
Withholding (glossary term), 297
Workers' compensation insurance, 9–10
Workflow
    analysis, 199–200
    components (health care delivery model), 200, *201*
    patient check-out, 205
    patient self-check-in, 203–204
    transformation in IT conversions, 199–206
Write down (glossary term), 297
Write off (glossary term), 297

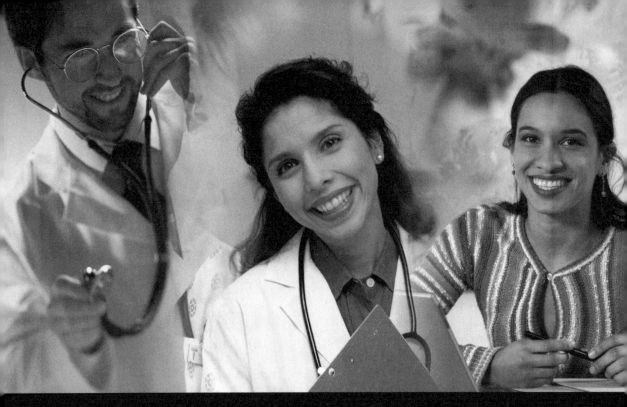

AMERICAN MEDICAL ASSOCIATION

Critical resources for today's demanding practice environment

With more than 40 years of experience, there's no better resource to learn from than the source of Current Procedural Terminology (CPT®), the American Medical Association (AMA). As the world's foremost scientific publisher, the AMA offers a broad range of authoritative resources that can help physicians and their staff run a more efficient practice. Also of interest to health care providers is our line of annual medical education and physician statistics directories.

To learn more visit
www.amabookstore.com
or call (800) 621-8335.

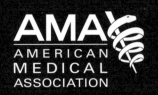

www.ama-assn.org | TOGETHER WE ARE STRONGER

Stay compliant in today's busy physician practice

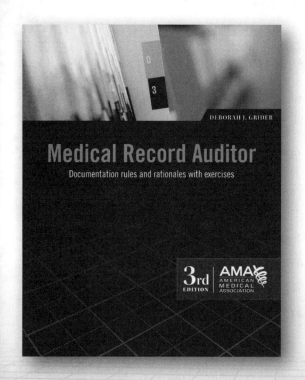

Newly updated and revised, the third edition of *Medical Record Auditor* offers an in-depth discussion of how the medical record is structured and how to review medical record documentation to determine level of service. In addition to reviewing the documentation and coding guidelines used today, this resource provides chart-auditing fundamentals, case studies, and other helpful examples to guide and enhance your understanding.

Designed to help navigate the important topic of record auditing, this book will assist the physician practice in maintaining compliance with the government, insurance carriers, and other agencies that review medical records.

Tools are provided to aid in the proper audit of medical records, as well as instruction on analyzing and reporting results of an audit. Chapter exercises are included to test the reader's comprehension of the material, and include a new chapter and PowerPoint® presentation on regulatory guidance.

Visit www.amabookstore.com for more information or call (800) 621-8335 to order!

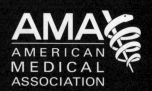

www.ama-assn.org | TOGETHER WE ARE STRONGER

UNLOCK
THE SECRETS OF NCCI
Learn to Code with Confidence

Learn the logic behind Medicare's National Correct Coding Initiative (NCCI) coding system and code with confidence. With hundreds of thousands of NCCI code pairs to search through, *Understanding Medicare's NCCI* teaches the reader how to make quick coding decisions to save time. Explanation and analysis of Medicare's NCCI edits will improve coding accuracy for those who use the Current Procedural Terminology (CPT®) and HCPCS code sets for reimbursement. In addition to walking coders, providers, and payers through the logic behind the NCCI coding system, this book teaches the reader how to make the correct determination regarding bundling vs billing separately for edited services.

Expanding on Medicare's basic guidelines, *Understanding Medicare's NCCI* features:

- ***Chapters organized by CPT codebook section***—offer the rules behind the edits, and guides the reader through each of the CPT codebook sections by reviewing and analyzing the guidelines

- ***Modifier application explanations***—detail when the appropriate modifier can be appended, such as modifier 25 and 59, to decrease confusion about modifiers that may be used to bypass edits

- ***CPT Coding, Documentation, and Learning Break Tips***—offer pointers on CPT coding, proper documentation requirements, and when it is appropriate and inappropriate to bypass edits for mutually exclusive edits (MUES)

Visit www.amabookstore.com
or call (800) 621-8335 to order

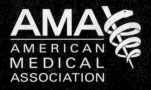

AMA
AMERICAN MEDICAL ASSOCIATION

Start now.

The earlier you familiarize yourself with the ICD-10-CM code set, the easier the transition will be!

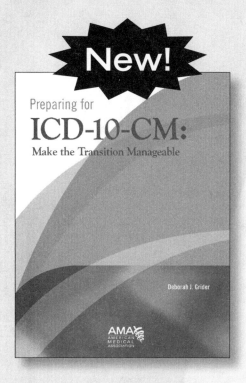

Be ready when the next generation of codes comes—rely on this helpful resource to make the transition between the ICD-9-CM and ICD-10-CM code sets easier.

Designed to help you prepare for the switch, *Preparing for ICD-10-CM*, includes

- Easy-to-understand explanations of how the change to ICD-10-CM will effect your medical practice

- Explanations describing the differences between the ICD-9-CM and ICD-10-CM code sets

- Detailed code set overview with helpful Q&A sections by chapter, ICD-10-CM conventions and resourceful tables and guidelines throughout

Order today!

Call (800) 621-8335 or go to:
www.amabookstore.com

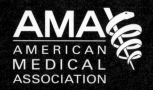